Early praise for
Handbook of Motivation and Change:
A Practical Guide for Clinicians

"Alcohol and substance abuse disorders change the brain's motivational system—but motivation is crucial to the care of these common and devastating conditions. And how does the busy clinician learn to instill and support that crucial motivation? By reading this clear, comprehensive, concise, and thoroughly enjoyable book."

Nada Stotland, M.D., M.P.H., Professor of Psychiatry, Rush Medical College, Chicago, Illinois

"How do you deal with patients when their very disorder undermines their motivation for treatment? This book provides both theory and case examples for the clinician confronting this problem. Because of this, it is a valuable addition to the library of anyone who faces this quandary. So do make this book part of your library. You will have use for it."

Marc Galanter, M.D., Professor of Psychiatry and Director, Division of Alcoholism and Drug Abuse, New York University School of Medicine, New York

"Motivational Interviewing is increasingly recognized as a critical skill in the fields of substance abuse, mental health, and beyond. For every clinician who's ever wondered why your best advice was not always followed, this book is for you! How do we engage our patients, recognizing the extent of their willingness to change? What are the unique challenges of the life cycle and the integration of Motivational Interviewing with other interventions? The mix of insightful case vignettes, complemented by a sampling of popular movies and television series, is both thought-provoking and entertaining. Practitioners, teachers, and trainees alike will appreciate the engaging format."

Nady el-Guebaly, M.D., Professor and Head, Addiction Division, Department of Psychiatry, University of Calgary, Canada; Executive Medical Director, International Society of Addiction Medicine

"Motivational Interviewing, a directive relational style grounded in Rogerian and supportive psychotherapy, is an important skill that all clinicians should learn. This engaging book makes sound arguments as to why traditional paternalistic approaches to treatment engagement and adherence tend to fall flat—and how the hard work of increasing patients' intrinsic motivation for change using this evidence-based intervention pays off in a variety of situations. Unlike the typical, dry expository approach of clinical texts, Levounis and Arnaout have succeeded in engaging the reader to experience the continuum of motivational work using clinical situations that practitioners will recognize from their own experience—situations that the chapter authors address with clear expertise and which are anchored in the easily recognizable life experience of characters from film. This is an excellent textbook, which is actually fun to read."

Richard N. Rosenthal, M.D., Professor of Clinical Psychiatry, Columbia University College of Physicians and Surgeons; Chairman, Department of Psychiatry, St. Luke's Roosevelt Hospital Center, New York

"This is a wonderful, easy-to-read guide that will help any busy clinician whether he or she is a general psychiatrist, family practitioner, internist, or pediatrician who is interested in how to advise, counsel, motivate, and direct a patient into making a major life change. I highly recommend this book to any clinician seeing patients with a substance abuse problem or psychiatric disorder who are in denial of their illness. The physician is presented with an easy how-to method of providing proper motivation to change in patients who are in denial of their substance abuse problem or psychiatric disorder. This excellent book is filled with many case studies and practical suggestions on how to direct troubled patients through their various stages of change as originally presented in Prochaska and DiClemente's Stages of Change Model. As an added treat, the book is fun especially if you are a movie buff: in each chapter, the authors illustrate a clinical point through the presentation of a scene from a popular movie."

Nicholas A. Pace, M.D., Clinical Associate Professor of Medicine, New York University Medical Center, New York; Fellow of the American Society of Addiction Medicine; Diplomate of the American Board of Addiction Medicine

"Read this book and your clinical practice is certainly going to change—whether you treat addiction, depression, or any other psychiatric illness that requires motivation to change behavior. Motivational Interviewing is a wonderful technique, and it is even more fascinating when taught the way it is in this handbook. Superb structure, organization, and creativity seem to have magically come together in this little volume, making it an essential part of a clinician's library and a sheer delight to read."

Analice Gigliotti, M.D., President, Brazilian Association on Studies of Alcohol and Other Drugs

"Substance abusers who are ambivalent or not ready for change can be some of the most challenging clients, leaving clinicians feeling helpless and turning away patients, saying, 'Come back when you are ready.' However, this invaluable book offers a powerful tool for therapists to help their clients become ready. Drs. Levounis and Arnaout have written an invaluable guide to Motivational Interviewing. Modern-day theories and data-supported practices are explained in clear, approachable language, and clinical vignettes demonstrate practical solutions to clinical scenarios that therapists in the field actually see. This book should be required reading for any clinician who sees substance abuse issues in his or her practice."

Steven J. Lee, M.D., Addiction Specialist in Private Practice; Assistant Clinical Professor of Psychiatry, Columbia University College of Physicians and Surgeons, New York

"Levounis and Arnaout's *Handbook of Motivation and Change* is destined to become an indispensable guide in the navigational toolbox of all practitioners working with substance-abusing patients. The clinical examples in each chapter are frequently engaging and central to the Handbook's teaching narrative. Clearly and accessibly written, clinically illuminating and useful, this volume offers much of value to both seasoned and beginning therapists."

Jack Drescher, M.D., Clinical Associate Professor of Psychiatry, New York Medical College, Valhalla, New York

Handbook of
MOTIVATION
and **CHANGE**

A Practical Guide for Clinicians

Handbook of
MOTIVATION
and **CHANGE**

A Practical Guide for Clinicians

Edited by

Petros Levounis, M.D., M.A.
Bachaar Arnaout, M.D.

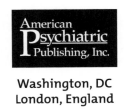

American Psychiatric Publishing, Inc.

Washington, DC
London, England

Copyright © 2010 American Psychiatric Publishing, Inc.
ALL RIGHTS RESERVED

Manufactured in the United States of America on acid-free paper
14   13   12   11   10   5   4   3   2   1
First Edition

Typeset in Adobe's ACaslon and The Mix

American Psychiatric Publishing, Inc.
1000 Wilson Boulevard
Arlington, VA 22209–3901
www.appi.org

Library of Congress Cataloging-in-Publication Data
Handbook of motivation and change : a practical guide for clinicians / edited by Petros Levounis, Bachaar Arnaout. — 1st ed.
     p. ; cm.
   Includes bibliographical references and index.
   ISBN 978-1-58562-370-9 (alk. paper)
   1. Motivation (Psychology) 2. Psychotherapy. I. Levounis, Petros.
II. Arnaout, Bachaar, 1974–
   [DNLM: 1. Behavior Therapy—methods. 2. Behavior, Addictive—therapy.
3. Health Behavior. 4. Interview, Psychological. 5. Motivation. 6. Substance-
Related Disorders—therapy. WM 425 H2368 2010]
   RC489.M655H36 2010
   616.89'14—dc22

                                                                          2010010620

British Library Cataloguing in Publication Data
A CIP record is available from the British Library.

Contents

Contributors

Michelle Acosta, Ph.D.
Assistant Professor of Clinical Psychology, Department of Psychiatry, Columbia University College of Physicians and Surgeons; Investigator, National Development and Research Institutes, Inc., Center for Technology and Health, New York, New York

Bachaar Arnaout, M.D.
Assistant Clinical Professor of Psychiatry, Yale University School of Medicine, VA Connecticut Healthcare System, West Haven, Connecticut

Ileana Benga, M.D.
Assistant Clinical Professor of Psychiatry, Columbia University College of Physicians and Surgeons; Medical Director, Opioid Treatment Program, The Addiction Institute of New York at St. Luke's and Roosevelt Hospitals, New York, New York

Benjamin Cheney, M.D.
Clinical Instructor, Department of Psychiatry, New York University School of Medicine; Director, Chemical Dependency Crisis and Detoxification Unit, Bellevue Hospital Center, New York, New York

Christopher Cutter, Ph.D.
Associate Research Scientist, Section of General Internal Medicine, Yale University School of Medicine, New Haven, Connecticut

David A. Fiellin, M.D.
Associate Professor of Medicine and Investigative Medicine, Yale University School of Medicine, New Haven, Connecticut

Georgia Gaveras, D.O.
Attending Psychiatrist, Comprehensive Adolescent Rehabilitation and Education Services, The Child and Family Institute at St. Luke's and Roosevelt Hospitals, New York, New York

Marianne T. Guschwan, M.D.
Clinical Assistant Professor of Psychiatry, New York University School of Medicine, New York, New York

Deborah L. Haller, Ph.D., A.B.P.P.
Associate Professor of Clinical Psychology (in Psychiatry), Columbia University College of Physicians and Surgeons; Director of Psychiatric Research, St. Luke's-Roosevelt Hospital Center, New York, New York

Jennifer Hanner, M.D., M.P.H.
Psychosomatic Medicine Fellow, New York University School of Medicine; Division of Consultation Liaison Psychiatry, New York University Langone Medical Center, New York, New York

Karen Ingersoll, Ph.D.
Associate Professor of Psychiatry and Neurobehavioral Sciences, Clinical Psychologist, University of Virginia School of Medicine, Charlottesville, Virginia

Gary P. Katzman, M.D.
Clinical Assistant Professor, Department of Psychiatry, Mount Sinai Medical Center, New York, New York

Petros Levounis, M.D., M.A.
Director, The Addiction Institute of New York; Chief, Division of Addiction Psychiatry, The St. Luke's and Roosevelt Hospitals; Associate Clinical Professor of Psychiatry, Columbia University College of Physicians and Surgeons, New York, New York

Steve Martino, Ph.D.
Associate Professor of Psychology (in Psychiatry), Yale University School of Medicine, Veterans Administration Connecticut Healthcare System, New Haven, Connecticut

Daniel McMenamin, M.D.
Clinical Instructor, Department of Psychiatry, New York University School of Medicine; Attending Physician, Department of Psychiatry, Bellevue Hospital Center, New York, New York

Edward V. Nunes, M.D.
Professor of Clinical Psychiatry, Columbia University College of Physicians and Surgeons, New York, New York; Principal Investigator, Long Island Node, National Institute on Drug Abuse Clinical Trials Network, New York State Psychiatric Institute, New York, New York

Paul J. Rinaldi, Ph.D.
Clinical Director, The Addiction Institute of New York at St. Luke's and Roosevelt Hospitals, New York, New York

Stephen Ross, M.D.
Assistant Professor of Psychiatry and Oral Medicine, New York University School of Medicine and New York University College of Dentistry; Director, Division of Alcoholism and Drug Abuse, Bellevue Hospital Center; Clinical Director, Center of Excellence on Addiction, New York University Langone Medical Center, New York, New York

Daryl I. Shorter, M.D.
Assistant Professor, Division of Alcoholism and Addiction Psychiatry, Menninger Department of Psychiatry and Behavioral Sciences, Baylor College of Medicine; Staff Psychiatrist, Michael E. DeBakey Veterans Administration Medical Center, Houston, Texas

Ramon Solhkhah, M.D.
Vice Chairman for Education and Director of Child & Adolescent Services, Department of Psychiatry, Maimonides Medical Center, Brooklyn, New York; Assistant Clinical Professor of Psychiatry, Columbia University College of Physicians and Surgeons, New York, New York

Jose P. Vito, M.D.
Attending Staff Psychiatrist, Department of Psychiatry, Bronx Psychiatric Center, Albert Einstein College of Medicine, Bronx, New York

Christopher Welsh, M.D.
Associate Professor, Department of Psychiatry, Division of Alcohol and Drug Abuse, University of Maryland School of Medicine, Baltimore, Maryland

Susan D. Whitley, M.D.
Clinical Instructor in Psychiatry and General Internal Medicine, New York University School of Medicine; Unit Chief, Opioid Addiction Treatment Program, Bellevue Hospital Center, New York, New York

Disclosures of Interest

The following contributors to this book have indicated a financial interest in or other affiliation with a commercial supporter, a manufacturer of a commercial product, a provider of a commercial service, a nongovernmental organization, and/or a government agency, as listed below:

Marianne T. Guschwan, M.D.   Affiliated with New York University School of Medicine as a faculty member; receives a salary from New York University School of Medicine for work done at Bellevue Hospital

Petros Levounis, M.D., M.A.   *Speakers' Bureau:* AstraZeneca, Pfizer

Susan D. Whitley, M.D.   *Speakers' Bureau:* Reckitt Benckiser

The following contributors to this book stated that they had no competing interests during the year preceding manuscript submission:

Michelle Acosta, Ph.D.; Bachaar Arnaout, M.D.; Ileana Benga, M.D.; Benjamin Cheney, M.D.; David A. Fiellin, M.D.; Georgia Gaveras, D.O.; Deborah L. Haller, Ph.D., A.B.P.P.; Jennifer Hanner, M.D., M.P.H.; Karen Ingersoll, Ph.D.; Gary P. Katzman, M.D.; Steve Martino, Ph.D.; Edward V. Nunes, M.D.; Stephen Ross, M.D.; Daryl I. Shorter, M.D.; Jose P. Vito, M.D.; Christopher Welsh, M.D.

Preface

The idea for writing *Handbook of Motivation and Change: A Practical Guide for Clinicians* came primarily from our clinical experience as psychiatrists working with patients who have substance use and other psychiatric disorders. Although there are several books that address motivation and change in our population of patients, we felt that a book based on case studies, practical suggestions, and movie ideas to enrich the clinical material—and written by busy clinicians for busy clinicians—was much needed. We hope that you will find this volume to be informative, useful, easy to read, and fun.

Our audience is primarily the general psychiatrist. However, we expect that this volume will also be helpful to family practitioners, internists, pediatricians, medical students, allied professionals, and anyone else who may be interested in issues of motivation and change—including physicians and other personnel of hospital emergency departments, where Motivational Interviewing can be particularly important in catalyzing behavior change. The book is written at a level that can be understood by clinicians who have an interest in this area but who do not have specialized knowledge or expertise in addiction treatment.

The main theoretical platforms for our book are two ground-breaking innovations in addiction treatment: Prochaska and DiClemente's (1984) Transtheoretical Model of Change, also known as the Stages of Change model, and Miller and Rollnick's (1991, 2002) Motivational Interviewing. We have based our clinical discussions on their ideas and are deeply grateful for the opportunity to expand on their seminal body of work. However, we have also opened the theoretic framework to include other ideas and techniques that the chapter authors have found helpful in their scholarship and clinical experience.

This book is organized into 16 chapters that discuss the clinical aspects of working with patients on issues of motivation and change, especially as these concepts relate to substance use disorders. In the opening chapter of this book, Edward V. Nunes, M.D., helps us place our work in the general context of addiction treatment. In the following seven chapters, we then present the fundamentals of motivation and change before detailing the stages of change as well as relapse—and how to treat our patients who struggle through those stages. The next four chapters outline the intersection of motivational work with other interventions from psychopharmacology to Alcoholics Anonymous. In the following two chapters, we turn to the unique challenges of treating patients throughout the life cycle: adolescents and older adults. Next, the chapter on changing the culture illustrates an application of clinical principles to the "outside world." The book concludes with a systematic review of the research on Motivational Interviewing. Although the reader may decide to follow the flow of the book and read it sequentially, we have given each chapter enough autonomy to be easily studied out of order.

In order to create a somewhat uniform and as-readable-as-possible book, each chapter (except for the first two chapters and the last) follows the following format:

- **Introduction:** We begin each chapter by setting up the specific subject in the context of the overall framework of motivation and change.
- **Clinical Case:** The cases in this book are composites of several clinical (and sometimes nonclinical) experiences of the authors; the settings have been changed, all names are fictional, and every effort has been made to conceal any identifying information.
- **Discussion of the Clinical Case:** Here we discuss the specifics of the case as they pertain to the educational objectives of each chapter.
- **Suggestions for Treatment:** This section is the focus and centerpiece of each chapter; it provides practical information about helping people change.
- **Suggestions for Teaching and Supervision:** This is a short list of suggestions for supervisors and other educators to facilitate teaching and learning.
- **Movie/Television Series:** We present scenes from a popular movie or television series that illustrate a clinical point for discussion and briefly explain how each scene relates to the chapter material.
- **Key Clinical Points:** Bulleted points summarize the most essential take-home messages of each chapter.
- **Multiple-Choice Questions:** We provide five multiple-choice questions at the end of each chapter, with explanations of the correct answers in the Answer Guide at the end of the book. We fully appreciate, expect, and welcome that sometimes the reader will disagree with the wisdom, clinical judgment, and idiosyncrasies of the authors.
- **References:** Except for the first two chapters and the last, which review in detail the context and evidence base of Motivational Interviewing, chapters are not intended to provide extensive literature reviews; we have tried to keep the number of references at the end of each chapter to a minimum.

At the end of the book, we have included some helpful appendixes for readers. Appendix 1 contains a list of movies that could be used in the teaching of a wide range of addiction-related topics. And with the explosion of information over the Internet (readily available to both clinicians and patients), we have suggested helpful Internet sites in Appendix 2.

We are deeply indebted to our colleagues who contributed to this volume for their wonderful clinical insights and imaginative approach to treatment. We are also grateful to our teachers, who have shaped our understanding and compassion throughout the years. Finally, we couldn't have completed this book without the support of our families and friends who, at times, were really hoping to motivate us to change our attitude and go to the movies instead of write about them.

Petros Levounis, M.D., M.A.
Bachaar Arnaout, M.D.

References

Miller WR, Rollnick S: Motivational Interviewing: Preparing People to Change Addictive Behavior. New York, Guilford, 1991

Miller WR, Rollnick S: Motivational Interviewing: Preparing People for Change, 2nd Edition. New York, Guilford, 2002

Prochaska JO, DiClemente CC: The Transtheoretical Approach: Crossing Traditional Boundaries of Therapy. Homewood, IL, Dow Jones-Irwin, 1984

CHAPTER 1

Addiction Treatment in Context

Edward V. Nunes, M.D.

How do we talk with patients? As physicians and psychiatrists, having made a diagnostic assessment and a treatment plan, how do we get our patients to follow it? Surprisingly little in medical school or specialty training, even psychiatric training, teaches this—what would seem a rather fundamental clinical skill. The same may often be true in allied fields such as psychology, social work, and nursing. This is the focus of Motivational Interviewing and the focus of this introductory book.

Medical training and psychiatric training focus on biology, psychology, disease mechanisms, and treatment methods. The assumption is that patients, having received an explanation and a recommendation, will naturally fall into line and follow the recommended course of therapy. Yet, failure to adhere to recommended treatments is common in patients with a wide range of medical problems such as hypertension or management of cardiovascular risk factors (e.g., diet, exercise) and psychiatric disorders including substance use disorders. This book focuses on substance use disorders and how to motivate patients to stop using substances and adhere to specific treatments including medications and counseling or psychotherapy in its various forms. But, in a broader sense the methods and skills of Motivational Interviewing can be applied to any health behavior that the clinician is trying to get a patient to follow, be it giving up alcohol, giving up cigarettes, taking medication for hypertension or high cholesterol levels, or changing dietary and exercise habits. A large proportion of national disease burden in developed countries can be traced to such health behaviors. Yet as clinicians well know, these behaviors

1

are hard to change, and it is often not enough to simply tell patients it is time to quit alcohol or cigarettes, make other changes in their lifestyle, or adhere to treatments that may be cumbersome or uncomfortable in one way or another.

Since the 1970s, the development of new treatments for substance dependence has been an intensive focus of research, accelerated by a growing awareness of the morbidity and social costs of the addictions, including addiction to nicotine, alcohol, and other drugs. This investment in research has produced a number of promising medications and psychotherapeutic and behavioral treatments with solid evidence of efficacy from clinical trials. Medications include methadone, buprenorphine, and naltrexone for opioid dependence; disulfiram, naltrexone, and acamprosate for alcohol dependence; and nicotine replacement, bupropion, and varenicline for nicotine dependence. Behavioral approaches include various cognitive-behavioral approaches, 12-step facilitation, family therapy approaches, and contingency management using vouchers or prizes as rewards for abstinence. Further, important treatment approaches have developed out of experience and clinical work, including 12-step methods such as Alcoholics Anonymous and various residential treatment approaches such as the 28-Day Model and long-term therapeutic community treatment. The National Institute on Drug Abuse Clinical Trials Network has been engaged in testing evidence-based treatments when delivered by clinicians in real-world, community-based treatment settings and has found considerable support for the effectiveness of such treatments (e.g., Ball et al. 2007; Carroll et al. 2006; Peirce et al. 2006; Petry et al. 2005; Tross et al. 2008). All told, the scope of progress has been considerable.

Among all these treatment approaches, Motivational Interviewing is of special importance because it can be viewed as the essential clinical skill 1) for engaging patients in treatment and 2) for motivating patients to reduce substance use and to follow through with whatever specific behavioral or pharmacological treatments are recommended. Motivational Interviewing is also challenging to master: it requires learning sophisticated new skills (e.g., complex reflection and the tactical combination of open-ended questions and reflections to move the patient toward change) and unlearning of the prescriptive stance (e.g., closed questions, persuasion, and confrontation) that is often second nature to clinicians.

Efficacy of Motivational Interviewing

There is extensive evidence of efficacy for Motivational Interviewing from controlled trials in treating alcohol use disorders (e.g., Bien et al. 1993; Borsari and Carey 2000; Marlatt et al. 1998; Martino et al. 2000; Miller et al. 1993; Project MATCH Research Group 1997) and drug use disorders (Babor et al. 1999; Ball et al. 2007; Carroll et al. 2006; Saunders et al. 1995; Swanson et al. 1999). Two meta-analyses of clinical trials of Motivational Interviewing for alcohol abuse, drug abuse, and other problem health behaviors confirm overall effect sizes in the medium range. The meta-analyses also highlight variability of effect across populations, settings, and types of clinicians (Burke et al. 2003; Hettema et al. 2005), suggesting the need to better understand the underlying mechanisms of Motivational Interviewing and to develop training methods in order to maximize effectiveness (Miller and Rollnick 2002b).

Efforts to delineate the underlying mechanisms of Motivational Interviewing have examined the relationship between particular therapist behaviors or skills and the ability to engender change in patients, and these have direct implications for how to design training methods for Motivational Interviewing. A seminal finding has been that when a patient makes statements during a Motivational Interviewing session committing to changing his or her behavior (also known as *commitment language* or *change talk*), this is associated with improved substance use outcomes at follow-up (Amrhein et al. 2003; Moyers et al. 2007). Further, evidence suggests that therapist behavior consistent with Motivational Interviewing is more likely to engender change talk, whereas Motivational Interviewing–inconsistent behavior (e.g., directing, confronting) is associated with expressions of resistance to change (*counterchange talk*) (Moyers and Martin 2006; Moyers et al. 2007). Other studies (Boardman et al. 2006; Moyers et al. 2005) have examined the relative importance of clinicians having specific Motivational Interviewing–consistent behaviors and skills (e.g., affirming, asking open-ended questions, making reflections) versus having a more global interpersonal style or the spirit of Motivational Interviewing (e.g., collaborativeness, empathy). These findings have tended to show that the global style and spirit of Motivational Interviewing may be more powerful than the specific skills in engendering client engagement and treatment alliance, although these latter studies did not assess change talk among patients. The implications for training include these points:

1. It is important to teach clinicians Motivational Interviewing–consistent behaviors and to minimize Motivational Interviewing–inconsistent behaviors, although emphasis should also be placed on teaching the global style and spirit of Motivational Interviewing.
2. Clinicians should be trained to recognize and reinforce their patients' change talk.

Theory and Basic Concepts of Motivational Interviewing

In medical school and residency training, physicians learn to conduct diagnostic evaluations, order tests, and prescribe medications and other treatments. In a sense, the emphasis is on a model of the physician, bedecked with white coat, as the authority. And, after so many years of training, why not? The same may apply to training in psychology and our other allied health fields. Even in clinical training, such as psychiatric residency, where psychotherapy is taught, many of the specific psychotherapeutic techniques can take on the same authoritative stance. In Cognitive-Behavioral Therapy (CBT), for example, the therapist is providing formulations regarding patterns of thought and behavior that need to be changed and is giving out homework assignments. It is clinician as teacher.

Motivational Interviewing (Miller and Rollnick 2002b) is founded partly on the clinical intuition of its founders and partly on psychological research, which shows that when a person is ambivalent about making a particular change in his or her behavior, a prescriptive approach is likely to engender resistance and to decrease the probability of change. Hence, giving orders and prescribing changes in behavior, as clinicians have been taught to do, may often be countertherapeutic. Instead, people are more likely to change if they feel it is their own free decision, for reasons that they have determined and endorsed.

Motivational Interviewing is also founded on the theory of cognitive dissonance. When a person holds conflicting ideas in his or her mind, it creates dissonance, and there is a tendency to resolve the conflict in one direction or the other. For a patient with drug or alcohol dependence, there are usually many unpleasant facts about the consequences of the substance use, which, if viewed starkly, are at odds with the person's values about himself or herself and what he or she cares about. The effort in Motivational Interviewing is to help the patient view such facts starkly, while at the same time eliciting the patient's deeply held values, in order to elicit and amplify the cognitive dissonance between the two and create drive for change. This resolution of cognitive dissonance could go either way in the sense that the person could decide to change his or her behavior and stop using substances or, conversely, to reframe or minimize the facts and continue using substances. The skill of the therapist is to guide the patient toward change.

Thus, Motivational Interviewing is founded on the following: *collaboration*, *evocation*, and *autonomy* (Miller and Rollnick 2002b):

- **Collaboration:** The patient should be approached as a partner in a consultative manner. The emphasis is on working together with the patient to arrive at decisions as to what to do and how to proceed. This is the opposite of the classic authoritative, prescriptive stance that we clinicians tend to inherit from our basic training.
- **Evocation:** The clinician should ask the patient about what is important to him or her, and what he or she values, then listen carefully and formulate more questions mainly to further draw out the patient's point of view. Thus, the emphasis is on open-ended questions, and active, *reflective* listening.

This is the opposite of the intensive fact-finding and closed-ended questions that are characteristic of the typical diagnostic interview.

* **Autonomy:** The patient is ultimately in charge of his or her care, and the clinician should respect the patient's decisions and freedom to choose. This is the opposite of the paternalistic stance of clinician as teacher and authority figure.

These are not entirely new ideas. For example, informed consent, which has emerged in recent decades as a cornerstone of medical care, holds that patients should be fully informed by their physicians and be a partner in making decisions about how to proceed with their care. This grows out of the medical ethical principle of "respect for persons" and respect for the autonomy of the individual. It is an ethical imperative, but there is also the recognition that patients are more likely to cooperate—and the clinical outcome is likely to be better—if patients are, in fact, active partners in their own care rather than passive recipients, as in the doctor-knows-best model. Indeed, this has probably been one of the basic components of a good bedside manner long before the articulations of medical ethics or Motivational Interviewing.

These principles are also familiar to any good salesperson. A good salesperson does not simply tell the customer what to buy. A good salesperson gets to know the customer, what the customer's interests are, and what he or she cares about. The salesperson can then describe his products in light of how they would fit into the customer's life. The salesperson guides the customer toward a decision to buy something, while the customer feels that the product is what he or she wants, and that it has been his or her own decision. The approach is Machiavellian perhaps, but effective. We are not taught salesmanship in clinical training, yet as clinicians we are often placed in the position of selling patients on treatments and lifestyle changes that they are not sure that they want.

It is important to recognize that Motivational Interviewing is neither just offering a sympathetic ear nor a client-centered approach where the clinician listens to the patient and helps the patient decide what to do. Rather, it is an active persuasion technique. The clinician has a definite agenda, a product to sell—namely, changing behavior in the direction of health (reducing or stopping substance use or some other unhealthy behavior). However, the sales technique is subtle.

Motivational Interviewing and the Tradition of Confrontation in Addiction Treatment

Denial and confrontation of denial are two concepts that have been fundamental to the clinical approach to the addictions. Patients often do seem to deny or minimize the problems caused by an addiction. The traditional idea was that this denial needs to be recognized and confronted. The patient needs to be shown the problems and be told what to do. If the patient does not take the advice, then perhaps the patient is not ready for treatment, and the clinician might ask the patient to "return when ready." However, it is likely that once a patient presents at the office of a psychiatrist or other clinician for consultation, more than a few friends and relatives (and perhaps other clinicians) will have already spoken in this way to the patient, perhaps ad nauseam. As noted earlier in this chapter, such an approach is likely to only stiffen the resistance to change. In contrast, Motivational Interviewing encourages the clinician in this situation first to listen to the patient and to hear the patient's point of view. The clinician may find that rather than dense denial, what is likely to emerge is ambivalence: the patient is aware of the problems caused by the addiction and wants to quit, but there are aspects of the substance and the taking of the substance that still attract the patient. Motivational Interviewing provides a way to help the patient resolve this ambivalence in the direction of abstinence and health.

At the same time, it is important to recognize that there are situations where the approach of Motivational Interviewing is not appropriate (Miller and Rollnick 2002a). Sometimes the situation is urgent and family members, friends, and clinicians need to force patients into therapy. A patient who is grossly intoxicated needs to be protected until his or her sobriety and judgment return. A patient who is acutely suicidal needs to be hospitalized, against the patient's will if necessary. Where to draw such a line with addicted patients can be less clear. When is the drinking or drug use of a minor teenager so out of control that the parents should exercise their legal authority and force the youngster into residential treatment? When should an adult patient be the subject of an intervention by friends and family? These are difficult judgments, of which a clinician needs always to be mindful.

Mastering Motivational Interviewing

Motivational Interviewing is not easy to learn. Physicians and other clinicians emerge from professional training (as noted previously in "Theory and Basic Concepts of Motivational Interviewing") with a lot of knowledge and a tendency to want to impart that knowledge—to teach and recommend and prescribe, and perhaps even confront. In contrast, the skills of Motivational Interviewing require that the clinician forbear and suppress all these tendencies. This can be surprisingly difficult.

In fact, new skills of all sorts can be surprisingly difficult to impart to clinicians. A substantial amount of literature on continuing medical education (CME) has shown that the usual methods of imparting new knowledge—grand rounds and other lectures, scientific papers, books, and even conferences and workshops—are generally ineffective at actually getting physicians to adopt new treatment techniques. Physicians tend to go back to their offices and clinics and do the same old things. More successful are training programs that incorporate not only such didactic training, but also practice with supervision and feedback (Davis 1998; Davis et al. 1992, 1995; Grol 2001). There are two potential barriers: the new treatment is new, and it may be difficult. Motivational Interviewing is both new and difficult.

Research comparing the effectiveness of training methods for substance abuse treatments has just begun to emerge. A review by Walters et al. (2005) located 17 such studies that evaluated training mainly for either Motivational Interviewing or CBT. The conclusions were that workshops may result in transient improvements in skill, but mirroring the findings from CME assessment, trainings that involve follow-up after a workshop, including various forms of practice with supervision or feedback, appear more effective in engendering lasting skills (Miller et al. 2004; Morgenstern et al. 2001a, 2001b; Sholomskas et al. 2005).

This has important implications for the readers of this book, namely that reading a book like this is only a start. It is important to learn about Motivational Interviewing didactically. This book is intended to serve as such an introduction. The authoritative text by Miller and Rollnick (2002b) is also recommended. That text provides a broad introduction to the theory and practice of Motivational Interviewing and is the basis for most formal workshops and training programs. The present book is especially geared toward the perspective of psychiatrists and other physicians.

However, to truly learn the skill of Motivational Interviewing it is important to get feedback and supervision. Workshops in Motivational Interviewing generally involve role-playing exercises with feedback from the instructor. This is a start, but even this is not the same as seeing patients and receiving feedback on and supervision of one's actual clinical interviewing. Thus, readers are encouraged to study this book, then to seek training that involves making audiotapes of one's interviews and having the opportunity to discuss the interviews with an expert supervisor. The Motivational Interviewing Network of Trainers is one place to start in locating such experts with whom to work: www.motivationalinterview.org/training/trainers.html.

The social costs of the addictions are massive in terms of the pain endured by patients and their loved ones, and the costs in adverse health effects and associated medical treatments, accidents, and lost productivity. The addictions represent only one example from a larger set of adverse health behaviors (poor diet, sedentary lifestyle, and lack of weight control being other examples). Our society now confronts spiraling costs of health care and needs to find a way to control them. Greater emphasis is needed on preventive health care, and on helping patients to give up destructive substance use and to make other changes toward healthier lifestyles. Thus, physicians and other clinicians need to be more adept at helping our patients to decide to make these changes and adhere to them. We need to be more effective at selling our patients on healthy behavior. Motivational Interviewing is, arguably, the essential skill for helping patients to change, and it should be part of the armamentarium of every clinician.

References

Amrhein PC, Miller WR, Yahne CE, et al: Client commitment language during motivational interviewing predicts drug use outcomes. J Consult Clin Psychol 71:862–878, 2003

Babor T, McRee B, Stephens RS, et al: Marijuana Treatment Project: overview and results (abstract). Symposium conducted at the annual meeting of the American Public Health Association, Chicago, IL, November 1999

Ball SA, Martino C, Nich C, et al: Site matters: multisite randomized trial of motivational interviewing therapy in community drug abuse clinics. J Consult Clin Psychol 75:556–567, 2007

Bien TH, Miller WR, Boroughs JM: Motivational interviewing with alcohol outpatients. Behav Cogn Psychother 21:347–356, 1993

Boardman T, Catley D, Grobe JE, et al: Using motivational interviewing with smokers: do therapist behaviors relate to engagement and therapeutic alliance? J Subst Abuse Treat 31:329–339, 2006

Borsari B, Carey KB: Effects of a brief motivational intervention with college student drinkers. J Consult Clin Psychol 68:728–733, 2000

Burke BL, Arkowitz H, Menchola M: The efficacy of motivational interviewing: a meta-analysis of controlled clinical trials. J Consult Clin Psychol 71:843–861, 2003

Carroll KM, Ball SA, Nich C, et al; National Institute on Drug Abuse Clinical Trials Network: Motivational interviewing to improve treatment engagement and outcome in individuals seeking treatment for substance abuse: a multisite effectiveness study. Drug Alcohol Depend 81:301–312, 2006

Davis DA: Does CME work?: an analysis of the effect of educational activities on physician performance or health care outcomes. Int J Psychiatry Med 28:21–39, 1998

Davis DA, Thompson MA, Oxman AD, et al: Evidence for the effectiveness of CME: a review of 50 randomized controlled trials. JAMA 268:1111–1117, 1992

Davis DA, Thompson MA, Oxman AD, et al: Changing physician performance: a systematic review of the effect of continuing medical education strategies. JAMA 274:700–705, 1995

Grol R: Improving the quality of medical care: building bridges among professional pride, payer profit, and patient satisfaction. JAMA 286:2578–2585, 2001

Hettema J, Steele J, Miller WR: Motivational interviewing. Annu Rev Clin Psychol 1:91–111, 2005

Marlatt GA, Baer JS, Kivlahan DR, et al: Screening and brief intervention for high-risk college student drinkers: results from a 2-year follow-up and natural history. J Consult Clin Psychol 66:604–615, 1998

Martino SM, Carroll KM, O'Malley SS, et al: Motivational interviewing with psychiatrically ill substance abusing patients. Am J Addict 9:88–91, 2000

Miller WR, Rollnick S: Ethical considerations, in Motivational Interviewing: Preparing People for Change, 2nd Edition. New York, Guilford, 2002a, pp 161–175

Miller WR, Rollnick S: Motivational Interviewing: Preparing People for Change, 2nd Edition. New York, Guilford, 2002b

Miller WR, Benefield RG, Tonigan JS: Enhancing motivation for change in problem drinking: a controlled comparison of two therapist styles. J Consult Clin Psychol 61:455–461, 1993

Miller WR, Yahne CE, Moyers TB, et al: A randomized trial of methods to help clinicians learn motivational interviewing. J Consult Clin Psychol 72:1050–1062, 2004

Morgenstern J, Blanchard KA, Morgan TJ, et al: Testing the effectiveness of cognitive-behavioral treatment for substance abuse in a community setting: within treatment and posttreatment findings. J Consult Clin Psychol 69:1007–1017, 2001a

Morgenstern J, Morgan TJ, McCrady BS, et al: Manual-guided cognitive-behavioral therapy training: a promising method for disseminating empirically supported substance abuse treatments to the practice community. Psychol Addict Behav 15:83–88, 2001b

Moyers TB, Martin T: Therapist influence on client language during motivational interviewing sessions. J Subst Abuse Treat 30:245–251, 2006

Moyers TB, Miller WR, Hendrickson SM: How does motivational interviewing work? Therapist interpersonal skill predicts client involvement within motivational interviewing sessions. J Consult Clin Psychol 73:590–598, 2005

Moyers TB, Martin T, Christopher PJ, et al: Client language as a mediator of motivational interviewing efficacy: where is the evidence? Alcohol Clin Exp Res 31 (10 suppl):40s–47s, 2007

Peirce JM, Petry NM, Stitzer ML, et al: Effects of lower-cost incentives on stimulant abstinence in methadone maintenance treatment: a National Drug Abuse Treatment Clinical Trials Network study. Arch Gen Psychiatry 63:201–208, 2006

Petry NM, Peirce JM, Stitzer ML, et al: Effect of prize-based incentives on outcomes in stimulant abusers in outpatient psychosocial treatment programs: a national drug abuse treatment clinical trials network study. Arch Gen Psychiatry 62:1148–1156, 2005

Project MATCH Research Group: Matching Alcoholism Treatments to Client Heterogeneity: Project MATCH posttreatment drinking outcomes. J Stud Alcohol 58:7–29, 1997

Saunders B, Wilkinson C, Phillips M: The impact of a brief motivational intervention with opiate users attending a methadone programme. Addiction 90:415–424, 1995

Sholomskas DE, Syracuse-Siewert G, Rounsaville BJ, et al: We don't train in vain: a dissemination trial of three strategies of training clinicians in cognitive-behavioral therapy. J Consult Clin Psychol 73:106–115, 2005

Swanson AJ, Pantalon MV, Cohen KR: Motivational interviewing and treatment adherence among psychiatric and dually diagnosed patients. J Nerv Ment Dis 187:630–635, 1999

Tross S, Campbell AN, Cohen LR, et al: Effectiveness of HIV/STD sexual risk reduction groups for women in substance abuse treatment programs: results of NIDA Clinical Trials Network Trial. J Acquir Immune Defic Syndr 48:581–589, 2008

Walters ST, Matson SA, Baer JS, et al: Effectiveness of workshop training for psychosocial addiction treatments: a systematic review. J Subst Abuse Treat 29:283–293, 2005

CHAPTER 2

Fundamentals of Motivation and Change

Bachaar Arnaout, M.D.
Steve Martino, Ph.D.

In this chapter, we explore the fundamentals of motivation and change, first by presenting prior commonly held views about motivation and change in addictions treatment, then by describing Motivational Interviewing and the Stages of Change model, and finally by examining what Motivational Interviewing and other psychotherapies have in common. We end with suggestions for teaching and supervision.

The concept of change is paramount in psychiatric practice and may be of special importance in behavior change models for substance users. The predominant past view of substance users had been that alcohol- and drug-addicted patients were inherently incapable of changing because of their rigid defensiveness in recognizing their problems, most embodied in the notion of their denial of addiction. This deficit in motivation for change was seen more as a personality trait than as a state subject to the patients' changing circumstances and self-perceptions. This view led to justification of the use of aggressive confrontational tactics that purported to break down resistance or bust through denial, accelerate the process of hitting bottom, and reshape the addict's personality (Miller and Rollnick 1991).

Over time these directly confrontational and authoritarian interventions have yielded to addiction treatments that are guided by more contemporary and humane models of how people with substance use disorders change. In particular, two models have become quite popular since the 1980s and are a natural fit for each other. The models are Miller and Rollnick's Motivational Interviewing (Miller and Rollnick 1991, 2002) and Prochaska and DiClemente's Stages of Change model (Prochaska and DiClemente 1984). Each model is described below in more detail.

Motivational Interviewing

Motivational Interviewing, first detailed in William R. Miller's landmark paper (Miller 1983) and then in Miller and Rollnick's books (1991, 2002), is deeply grounded in humanistic psychology, especially the work of Carl Rogers (1951). Miller and Rollnick propose that change is a natural and ubiquitous process that is intrinsic to each person and may occur without outside intervention, a concepts supported by research (Ellingstad et al. 2006; Schachter 1982). Motivational Interviewing seeks to hasten this natural change process by creating an interpersonal situation wherein the patient can engage in a collaborative dialogue that supports behavior change from the patient's perspective.

Fundamentally, Motivational Interviewing is not exactly a *method* or a bag of tricks, not something that can be done *to* someone, but something that is done *with* someone, a way to *be with* another person that increases the likelihood they will consider and become more committed to change. Clinicians adopt a style or *spirit* of interacting and communicating with patients such that they

- Respect the patient's views (*collaboration*)
- Elicit and build on the patient's resources and strengths that support change (*evocation*)
- Respect the patient's autonomy (*autonomy*).

This empathic stance conveys respect and acceptance of the patient and presumes that the resources for enhancing motivation reside within the patient. By creating a therapeutic atmosphere grounded in this spirit, clinicians help patients feel more open to exploring their ambivalence about change and feel empowered by the self-direction afforded to them.

From this spirit emanate the general principles of Motivational Interviewing, captured by the acronym **REDS:**

- **Roll with resistance:** The therapist handles resistance by acknowledging the patient's concerns and encouraging new perspectives.
- **Express empathy:** The therapist maintains a supportive, nonjudgmental, and respectful attitude and conveys understanding.

- **Develop discrepancy:** The therapist aims to help the patient consider how current behavior conflicts with important goals or values and how positive behavior change might resolve the discrepancies.
- **Support self-efficacy:** The therapist supports qualities and experiences that help the patient feel able to change and committed to a course of action.

Motivational Interviewing is not neutral in stance. It targets specific behavior changes that have a clearly positive direction (e.g., drinking less or not at all). Hence, clinicians who employ Motivational Interviewing strategically support and elicit from their patients statements that favor change. These patient statements are referred to as *change talk* and have been categorized to provide clinicians with a more nuanced understanding of factors that enhance the patients' motivation to address their substance use problems. Change talk includes statements that indicate a patient's desire, ability, reason, need, and commitment to change. The elicitation and elaboration of these types of statements during a session, in the context of the clinician's empathic spirit, is fundamental to how Motivational Interviewing works to induce behavior change (Amrhein et al. 2003; Miller and Rose 2009).

Developing areas of motivation not expressed in the patients' change talk provides direction in the session. For example, a patient may say why he or she needs to change (e.g., potential loss of child custody), yet not express an ability to stop using a substance of abuse. The clinician would be most effective by drawing out any experiences or skills the patient has that might develop the patient's confidence or self-efficacy to change. Through this attentive process of building motivation (often referred to as the first phase of Motivational Interviewing), the patient may become ready, willing, and able to change.

The second phase of Motivational Interviewing involves active efforts by the clinician to strengthen the patient's commitment to change. In this phase, the clinician helps the patient decide what he or she will do in the form of negotiating a change plan. Here again, careful attention to what the patient says is critical because the person's ambivalence may resurface when considering his or her commitments. If the clinician continues to pursue a change plan rather than attending to the patient's ambivalence, the patient will likely backtrack motivationally.

When people consider making a change, *counterchange talk* (statements that support not changing) typically emerges. Patients often have mixed thoughts and feelings about approaching change. Ambivalence is presumed to be a normal, expected part of the change process rather than a sure sign of the patient's wavering motivation. Skillfully handling ambivalence and addressing counterchange talk is another key feature of Motivational Interviewing. Clinicians view these statements as important communications by patients about what leads them to not change. Carefully listening to these issues without judgment (i.e., rolling with resistance) often provides therapeutic inroads to enhancing motivation (e.g., "I'm too depressed to stop using" signals addressing the patient's concerns about his or her mood as a pathway to not using). Moreover, this empathic and curious stance avoids arguing with patients about the merits of changing or, conversely, about the drawbacks of status quo behaviors—sidestepping the danger of creating a dynamic in which patients counterargue the clinicians' points, thereby contributing to a process in which patients talk themselves into not changing.

Importantly, counterchange talk is distinguished from resistance in that resistance is seen more as the style in which a patient might argue against change (e.g., negating, dismissing, arguing) rather than necessarily being an indicator of amotivation. For example, a patient referred to treatment as a term of probation might appear hostile toward a clinician during intake, yet simultaneously use change talk. This client might be motivated to change and at the same time, be disgruntled by the circumstances of his or her referral to treatment. In Motivational Interviewing, clinicians learn how to not let the resistance in a patient's stance blindside them into not hearing the change talk.

Clinicians use several treatment strategies or techniques in Motivational Interviewing. These strategies are intertwined throughout the session and include 1) fundamental patient-centered counseling skills and 2) strategies directed toward the goal of eliciting change talk and solidifying commitment. Fundamental strategies involve open-ended questions, affirmations, reflections, and summaries (OARS). Much emphasis is placed on the clinician's use of high-quality reflections and summaries that succinctly capture what patients have said and on maintaining a more reflective rather than questioning interviewing style in the session. Common change talk–eliciting strategies include the following:

- Direct efforts by counselors to develop discrepancies between the patient's preferred goals, values, and self-perceptions and the patient's substance use
- Strategic use of open-ended questions and reflections to evoke change talk
- Use of importance and confidence rulers that invite discussion about the presence of some motivation—rather than none at all—for change
- Change-planning discussions for strengthening commitment to a behavior change process.

Learning how to use these strategies well takes much practice and close supervision (see "Suggestions for Teaching and Supervision" later in this chapter).

The Stages of Change Model

Prochaska and DiClemente (1984) described the Stages of Change model, otherwise referred to as the Transtheoretical Model of Change, to signify that change is a process of progressive, fluid, and recurring stages rather than a singular event. These stages are applicable to the broad process of behavior change, including efforts that occur with and without professional assistance or treatment programs and across a wide range of behaviors. The stages of change are as follows:

- **Precontemplation:** The patient is unaware or does not believe that there is a problem or may believe that there is a problem but is not considering changing it.
- **Contemplation:** The patient is ambivalent about recognizing a problem and shies away from changing it.
- **Preparation:** The patient is ready to work toward behavior change in the near future and develops a plan for change.
- **Action:** The patient takes steps to implement specific behavior changes.
- **Maintenance:** The patient works to maintain and sustain long-lasting change.

Thus, the Stages of Change model posits that change occurs sequentially as patients move from being unaware of or opposed to addressing a problem, to considering the possibility of change, becoming more determined and planful, taking action, and then making these changes an enduring part of their lives.

The Stages of Change model proposes that each step involves multiple tasks and different strategies for advancing behavior changes. Tailoring interventions to a patient's stage of change is a hallmark of this model. For example, a patient in the precontemplation stage who is reluctant to change his or her drinking might be provided with information (e.g., blood test results documenting poor liver functioning) that may prompt consideration of drinking as a problem. Someone in the contemplation stage might be guided through a cost-benefit analysis of making a change. An individual in the action stage, fully committed to changing his or her substance use, might benefit most from learning coping skills to not use alcohol or drugs.

The strength of this model is that it provides clinicians with a practical paradigm of the change process by helping them match their interventions to a patient's current stage. This model also recognizes that relapse is possible as a patient's motivation wavers across stages and that patients may regress and recycle through the stages many times before they make enduring changes. This perspective is constructive in that relapse becomes an opportunity to increase support, learn from experience, and sharpen the patient's change effort rather than being a mark of failure.

Contrary to a common misconception, the Stages of Change model is distinct from Motivational Interviewing, although they naturally fit together. DiClemente and Velasquez (2002) clarify how Motivational Interviewing can be used to help clients move from one stage of change to another. First, Motivational Interviewing provides a way of working with patients in the early stages. The patient-centered counseling skills of Motivational Interviewing would work well with someone in the precontemplation stage and might provide a means by which the clinician could recognize potential sources of change talk. The skillful handling of ambivalence, a key feature of Motivational Interviewing, would be quite useful for contemplators who are stuck in indecision. Strategies for discussing change plans and strengthening commitment to this plan would be well matched to patients in the preparation stage.

Motivational Interviewing also can be useful in later stages of change when patients' motivation to change waxes and wanes as they take action or try to maintain changes in the face of stressful life circumstances. Furthermore, clinicians' continued incorporation of the accepting and understanding Motivational Interviewing style of communication may help sustain a good working relationship between the patient and clinician. Finally, because Motivational Interviewing is not a comprehensive treatment, clinicians likely will integrate it with other skills (e.g., Cognitive-Behavioral Therapy [CBT]) or recovery support–building treatments (e.g., 12-step facilitation) more appropriate for the action and maintenance stages. Hence, the Stages of Change model provides guideposts for helping clinicians know how to blend Motivational Interviewing with other therapeutic approaches.

Motivational Interviewing and Other Psychotherapies

As noted in the preface to this book, its objective is to provide a practical text written for clinicians by clinicians. All the authors of the book's chapters are seasoned addiction clinicians with different roles and theoretical backgrounds—some with a cognitive-behavioral background, others with a passion for psychodynamics or motivational interventions, and many avid psychopharmacologists. What unites them despite their theoretical differences is the ability to work with individuals toward behavior change and to write about the scenery they have explored during such journeys. Not uncommonly, advocates of different theoretical approaches strive to discredit one another's views or point out the deficiencies of other theoretical perspectives. In line with the gentle and nonjudgmental approach of humanistic psychology, we wish to do quite the opposite—that is, to point out what Motivational Interviewing has in common with other psychotherapies, which altogether form the rich and fascinating mosaic of the psychotherapeutic community.

The therapeutic relationship may be the element most central to all effective psychotherapies. The therapist's empathy, attunement, and acceptance of the patient enable the therapeutic dialogue to unfold, and the exploration of challenging detail about the person's life and goals to occur. This *empowerment through acceptance* can be viewed as essential to all successful psychotherapy and to change in general. As noted earlier in the "Motivational Interviewing" section, change can be viewed as natural and intrinsic to each person and is facilitated in psychotherapy by creating a supportive and accepting environment.

This dialectic of acceptance and change is most clearly stated in the serenity prayer and 12-step literature and is perhaps even more typically associated with Dialectical Behavioral Therapy. It is worth noting that acceptance does not mean indifference, but rather a way to slow down and take note of what is in the individual's mind. The confidence that acceptance brings gives the person the time to think and decide whether and how to respond to an impulse, rather than equating impulse with behavior. This ability to uncouple impulse from behavior is, in turn, a central component in CBT.

In psychodynamics, commonalities with Motivational Interviewing and humanistic psychology may be especially prominent in the interpersonal, relational, and intersubjective traditions. Psychodynamic work is often portrayed as a balancing of supportive (i.e., accepting) and expressive (i.e., challenging) components, well embodied by the words "I do enough psychotherapy [often seen as more supportive] to make psychoanalysis [often seen as more challenging] possible" (Stefan R. Zicht, personal communication, 2007). As disputable as the distinctions between psychoanalytical terms may be, this mental space that enables dialogue and makes change possible has been referred to differently by many authors, including *transitional space* (Winnicott 1971), *negotiation* (Pizer 1998), and *thirdness* (Benjamin 2004).

It is in this environment that the will of the individual is reified, empowering him or her to change. Empowering constitutes the opposite of what is often called *enabling*. Enabling creates an atmosphere where another dialectic—one of dominance and dependence, clinging and discarding, of push-pull relationships—fuels current patterns and hampers change.

Miller and Rollnick (1991, 2002) see Motivational Interviewing as consistent with other psychotherapeutic modalities. They also add that Motivational Interviewing can be used along with other modalities as a prelude to them, a permeating factor used alongside other approaches, or a fallback position whenever motivational issues reemerge in treatment (Miller and Rollnick 2002). In fact, some of Motivational Interviewing's most enduring treatment effects have been found when it has been used as a prelude to more intensive standard treatment programs (Burke et al. 2003; Hettema et al. 2005). This has been applied in clinical practice, where blends of Motivational Interviewing with other psychotherapeutic modalities, such as CBT, and with 12-step facilitation are often used. Motivational Interviewing and CBT are particularly often seen as complementary, as the former focuses on the *why* and the latter on the *how* of change (Carroll 1998). In research this has been applied in the Combined Pharmacotherapies and Behavioral Interventions (COMBINE) study, where components of Motivational Interviewing, CBT, and 12-step facilitation as well as support system involvement targeting alcohol dependence were blended into the combined behavioral intervention (Anton et al. 2006).

Suggestions for Teaching and Supervision

Teaching Motivational Interviewing can be a very gratifying experience. The difficulty, however, often lies in Motivational Interviewing being a *methodless* method, one that places an emphasis on spirit and attitude before technique. Although the theory and technique of Motivational Interviewing can be fairly easily intellectually grasped, the shift in attitude that Motivational Interviewing welcomes is a lengthier process.

The medical profession trains its students to gather extensive histories with focused and detailed accounts of patients' complaints and symptoms. Thus, not infrequently, students shower patients with a litany of closed-ended questions and find it difficult to ask open-ended questions and to then follow them with reflections. Another barrier is the illusion that the clinician can, and in fact *has to*, change patients by convincing them and giving extensive expert advice. Perhaps the high stress and expectations inherent in the medical profession are often dealt with through an excessive need to control, especially among junior physicians and medical students. Although there certainly is a place for closed-ended questions, gathering detailed data, and assured expert advice and recommendations, it is valuable to encourage students to try to adopt the spirit of collaboration, evocation, and autonomy that Motivational Interviewing invites.

This shift in attitude is likely better taught by demonstration, wherein the teaching itself is conducted in this spirit. After explaining the basic tenets of Motivational Interviewing, the teacher engages the students in a discussion in the spirit of Motivational Interviewing, embodied by using OARS as a teaching tool and empowering students by accepting their views even when they differ from the teacher's. This can be followed up by the teacher playing a patient while the students practice the acquired skills in a role-play.

Another key aspect of teaching students Motivational Interviewing is having them learn it using experiential activities that sequentially build their skills over time. Miller and Moyers (2006) have described eight steps and associated skills by which clinicians become increasingly proficient. Training begins with helping clinicians become open to the assumptions and principles of Motivational Interviewing and grasping the Motivational Interviewing spirit as a style of interacting with patients (step 1). Training then moves toward teaching and honing clinicians' patient-centered counseling skills (step 2). Next, clinicians learn how to recognize, elicit, and reinforce change talk, and handle resistance skillfully (steps 3, 4, and 5). Shifting to change planning and strengthening commitment to change follows (steps 6 and 7). Finally, with Motivational Interviewing skills solidified, clinicians learn how to flexibly shift back and forth from Motivational Interviewing to other approaches (step 8). Providing students multiple learning activities in each of these areas is helpful. David Rosengren's (2009) book, *Building Motivational Interviewing Skills*, is an excellent resource for these types of training activities.

Eventually students need to conduct Motivational Interviewing with real patients and with supervision, where the interaction between the patient and supervisee is paralleled by the interaction between supervisee and supervisor. Taping sessions after gaining the patient's consent offers a more fine-grained assessment of the session and can be very beneficial to master the therapy. This type of direct observation of the student's session is critical in that clinicians learning Motivational Interviewing have been shown to overestimate their abilities (Martino et al. 2009). Moreover, supervisors can rate the students' Motivational Interviewing skills using established rating systems (Martino et al. 2008; Moyers et al. 2005) that then can provide the basis for providing students feedback and coaching. The combination of repeated direct observation, feedback, and coaching following didactic and workshop training is the only method to date that has been shown to significantly develop clinicians' skills in Motivational Interviewing (Miller et al. 2004).

Making this process collaborative and positive rather than solely supervisor driven is important. One of the writers (B.A.) had a supervisor who encourages students' self-evaluation during supervision, whereby the student is asked to identify three skills that were utilized well during the therapeutic session with the patient, and balance them with one area that the student feels needs improvement. Students are often amused by this ratio of 3:1, and at times are more ready to engage in self-criticism than to name what skills they have actually mastered.

An often-voiced concern among teachers is that some students are natural motivational interviewers whereas others are not. In our experience, it is valuable to always draw on the positive and affirm students wherever they may be on their learning journey. Overall, good teachers and supervisors are able to roll with students' resistances and certainly avoid arguing and attempting to convince students to drop reservations they have about Motivational Interviewing.

Movie: *Malcolm X*

Spike Lee's 1992 film *Malcolm X* illustrates the concept of change as a natural and human process. In this film, the protagonist engages in a journey of perpetual change and self-discovery, from involvement in crime, gambling, and substance abuse to becoming Malcolm X—beacon of discipline, charismatic leader, and visionary and human rights activist. What is remarkable in the life of Malcolm X was his ability to endlessly reconsider and rework his life and his preferences and to expand his views and influences. We believe that this potential for change lies at the core of every human being.

Key Clinical Points

- Change is natural, is intrinsic, and can be hastened by a supportive yet directive approach.

- Motivational Interviewing is a contemporary treatment approach for developing the patient's intrinsic motivation for positive behavior change by using a style of communication that blends patient-centered listening skills with methods directed at eliciting the patient's motivation and commitment to change.

- The clinician adopts a spirit of interacting with the patient marked by collaboration and evocation of the patient's resources and motivation for change, while supporting the patient's autonomy.

- The clinician's ability to recognize and elicit change talk (i.e., the patient's desire, ability, reason, need, and commitment to change) in the context of the spirit of the approach is the main mechanism by which Motivational Interviewing is presumed to work.

- Motivational Interviewing strategies include 1) use of fundamental patient-centered listening skills known as OARS (open-ended questions, affirmations, reflections, and summaries) and 2) methods directed at strategically eliciting change talk.

- The five stages in the Stage of Change model are

  1. Precontemplation
  2. Contemplation
  3. Preparation
  4. Action
  5. Maintenance.

- Tailoring interventions to a patient's stage of change is a hallmark of the Stages of Change model.

- Motivational Interviewing is seen as a natural fit in the early stages of change and can be used as needed when motivational issues arise in the later stages.

- Relapse is viewed as an opportunity for further support, exploration, planning, and progress in recovery.

- Motivational Interviewing has many parallels with other modes of therapy, and the ability to provide change-oriented therapy is seen as common to many schools of psychotherapy.

- Teaching and supervision are effectively done in a supportive and collaborative manner that is consistent with the spirit of Motivational Interviewing. Skills can be mastered and applied with adequate instruction and supervision. Change in trainees is natural.

Multiple-Choice Questions

For the correct answers to these questions, including explanations of answers, please see the Answer Guide at the end of this book.

1. Motivational Interviewing is most closely related to:
   A. Psychoanalysis.
   B. Behaviorism.
   C. Humanistic psychology.
   D. The 12-step tradition.

2. The spirit of Motivational Interviewing lies in:
   A. Criticism, elucidation, and analysis.
   B. Creativity, expansion, and advocacy.
   C. Confrontation, education, and authority.
   D. Collaboration, evocation, and autonomy.

3. A clinician who has mixed feelings about seeking supervision for Motivational Interviewing and has not yet planned to contact a supervisor is likely to be in which of the following stages of change?
   A. Precontemplation.
   B. Contemplation.
   C. Preparation.
   D. Relapse.

4. Motivational Interviewing often can be successfully combined with other therapeutic modalities. This statement is:

   A. False, because any association with other therapies will confuse the patient.
   B. True, because Motivational Interviewing is compatible with many approaches.
   C. Dangerous, because clinicians should always be passionate advocates of only one psychotherapeutic school.
   D. Irrelevant, because competent clinicians spontaneously know what to do without the need to learn Motivational Interviewing.

5. Teaching and supervision of Motivational Interviewing:

   A. Is best done in an accepting and collaborative manner.
   B. Is best done through confrontation to emphasize contrast with the style of Motivational Interviewing.
   C. Requires that the student undergo his or her own motivational therapy.
   D. Should focus on convincing the student that Motivational Interviewing is better than other therapies.

References

Amrhein PC, Miller WR, Yahne CE, et al: Client commitment language during motivational interviewing predicts drug use outcomes. J Consult Clin Psychol 71:862–878, 2003

Anton RF, O'Malley SS, Ciraulo DA, et al; COMBINE Study Research Group: Combined pharmacotherapies and behavioral interventions for alcohol dependence: the COMBINE study: a randomized controlled trial. JAMA 295:2003–2017, 2006

Benjamin J: Beyond doer and done to: an intersubjective view of thirdness. Psychoanal Q 73:5–46, 2004

Burke BL, Arkowitz H, Menchola M: The efficacy of motivational interviewing: a meta-analysis of controlled clinical trials. J Consult Clin Psychol 71:843–861, 2003

Carroll KM: National Institute on Drug Abuse Therapy Manuals for Drug Addiction: A Cognitive-Behavioral Approach: Treating Cocaine Addiction (NIH Publ No 98–4308). Rockville, MD, National Institute on Drug Abuse, 1998

DiClemente CC, Velasquez MM: Motivational interviewing and the stages of change, in Motivational Interviewing: Preparing People for Change, 2nd Edition. Edited by Miller WR, Rollnick S. New York, Guilford, 2002, pp 201–216

Ellingstad TP, Sobell LC, Sobell MB, et al: Self-change: a pathway to cannabis abuse resolution. Addict Behav 31:519–530, 2006

Hettema J, Steele J, Miller WR: Motivational interviewing. Annu Rev Clin Psychol 1:91–111, 2005

Martino S, Ball SA, Nich C, et al: Community program therapist adherence and competence in motivational enhancement therapy. Drug Alcohol Depend 96:37–48, 2008

Martino S, Ball SA, Nich C, et al: Correspondence of motivational enhancement treatment integrity ratings among therapists, supervisors, and observers. Psychother Res 19:181–193, 2009

Miller WR: Motivational interviewing with problem drinkers. Behavioural Psychotherapy 11:147–172, 1983

Miller WR, Moyers TB: Eight stages in learning motivational interviewing. Journal of Teaching in the Addictions 5:3–17, 2006

Miller WR, Rollnick S: Motivational Interviewing: Preparing People to Change Addictive Behavior. New York, Guilford, 1991

Miller WR, Rollnick S: Motivational Interviewing: Preparing People for Change, 2nd Edition. New York, Guilford, 2002

Miller WR, Rose GS: Toward a theory of motivational interviewing. Am Psychol 64:527–537, 2009

Miller WR, Yahne CE, Moyers TE, et al: A randomized trial of methods to help clinicians learn motivational interviewing. J Consult Clin Psychol 72:1050–1062, 2004

Moyers TB, Martin T, Manuel JK, et al: Assessing competence in the use of motivational interviewing. J Subst Abuse Treat 28:19–26, 2005

Pizer SA: Building Bridges: The Negotiation of Paradox in Psychoanalysis. Hillsdale, NJ, Analytic Press, 1998

Prochaska JO, DiClemente CC: The Transtheoretical Approach: Crossing Traditional Boundaries of Therapy. Homewood, IL, Dow Jones-Irwin, 1984

Rogers CR: Client-Centered Therapy. Boston, MA, Houghton Mifflin, 1951

Rosengren DB: Building Motivational Interviewing Skills: A Practitioner Workbook. New York, Guilford, 2009

Schachter S: Recidivism and self-cure of smoking and obesity. Am Psychol 37:436–444, 1982

Winnicott DW: The use of an object and relating through identifications, in Playing and Reality. London, Tavistock, 1971, pp 101–121

CHAPTER 3

Precontemplation

Paul J. Rinaldi, Ph.D.

In this chapter, I explore the concept of precontemplation as it applies to substance use treatment. I define the concept and look at applications in both the preclinical and clinical realms.

The precontemplation stage is marked by the individual not yet acknowledging that there is a problem behavior that needs to be changed. However, this commonly used definition is accurate yet limited: it is accurate in its context, but it is important to recognize that the context is one of addiction. The Stages of Change (Prochaska et al. 1994) is a transtheoretical model that has as one of its bases the idea of bringing to consciousness the decisional balances that exist in all behavioral acts. We are constantly making positive and negative lists in our heads in making decisions about how to act. These are usually made at such a speed as to be imperceptible unless focused on purposefully. In the continuum of substance use—from occasional social use to physical and psychological dependence—countless decisions are made that are relevant to every chapter of this book. However, prior to the exploration of that continuum is the person's original decision to take the first drink or drug of his or her life.

Precontemplation is not only relevant in the context of making the decision to treat a maladaptive pattern of use: a person is also in this stage before having that first substance. Children and teens are the majority of the individuals in this stage. The exposure of children to substance use or abuse differs depending on the context in which the person lives. During this time, there may be protective factors that will serve to help a person successfully navigate his or her relationship to substances. These protective factors might include positive parental and family relationships, positive peer relationships, social and academic involvement, and other prosocial behaviors that all reinforce self-efficacy.

Although these can serve as protective factors in avoiding substance abuse, they are not guarantees of success in avoiding problems with substances. There are many families who are shocked when one child develops a problem with substances while the other children and adults in the family have not had issues. When presented with such a case, it is important to understand the context in which the substance user developed a problem. It is important to understand the context in order to appreciate the etiology of the problem, and it is equally important in planning treatment. If the clinician does not consider the context in which a client is receiving treatment, that planning is lacking an important dimension. However, the importance of context does not diminish the importance of taking a detailed history over the course of treatment, because historical context is important in aiding a client to understand his or her substance issue. If a client lives in a housing project in a large city that is known to be drug infested, the clinician might choose to focus on the development and reinforcement of *refusal skills*, which refer to ways of being able to refuse substances when confronted with them. By doing so, the clinician is tailoring the treatment based on the individual context and potential vulnerability of the client.

People who are using substances are frequently in the precontemplation stage of change for long periods. In the context of being precontemplative about changing substance use behavior, people are not intent on changing a problem behavior. They may be unaware that the behavior is problematic or, if they are aware, they might see more reasons to support continuing the behavior than to support changing the behavior. The decisional balance is tipped toward not changing. Once a person's substance use has been labeled as problematic, the precontemplator is someone who is frequently described as being resistant or in denial. Precontemplators might even seek treatment for their use, but they only do so to placate others, not because of intrinsic motivation to change. They might be the clients who grudgingly attend group therapy at a treatment center but do not engage with the therapist or other group members.

In describing the precontemplator, DiClemente (1991) discuss the individual's resistance to change as the four *R*s: reluctance, rebellion, resignation, and rationalization. These patterns serve to keep precontemplators from changing.

Reluctant precontemplators are those who, through ignorance or inertia, do not want to consider change. They might be thought of as preconscious in that they are truly unaware of the effect of their problem. They often require patience and a particularly gentle approach because they are not feeling uncomfortable with their behavior and might not want to assume the risks associated with change.

Rebellious precontemplators might have a great deal of knowledge about the behavior that is considered problematic but might have an investment in maintaining the behavior. They do not like being told what to do and might present as hostile and argumentative. These are the clients that are often the most challenging to clinicians because they are frequently the most difficult to engage. They employ defenses that are challenging and sometimes hostile.

Unlike the rebellious precontemplator, the *resigned* precontemplator is marked by a lack of investment and energy. This client often presents as feeling that he or she is unable to change. This type of client might see himself or herself as beyond hope or help and therefore be unmotivated to try to effect changes in the problematic behavior. It is important for the clinician to strongly convey a sense of hope and faith in the client's ability to change if that is what the client desires.

Rationalizing precontemplators do not want to change because they have calculated the odds of risk and believe that their current state is best, or they might feel that the problem is not theirs but one belonging to others. They might project blame on the person who is pressuring them to get help. This type of precontemplator is resistant in a cognitive manner rather than in an emotional manner as the rebellious precontemplator is. These clients relish engaging in an intellectual debate about the reasons that they are choosing to use substances in what others consider to be a problematic pattern. It is important for the clinician to disengage from the debate that the client desires. Instead of engaging in emphasizing the cons of substance use, the clinician should clearly summarize the decisional balance faced by the client.

Clinical Case and Discussion of the Case

Troy is a 12-year-old boy who is in seventh grade and lives with his parents, brother, and sister in a middle-class suburb of New York City. He is a good student, is active in sports and music, and has stable, close friendships. He has never tried alcohol or drugs.

Is Troy at high risk for a substance use problem? I think most would agree that Troy is at very low risk for a substance use problem because he has inoculating factors that have been shown to influence the development of future substance use problems (National Institute on Drug Abuse 2002). His stable family and social relationships, his positive academic performance, and his extracurricular activities are all factors that can help Troy avoid future problems with substances. One way of understanding the relationship between these inoculating factors and substance use is to think of Troy as being in denial of the fact that drugs and alcohol are probably in his immediate world and could be available to him. He has not noticed their availability because he has no need to be seeking drugs or alcohol, and he has not been presented the opportunity explicitly up to this point in his life. Troy is ignorant of the behavior's existence. His environment supports his not engaging in the behavior. His context provides protective rather than risk factors. This example of precontemplation is rooted in a preventive model in addressing substance use. From that perspective, the goal would be to work on reinforcing those protective factors in order to continue the ignorance that Troy has of substances. How does this model of ignorance predict Troy's future relationship with substances?

> When Troy turns 14 and enters high school, his social environment expands. He is now a freshman in a large, middle- to upper-middle-class suburban high school. His pattern of overall success has continued. He has grown considerably over the past year and has matured physically and emotionally. He has a very active social life and is quite popular with both boys and girls. He does very well in school and is part of a "cool" crowd in school who are all good students and social leaders. In attending social functions, he has now been exposed to alcohol and marijuana smoking, although he and his friends have not used any substances.

Those factors that were protective earlier have continued to help protect Troy from problematic use but will not necessarily protect him from some use (Carroll 1997). By virtue of Troy's positive engagements in his life including school and family, he is likely to have a fairly high level of self-efficacy. Most people who develop substance use disorders do not have high levels of self-efficacy, so we can guess that Troy's high level of self-efficacy will also serve as a protective factor. It seems that an individual's context can outweigh the pull of protective factors. Perhaps those protective factors are resilient and serve purposes as determined by the individual's developmental tasks at any given time. Troy's protective factors worked to help him avoid substances in the context of grade school and middle school.

We can guess that given his social context, Troy is now at significant risk of *experimenting* with alcohol and/or marijuana. Although he has proven protective factors, social context is a powerful force, particularly for adolescents.

> As Troy progresses through high school, he does in fact use alcohol in the context of parties and social gatherings where his peers are also drinking. As he prepares to graduate high school, he has done well academically, landing in the top 10% of his class and being an accomplished soccer player and musician. He is among the popular people in school and is a student leader. He is successful in all realms and has offers to several prestigious colleges. During his senior year, he parties most weekends with other students. At those times, he and his friends typically drink beer, sometimes to excess. Troy has been drunk twice but has never driven when he has been drinking. He has had no negative consequences associated with drinking. He tried marijuana once while in high school but felt nothing and did not enjoy the experience.

Although we have talked about Troy's protective factors, we have not considered other potential risk factors. Troy has had good, strong family relationships, but it is important to consider other contexts beyond the immediate social realm. When considering Troy's current use of alcohol, it is important to understand the family's history regarding substance use. What is the family's relationship with alcohol and what is its role in the life of the family? Troy's parents are very similar to him: they both are leaders in the community in that they have been heavily involved in school activities with Troy and his younger sister, who is also involved in athletics and music. His parents are both educated professionals who are socially popular in the community, regularly attending parties. Both of Troy's parents drink regularly at home but not to excess. They might have a glass of wine with dinner or a cocktail. They drink more heavily at parties and, like Troy, are known to be fun and to be "partiers." They are aware that Troy and his friends drink together. They do not approve of it, but they have not imposed any restrictions on Troy because of his drinking. They accept it as a normal part of growing up and tolerate it as long as Troy and his friends always have a designated driver and do not drink to excess—and as long as Troy continues to be a successful student.

The family history is significant in that Troy's maternal grandfather, who died when Troy was 13, had been an alcoholic without ever undergoing treatment or self-help. Several relatives including an uncle and cousins are alcohol abusers, some of whom have had serious consequences including jail and mandated treatment. Troy's parents are outliers in both of their families by having gone to college and having professional careers.

Let us return to Troy's development:

> Troy graduates from high school and begins studies at an elite Ivy League university. He has some difficulties adjusting to college life. He was comfortable in his high school, where he was a leader. He find that college is more challenging; whereas he had stood out in high school for his academic, social, and athletic prowess, in the realm of an elite university his performance is average. He continues to be socially engaged and popular, but he does not get recruited for varsity soccer and chooses to play on an intramural team rather than in competition.
>
> Troy has a reasonably successful freshman year at college. His grades are average, which is a disappointment to him and to his parents. Throughout his first year, he develops a pattern of drinking on Thursday, Friday, and Saturday nights. He and some of his friends do not have Friday classes, so they begin the weekend early with happy hour on Thursdays at the fraternity house where some of Troy's friends live. Troy consistently drinks to inebriation on all 3 nights each week. He does not drink alone and has had no outstanding incidents associated with alcohol (fights, arrests, illnesses, and so forth). When registering for the second semester, Troy makes sure to maintain his schedule with no classes on Fridays. Most of his freshman peers have Friday classes, so during the spring semester he begins to be better friends with upperclassmen rather

than his immediate peers. He joins a fraternity and makes plans to move into the fraternity house in his sophomore year. His grades for the second semester continue to be average. During the summer, he lives with his family and works at a local pool as a lifeguard. He reconnects with high school friends with whom he drinks at times, but not to excess because he has to be at work early in the morning 6 days per week.

On returning to college, Troy moves into the fraternity house and resumes his pattern of heavy drinking 3 nights per week. He is very active in fraternity life and begins playing club rugby. During the fall semester his grades slip, which creates conflict with his parents. While at home for the holidays, Troy socializes and drinks frequently over the 3 weeks that he spends at his family's home. His parents comment on his drinking but are struck mainly by Troy's overall surly demeanor.

During the spring semester, Troy becomes increasingly involved in his fraternity and begins to frequently miss classes. He is increasingly known for his reputation as a heavy drinker and a guy who is always ready for a party. He gains a great deal of satisfaction from being popular and being everyone's friend. He continues to drink heavily 3 nights per week but he also has one to four beers on the other days. He is known as someone who can hold his liquor and generally has more to drink during an evening than the majority of his friends. When drinking he usually is the life of the party, although there is one incident that semester in which he gets into a minor shoving match with an acquaintance in a bar. When speaking to his parents, he sounds happy and consistently reports that everything is going extremely well. He decides to spend the summer working in a restaurant at the New Jersey shore with friends from school and living in a shared house. He has a summer filled with parties and drinking but without any trouble for Troy.

In the fall he returns to school but is soon put on academic probation due to failing two courses and withdrawing from others. His parents are notified and they are extremely upset with Troy. The university requires Troy to meet regularly with a dean for academic counseling. Troy is unable to point to a particular reason for his poor performance except to admit to feeling "unmotivated." He dismisses his parent's suggestion that his social life is having a negative impact on his academic performance. During the course of the semester, Troy meets his responsibilities in going to classes and meeting with the dean, but he continues to drink heavily and frequently. In April Troy attends a fraternity party during which there is very heavy drinking by many in attendance. He loses count of how much he drank and his memories of the night stop at a certain point. He has flashes of remembering leaving the party and being in a bar. He next remembers waking up in a jail cell having been charged with public intoxication and disturbing the peace. Troy was being disruptive while walking on campus and proceeded to become verbally threatening to the university security guard; the guard called the police, who then arrested Troy.

He is allowed to remain in school under the condition that he be followed by the student counseling services staff and comply with whatever recommendations they make. His parents insist that he move out of the fraternity house and into a regular dormitory, but the school does not allow him to be in the dormitories, so he remains in the fraternity house. The counseling services staff feel that he needs to be in substance abuse treatment but he does not agree that he has a problem with alcohol; everyone involved agrees that he should go to individual psycho-therapy with a substance abuse specialist. Troy agrees to go but does not agree that he needs his alcohol use evaluated. He feels that everyone involved is overreacting and that the situation should be resolved by his apologizing to the security guard. His legal case is quickly settled, with Troy put on probation for 1 year after which his record will be expunged in the absence of any further offenses.

Troy attends the first session of therapy after being referred by the student health service. He is on time for his appointment and presents in a friendly yet anxious manner. He gives a history of what has occurred that is consistent with the information obtained from the referring clinician. When asked about his understanding of why he was referred, he is very honest in stating that he disagrees with the reason for referral and sees no reason for him to be there. He understands why all of the adults involved think it is a good idea but he feels that they are wrong and wasting his time and their money.

This is a common scenario in the engagement process of a precontemplator. It is important to remain focused on helping the client understand that he or she has made choices both good and bad and to help him or her "own" these choices. The first area in which to explore this choice lies in the common conclusion that the client truly had no choice but to attend. Even a court-mandated client has made a choice to attend. The alternatives for such a client might all hold negative consequences (e.g., going to jail, expulsion from school) but a choice has been made nonetheless. In Troy's case, I asked him about his decision to commit to therapy. At first, he angrily said that it was not his choice and that he was forced to attend. I calmly told him that in my view, he had several options and he chose the option to remain in school and attend therapy sessions. Again, it is important to always validate the client's reality. In Troy's case that meant explaining the alternatives and that in fact, he did make a choice although he felt that he had no real volition. It is imperative to consistently help clients to understand their choices in order to help the client work toward self-efficacy. Clients who have problematic substance use behavior usually feel impulses and proceed to action, leaving out the cognitive processes that often mediate our impulses. In my experience with clients, they often assume that those people without substance use problems do not experience impulses; they confuse impulsive *thoughts* with impulsive *behavior*. Therefore, it is important to help the client understand that we all have impulses, but we are able to mediate the behavior that follows through cognitive processes in which we decide whether or not to act.

During the first session, I asked Troy what his goal was regarding his alcohol use: remaining the same, reducing his use, or abstinence. He was certain that he did not want to work toward abstinence but was not sure of what goal he might have. Because my goal for this session was engagement, it was important to not challenge him but to try to engage him. I commented that I certainly believed that he was not necessarily partying more or less than many of his peers but that, somehow, he ended up sitting here and his friends did not have their use highlighted. I engaged him in the question of why that happened; given that his use was not different than the use of his peers, what was a difference that ultimately landed him in my office? He was able to connect to this on an intellectual level and agreed that trying to better understand his behavior when drinking was a goal for therapy.

This illustrates that as clinicians, we must work to suspend our judgments and carefully consider what our goals are and how appropriate such goals are to the therapy. As I stated, my sole goal was engagement of Troy. We often enter the consultation room with a well-meaning bias that we are going to help this person "get clean" and forget that the danger associated with that bias is that the client might not share that goal. By engaging Troy in the goal of simply exploring his use and behavior associated with it, I was able to get him to engage in the session and feel less defensive than he was feeling with his dean and parents. His anger was easily diffused. In other cases, mandated clients like Troy are sometimes more angry. One tactic that can be useful is to simply tell angry clients that although they were mandated to be in my office, they made the choice to attend. Further, now that they have made this choice, another choice they have is how to use the sessions. They can use them to vent, to sit silently, or to talk about things happening in their life. Again, the language used is geared toward the client feeling an increased sense of autonomy and self-efficacy.

> Troy continues to attend treatment weekly throughout the school year. He struggles with his use and has a few alcohol-related incidents that pique his interest in exploring his drinking further. In one instance, he was in a bar with friends and got beaten up after making a pass at the assailant's girlfriend. Troy's friends confirmed to him that he acted in a rude and forward manner toward the woman. Troy was quite upset by this because he prides himself on his good manners and his high standards in the treatment of women. This incident marks a shift in Troy's treatment. He becomes more focused on understanding his use patterns and begins to understand himself, not as an alcoholic, but as a young man who has the potential for alcohol to become a larger problem in his life. He continues in therapy for the remainder of his college career during which he struggles at times with drinking, but he graduates and becomes employed following graduation. Although his mandate for treatment is behind him after graduation, he chooses to remain in therapy. He stops therapy when he moves to another city for a job.

Suggestions for Treatment

In substance abuse treatment, it is common for clients to attend the first session under duress, thus reluctantly. When working within a Motivational Interviewing frame in therapy, the clinician tries hard to meet clients where they are at that time and not impose his or her own goals and wishes on clients. However, it is perfectly reasonable for the clinician to have some goals for sessions with clients if not for the outcomes of the treatment. The primary goal of the early sessions is to engage the client, providing an atmosphere that is considered empathic and nonjudgmental. A working alliance between the therapist and client then can be fostered, which is essential to progress in treatment.

It is important to stop and evaluate how we define terms because often we apply different meanings to the same words or terms; thus, what does *progress in treatment* mean? In a Motivational Interviewing paradigm, progress is understood as movement toward a goal or set of goals that is determined by the client and made explicit in the therapy.

How does the clinician engage a reluctant, sometimes hostile client who clearly does not want to be in the session? The first way is to be clear about what the clinician's role is and what is realistic to expect from a session. In working with a Motivational Interviewing approach, the clinician always seeks to encourage the client to talk by asking focused open-ended questions rather than yes-or-no questions. The interviewer should try to bring the client back to the reason for the referral and the goals of the session. The clinician should engage the client in a process of goal setting from the start. Often, angry or resistant clients eschew the notion of goal setting because they think that it requires buying into the notion that they require treatment. The clinician can point out that an example of a goal might be to not have to be sitting in his or her office. From there, the clinician can help the client compile a list of possible ways to reach that goal. By doing so, the clinician is beginning to establish the idea that the client, even the mandated client, has choices. The clinician is also reinforcing the client's locus of control. From there, the clinician can establish a framework from which the therapy builds. At each stage of change with a client, the therapist is reinforcing behaviors that promote the client's locus of control.

I would be remiss if I failed to address the very real situation that many clinicians face when the client is angry and bordering on being abusive because the clinician is perceived as part of the system that is "forcing" the client to attend treatment. It is imperative that the clinician continuously reflect back to the client that he or she does still have choices to make. For example, when a client is told to attend therapy due to a traffic stop and faces the resulting charge of driving while intoxicated, the client might see the clinician as connected to the court system and may be defensive when reporting his or her use patterns. The client understandably feels disempowered and that no choice exists but to sit with the clinician. The clinician must help the client see that there are choices to be made, even if all the choices available seem unattractive. When a clinician is facing rage from clients, it is important to process with them the choices that they have. For example, I might say to a client that he or she has chosen to attend the session because the alternatives are less attractive. The client having made that choice, another choice is how to use the sessions. Thus, clients are helped to feel some sense of empowerment when they feel that they have no choices or autonomy. I have often given the client a menu of choices in how to use the sessions, which include sitting in silence. Of course, I am always explicit in telling the client what I am required to report to an outside agency based on the agreement the client has made with that authority. By doing so, there can be discussion with the client, and the client can be helped to make conscious decisions about treatment.

Suggestions for Teaching and Supervision

1. Continuously help the therapist focus on the fact that the primary goal of treatment with the precontemplator is *engagement*.
2. It is important to help the therapist to manage his or her reactions to clients by focusing on the principles of Motivational Interviewing, which promote helping clients to assume responsibility for their choices.
3. There are times that as clinicians, we are confronted with clients who are in the precontemplative stage and are angry. They might present in emergency rooms (particularly psychiatric emergency rooms) or be mandated by outside agencies to receive substance use evaluation and treatment. Working within a Motivational Interviewing frame helps the clinician to diffuse the anger through refocusing clients on the realities of their situation that resulted in the meeting. As a clinician you should be constantly refocusing yourself on the engagement process while remembering that it is the client—not you—who holds the responsibility for the two of you meeting.

In my experience, clinicians (regardless of their specialty) are most derailed by their own reactions to clients who are provocative and angry. As supervisors, helping the supervisee to continuously return to the principles of Motivational Interviewing can serve to neutralize the countertransferential issues that are stoked by the clinician-client interaction. By definition, precontemplators are resistant to treatment because they do not understand or accept that they might have a problematic relationship with the substance at issue. It can be very frustrating to be faced with a client who has evidence of issues but is unable to accept responsibility for his or her actions and consequences.

Television Series: *Mad Men*

Mad Men is a television series that is set in New York City in the early 1960s. John F. Kennedy had been elected president, and there was great hope and optimism in the country. The series is set in an advertising agency and has been critically acclaimed for its accurate portrayal of life during this time. Drinking and cigarette smoking are prominently featured in the series. In the early 1960s, business was frequently conducted over cocktails and lunch, hence the term *the three-martini lunch.* In the series, business meetings in the office are often held with drinks poured and most people smoking. It is difficult to imagine such drinking and smoking during business being so normal. In this context, the drinking and smoking were consistent with social norms and not seen as culturally deviant in any way. Today, if someone routinely drank at lunch, it is likely that the person would be identified as being a problem drinker. Again, it is imperative to understand a person's cultural and social context in evaluating substance use.

During one episode of *Mad Men,* the main character, Don Draper, is visiting his physician, who tells him to slow down and that he is drinking too much. That is the only time that alcohol is mentioned as being problematic. The doctor did not discuss whether Don's drinking was a problem for him except to relate it to hypertension. Assuming that Don was in a precontemplation state, he would likely leave that appointment thinking that his drinking might be contributing to hypertension but not considering whether his medical consequences might be indicative of a problem with addiction.

An alternative to the above scene would be for the doctor to gently raise questions for Don about his drinking: How much does he drink? How frequently? When does he take his first drink of the day? Has he ever gone for more than 24 hours without drinking, and if so, how did he feel? By asking such questions, the doctor would begin the process of creating discrepancy in Don's thinking about drinking.

In another episode of *Mad Men,* an account executive named Freddy Rumsen is working on an ad campaign for an important client. He is leading a creative team of three people. Freddy has been with the agency for many years and is portrayed as a well-liked and friendly guy. As the creative team prepares for a business meeting where they will pitch their advertising campaign to the client, Freddy is not in attendance. When the other two team members go to his office, they find him asleep. When they rouse him and he stands up, it is clear that he has urinated on himself and that he is drunk. He does not attend the meeting and he is let go from his job.

Although the culture in which this episode takes place is highly tolerant of drinking, Freddy violated a cultural norm by having his drinking interfere with business in a way that could have embarrassed the firm. The story line with Freddy shows that when cultural norms are violated, the one who violates these norms is shunned rather than participants in the culture critically assessing those norms. Freddy's intoxication might have proved a threat to the culture of heavy drinking that was normative in many social strata at that time.

This episode is an example of a precontemplation state that is contextually defined. Freddy lives in a culture that is highly tolerant of heavy drinking. However, even in such a context, he crosses a culturally defined line and is exiled for that lapse.

Key Clinical Points

- Precontemplation refers to two phenomena: 1) when a person (often a child or adolescent) is naive to substances; and 2) after exposure (and possibly experimentation), when a person stays in a precontemplative state even when there is evidence to suggest that there is a problem.

- A Motivational Interviewing approach to working with the precontemplator focuses on the process of engaging the client in treatment.

- Because precontemplators do not accept that substance use is an issue, it is important to not take a confrontational approach.

- As a clinician, it is important to normalize ambivalence when working with a person in the precontemplation stage.

- When working with the precontemplator, the clinician needs to work toward helping the client to develop discrepancy between where the client's life is currently and where the client would like his or her life to be in the future.

Multiple-Choice Questions

For the correct answers to these questions, including explanations of answers, please see the Answer Guide at the end of this book.

1. The primary goal of working with a client in the precontemplation stage of change is:
   A. Breaking down the client's denial through confrontation.
   B. Engaging the client in the treatment process.
   C. Helping the client to identify triggers.
   D. None of the above.

2. Which of the following statements is false?
   A. Motivational Interviewing does not rely on a confrontational style.
   B. When working with a client in the precontemplation stage, the clinician should focus primarily on engaging the client.

    C. One should ask yes-or-no questions when using Motivational Interviewing.

    D. Motivational Interviewing should reinforce the client's locus of control.

3. When using a Motivational Interviewing approach to treating substance use issues, the clinician should:

    A. Encourage the client to accept responsibility for his or her successes and failures.

    B. Help the client identify goals.

    C. Focus on helping the client move toward a greater sense of self-efficacy.

    D. All of the above.

4. Which of the following statements is true of clients in the precontemplation stage?

    A. By definition, people in this stage do not seek treatment.

    B. When in this stage, people might seek treatment due to pressure from outside sources.

    C. People in this stage usually move to another stage quickly.

    D. None of the above.

5. In the precontemplation stage, resistance to change can be characterized by:

    A. Reluctance.

    B. Rebellion.

    C. Resignation.

    D. All of the above.

References

Carroll K: Compliance and alcohol treatment: an overview, in Improving Compliance With Alcoholism Treatment (Project MATCH Monograph Series, Vol 6; DHHS Publ No 97–4143). Edited by Carroll K. Rockville, MD, National Institute on Alcohol Abuse and Alcoholism, 1997, pp 5–12

DiClemente CC: Motivational interviewing and the stages of change, in Motivational Interviewing: Preparing People to Change Addictive Behavior. Edited by Miller WR, Rollnick S. New York, Guilford, 1991, pp 191–202

National Institute on Drug Abuse: NIDA Notes: Drug Abuse Prevention Research Update, Volume 16, Number 6 (February 2002). Available at: http://www.drugabuse.gov/NIDA_Notes/NN01Index.html. Accessed March 5, 2010.

Prochaska JO, Norcross JC, DiClemente CC: Changing for Good: A Revolutionary Six-Stage Program for Overcoming Bad Habits and Moving Your Life Positively Forward. New York, Avon, 1994

CHAPTER 4

Contemplation

Christopher Welsh, M.D.

According to *The Merriam-Webster Dictionary* (2005), the word *contemplate* means "to view or consider with continued attention." *Contemplation*, besides being the noun derivative of the word contemplate, is also the second stage in the Transtheoretical Model of Change originally proposed by Prochaska and DiClemente (1984), also known as the Stages of Change model. It generally refers to the period when an individual begins to realize that he or she has a problem. It may or may not also include the early consideration that the individual feels that he or she would like to do something to address this problem. In the research performed by Prochaska and DiClemente, the term *contemplation* was used to define individuals who were "seriously considering stopping the addictive behavior in the next six months" (DiClemente 2003, p. 140; Prochaska and DiClemente 1983, 1984).

This stage may last for varying amounts of time, from minutes to years. Because many individuals with substance dependence are impulsive and easily frustrated, it may be difficult for them to stop and consider potential problems or change for any significant amount of time. On the other hand, for various reasons, the individual may recognize that he or she has a problem and continue to think about changing it but not take the next step in preparing to actually make a change. In some cases, the individual would like to change the behavior but feels that he or she is unable to make the change. In other cases, he or she may realize that there is a problem but ignore the immediacy of the consequences of the behavior, leading to procrastination and avoidance of addressing the problem. Still others may perceive the thought of giving up the lifestyle associated with the problematic behavior as though it were the loss of a loved one. They may experience grief and require a period of mourning before actually moving to make a change. Regardless of the reason, the contemplation stage may continue for years with the individual's good intentions never actually resulting in behavior change.

The process of contemplation involves the unconscious and conscious gathering and examination of information in order to make a decision to change. In order to do this, all information, both for and against behavior change, must be considered. This often leads to a considerable amount of *ambivalence*. Being conflicted about a behavior is normal, even with the most destructive of behaviors. Often, in the early stages of substance *use* (before the development of substance abuse or dependence), significant benefits are gained from the use. Some examples are facilitation of socialization for a shy individual, increased acceptance by peers, reduction of anxiety, and escape from a traumatic (current or past) situation. Even though a behavior becomes extremely destructive, the original and current positive aspects still exist.

In addition, the positive effects of substance use, though generally brief, are often immediate and predictable (relaxation, increased energy) whereas the negative effects are often delayed (cirrhosis, hepatitis) and less predictable (driving while intoxicated dozens of time without being arrested or having an accident). Conversely, many of the positive effects of cessation of use are often delayed (e.g., improved health) whereas the negative effects are generally more immediate (e.g., opioid withdrawal symptoms). This inequity often contributes to the user's ambivalence.

The concept of a *decisional balance* (Figure 4–1) is a useful, simplified construct to help understand the internal psychic process (referred to by Baumeister as "crystallization of discontent"; Baumeister 1994) that leads to behavior change. The decisional balance was originated by Janis and Mann (1977), who postulated that the decision to change a behavior is based on the perceived difference between the anticipated gains and anticipated losses. They categorized these perceived differences as 1) utilitarian gains and losses for self, 2) utilitarian gains and losses for others, 3) self-approval or self-disapproval, and 4) approval or disapproval from significant others. This concept has been further expanded by Miller and Rollnick and is a useful tool for conveying the core issue (Miller and Rollnick 2002).

The decision to change a behavior is a very personal one. It is important to remember that not all pros and cons are created equal. The consideration of information necessary to make a change is unique to each individual. Personality, historical factors, and current social circumstances all contribute to this variability. Even the threat of incarceration may be extremely motivating for one individual and yet have a minimal effect on another.

Equally important is the idea that all decisions have a logical, rational component and an emotional, experiential component. In many cases of behavior

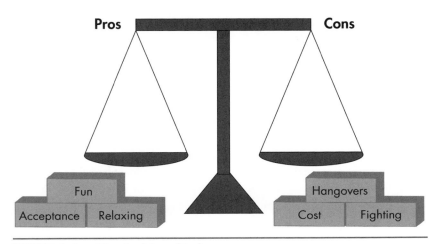

Pros   Cons

Fun   Hangovers

Acceptance   Relaxing   Cost   Fighting

FIGURE 4–1. The decisional balance.

change, knowledge is not enough to lead to significant, lasting change. As indicated above, the relative intellectual and emotional importance of a given factor varies with each individual. A seemingly minor factor, from an objective standpoint, may hold significant emotional importance for a given individual. For long-lasting behavior change to occur, both aspects must generally be acknowledged and addressed. It is important that contemplation involve heightening of awareness as well as arousal of emotions. Generally, this occurs through an evaluation of both internal factors (e.g., values, beliefs, and opinions) and external situations (e.g., relationships, employment, education, public safety, and legal issues) that are affected by the behavior.

It can often be helpful for the individual to consider both the pros and cons of changing the behavior and the pros and cons of not changing the behavior. Although these may seem simply to be the opposites of each other, they often are not, and the distinction may lead to different insights. As the individual begins to move through the contemplation stage and truly consider changing the behavior in the future, he or she may look at potential gains and losses. These may be concrete or material (e.g., jobs, money, freedom from incarceration) or less tangible (e.g., approval and disapproval from significant others).

Also important to remember is that harmful behaviors and behavior change do not occur in a vacuum. Once a behavior is established in an individual's life, it may begin to serve multiple purposes. Although not a great coping mechanism, it may, for brief periods, be better than some of the individual's preexisting mechanisms. Unless the individual begins to develop other means of coping, it may be difficult for him or her to do more than briefly contemplate change because the thought of going without the behavior becomes overwhelming. It is important for significant others and clinicians working with the individual to recognize this and assist the individual in developing new coping strategies. Similarly, if the patient is using substances as an imperfect means of coping with an underlying psychiatric disorder, a good evaluation and proper treatment (both pharmacological and psychotherapeutic) are often essential for the patient to be able to contemplate letting go of the substance use.

Similarly, others around the affected individual often change their behavior in response to the dysfunctional behavior. A spouse may gain confidence and reinforcement from the act of caring for the affected individual. The family of a prominent lawyer may cover up consequences of addiction in order to preserve the family's reputation and income. A physician parent may be in denial about her son's substance use, feeling that it could not be occurring with her child. Over time, this situation may fulfill needs (conscious and unconscious) of these individuals as well. Attempts to help the affected individual recognize and act on his or her addiction often upset the dynamic of the relationship that has adapted to the dysfunctional behavior. Sometimes, these issues must be addressed in addition to the primary addictive behavior in order for any change to be considered.

Yet another important factor to consider is that even when an individual does recognize that he or she has a problem that needs to be changed, the individual may not always move from the contemplation stage to the preparation stage because the individual *feels unable* to make the change. Because no one can make another individual change, a feeling of self-efficacy is essential in order for long-lasting change to occur.

Clinical Case

John is a 24-year-old second-year medical student. He began drinking in his sophomore year of high school, and being shy and extremely inhibited in social situations, he found that alcohol helped him to relax and feel more at ease when meeting people.

He enjoys going out with his classmates after exams (and several times per week in between) and enjoys a reputation of being the life of the party. He typically has 10–12 drinks on these occasions and usually gets intoxicated. Though he generally takes a cab or walks home from the bars following these outings, he occasionally does drive while intoxicated. He also has occasionally had unprotected sex with women he meets in the bars. He often has blackouts for much of the events of the evening, and on one of these occasions, he did not remember having sex with a classmate. This led to very uncomfortable interactions in class over the following few weeks as she thought that she might be pregnant. He rarely makes it to class the morning after these binges. He has missed required small group sessions during which attendance is taken. On another occasion, feeling anxious before giving an oral presentation in front of the entire class, John sneaked into the bathroom and consumed two miniature bottles of vodka in an attempt to feel calm during the presentation. Once while John was practicing the physical exam on a patient in the teaching hospital, the patient commented that John smelled of alcohol. John, thinking quickly, explained that it was the hand sanitizer and the patient seemed to accept the explanation.

One night, arriving home from a bar very intoxicated and having lost the keys to his house, John fell through a window of his house as he tried to force the window open. His housemates awoke to find him lying on the floor with multiple cuts. The stove was on (John had apparently attempted to cook a late-night snack before passing out). They encouraged him to go to the hospital but he refused, insisting on being left alone. The housemates tried to talk with him about his drinking problem but he got angry and locked himself in his bedroom, leaving his friends to clean up the mess. The following day, John awoke with a hangover and no memory of the events of the previous night, and was surprised to see a piece of cardboard taped over the kitchen window. His housemates had left him a note saying that they needed to talk with him that afternoon after class.

That afternoon, the housemates met with John, who was still slightly hung over and had not had anything to drink. They explained that they were concerned about his alcohol use and that it seemed to be causing more and more problems in his life. John countered that although he did not go to class when hung over, he felt that he was always able to catch up on the missed material. He also felt that the alcohol helped him to relax and be less self-conscious in social situations. One of the housemates, a classmate who had just had a lecture on Motivational Interviewing (which John had missed), encouraged John to make a chart listing the pros and cons of his drinking and the pros and cons of stopping or significantly reducing his drinking (i.e., a decisional balance sheet, discussed later in the section "Suggestions for Treatment"; see also Figure 4–4).

Continue current alcohol use

Pros	Cons
More social	*Hangovers*
More accepted	*Lower grades*
Easier to talk in front of people	*More injuries*
	Possible disciplinary action from school
	Possible driving while intoxicated
	Possible car crash
	Possible sexually transmitted disease
	Possible fathering of a child
	Cost

Stop current alcohol use

Pros	Cons
Fewer hangovers	*Less fun*
Improved grades	*Fewer women*
Fewer injuries	
Save money	

John and his housemates then discussed the various items on the chart, focusing on the list for continuing his current alcohol use. John argued that despite the higher number of items in the second column (cons), most of these things were rare and unlikely to ever happen. He also expressed that the more common things (such as hangovers) really weren't that bad and that the pros in the first column were much more tangible and predictable. After acknowledging that these benefits were obviously very important to John, the housemates again brought up the fact that John had missed some mandatory small group sessions and that his grade might be affected. John got very defensive and resistant to further discussion. His classmate, remembering the general principles of Motivational Interviewing, decided to roll with John's resistance and encourage him to think about his goal of being a neurosurgeon. John got even more angry and stormed out of the house. The housemates decided that given the events of the previous night and concern for their own safety as well as John's worsening behavior, they would need to give him an ultimatum that he would need to move out of the house if he did not seek some sort of help for his problem.

Discussion of the Clinical Case

As the above scenario demonstrates, decisions to change behavior are rarely black and white. Most learned behaviors, no matter how problematic they become, have both positive and negative aspects. Many of these aspects are subconscious and will not be obvious to the individual. Though it did not immediately lead to the revelation that he clearly has a problem, the act of listing pros and cons of the drinking may lead John to further contemplation of the issue and possible future insight.

The scenario also highlights the fact that the benefits of behavior change often seem much less immediate and tangible than those associated with continuing the behavior. John's possible untreated social anxiety disorder leads him to find some benefit from alcohol's anxiolytic effects. The increased self-confidence and feeling that he is the life of the party can cause a great deal of ambivalence about stopping his drinking and may outweigh the various actual or potential negative consequences of his drinking.

Given that ambivalence is generally present and that the individual with the problematic behavior often does not consciously recognize the consequences of the behavior, it is often the case that motivation for change starts externally, such as when significant others (or employers or the legal system) provide an ultimatum that there will be a consequence unless the behavior is addressed. The hope is that the source of motivation for change will change from external to internal.

Suggestions for Treatment

Some individuals are able to recognize and change problematic behaviors on their own or with the assistance of self-help books or television shows, such as Oprah Winfrey's talk show. For them, *intrinsic factors* are enough to force them to realize that their behavior is problematic and take steps to change this behavior. However, many others, due to denial and other unconscious processes, do not realize that their behavior is problematic. For them, *extrinsic factors* are initially needed for them to recognize the harmful impact that their behavior has on themselves and others. These pressures serve the purpose of setting up circumstances that assist the individual in taking a look at his or her behavior. The hope is that with time, extrinsic factors, which can lead to short-term behavior change, will give way to insights and emotional changes that promote *internal motivation*, which is generally needed for long-lasting change. Extrinsic factors may be supplied by caring significant others, bosses, school administrators, religious groups, the criminal justice system, or…health care professionals.

The primary goals of the clinician when a patient is in the contemplation phase are to help the patient:

1. Decrease the desirability (*pros*) of the problematic behavior
2. Recognize the costs (*cons*) of the behavior
3. Recognize the benefits of change
4. Recognize and work through ambivalence
5. Anticipate barriers to initial and ongoing change
6. Achieve a sense of self-efficacy.

There is no one method that works for everyone. It is useful for the clinician to be familiar with various techniques that can be used for different patients or with the same patient over time (Table 4–1). It is also important for the clinician to remember that for many patients, the contemplation stage takes a considerable amount of time and that unhealthy behaviors may continue during this time despite the best efforts of the clinician and others involved with the patient.

Once the patient does realize that he or she has a problem, the clinician can be helpful in assisting the patient in feeling that he or she can change the behavior, helping to *increase self-efficacy*. In this effort, it is important that the clinician emphasize that the patient has a choice to address the problem. As with

TABLE 4–1. **Approaches to encourage contemplation**

1. Self-observation

    Behavior chart

    Timeline followback

    Parallel-timeline followbacks

2. Provision of information

3. Testimony from role models

4. Feedback

5. Decisional balance sheet

6. Standardized scales (University of Rhode Island Change Assessment [URICA], Stages of Change Readiness and Treatment Eagerness Scale [SOCRATES][a])

7. Rollnick's Readiness Ruler (Miller and Rollnick 2002)

8. Sobell and Sobell's (1993) Two Questions

9. Goal setting

10. Ultimatums

[a]URICA and SOCRATES are in the public domain and are located in the appendixes at the end of this chapter.

diabetes, hypertension, or other medical conditions, regardless of how the individual develops the problem (genetics, surgery, and so forth), it is the individual's choice and responsibility to make the changes necessary to deal with the problem. The clinician can assist the patient in feeling hopeful that he or she can make changes. Supportively honest and affirming statements based on careful listening can help patients feel more confident about their ability to change. Because self-efficacy changes over time and will increase or decrease with each small step toward change, it is important that the clinician be encouraging of any movement toward positive change. Through the process of Motivational Interviewing (see Chapter 2, "Fundamentals of Motivation and Change"), the clinician can elicit *self-motivational statements* from the patient, such as "Maybe this is more of a problem than I thought."

Much of the clinical interactions can be carried out in the context of Motivational Interviewing (see Chapter 1, "Addiction Treatment in Context," and Chapter 2, "Fundamentals of Motivation and Change"), using the principles outlined by Miller and Rollnick (2002) and expressed in the acronym *REDS*: **R**oll with resistance, **E**xpress empathy, **D**evelop discrepancy (i.e., discrepancies between the patient's present behavior and future goals), and **S**upport self-

Time of behavior	Duration of behavior	Situational factors (e.g., place)	Thoughts at time of behavior	Feelings at time of behavior

FIGURE 4–2.   Sample behavior chart.

efficacy. The patient's concerns, complaints, and problems can be heard and addressed in a compassionate, nonconfrontational manner that helps guide him or her toward recognition of the problematic behavior and the benefits of changing the behavior. This can occur in the context of a several-minute, *brief intervention* or an ongoing, multisession interaction.

The process of *self-observation* can be very important in the early stages of contemplation. Some individuals may not be aware of the extent of their problematic behavior or how pervasive it has become in their life. For some, the simple act of monitoring the behavior may lead to an increased awareness of the extent of the behavior and to subsequent change. This can be a therapeutic intervention in itself. The clinician can have the patient construct and maintain a *behavior chart* (Figure 4–2) in which various aspects of the addictive behavior are recorded (e.g., amount, frequency, duration, intensity, situation, associated thoughts, and emotional factors). The specific components tracked in the chart may vary, depending on the behavior. A daily or weekly calendar might also be adapted for this.

A related intervention is the use of the *timeline followback* (Sobell and Sobell 1996). With this technique, patients use a calendar to look back at appointments, work trips, holidays, newsworthy events, established social patterns (such as drinking every Monday night while playing pool), and social milestones (such as graduation, marriage, loss of a job, incarceration) to try to estimate the quantity of past substance use. This retrospective estimate provides a rough number and temporal pattern that can be used for further intervention. It can be assigned or "prescribed" as homework and reviewed with the clinician at the next visit.

An extension of this technique uses multiple, *parallel-timeline followbacks* to try to correlate substance use with other events. In this, the clinician and patient together construct a grid (Figure 4–3) with a variable timeline, from 1 week to many years, and try to align various events or physical and mental health problems with substance use. As this is being done, the clinician can use motivational techniques to help the patient see the relationship of the substance use to these events or symptoms. The simple visualization of the temporal relationship may be enough for some individuals to recognize that the substance use behavior is problematic.

Some patients may be helped by the simple *provision of information* that affects their perception of personal or social norms with regard to the behavior. An individual may believe that "everyone drinks five drinks per occasion" or that "there is no harm from alcohol use if I don't drink every day." The clinician can talk to the patient about typical drinking behaviors as outlined by the National Institute on Alcohol Abuse and Alcoholism (2005) and compare those behaviors to those of the patient. For some, the objective knowledge that his or her behavior is not "normal" or "average" may be enough to help the patient consider changing the behavior. This may be particularly powerful coming from a nonjudgmental clinician (as opposed to a nagging spouse).

Inaccurate normative perceptions may also be influenced by *testimony from role models* or other nonsignificant others who can talk with the patient about his or her experience with the behavior. At the same time, these other individuals can help *normalize* the ambivalence that may be confusing and shameful to the patient. Mutual-help meetings such as those of Alcoholics Anonymous can be a good source for normalizing ambivalence but may appear intimidating and threatening to someone early in the contemplation stage. It can often be useful for a clinician to have a list of several individuals who have changed a given behavior and who are willing to talk with others about the behavior. Celebrities who speak about their own struggles with substance dependence may serve a similar function. Even the substance-related death of a celebrity may lead some individuals to contemplate risks associated with their substance use. Again, for some, this approach may have far more effect on challenging the patient's perception of what is "normal" than similar statements from family members or friends.

Feedback is another useful technique that can often facilitate the process of contemplation of behavior change. The feedback can come from significant others or the clinician. The primary goal of the provision of feedback is to help the patient become aware of the effect of the behavior on others with the hope that the emotional component of the process of contemplation will be affected. It is generally most useful if the feedback is accurate, factual, specific to the patient and the individual providing the feedback, and delivered in a relatively calm manner. If statements are exaggerated ("You are *always* drunk!"), hypothetical ("Everyone who drinks like you *will end up* with liver failure!"), generalized ("Your drinking *bothers people!*"), or delivered in anger ("Stop drinking,

Jan Feb Mar Apr May Jun Jul Aug Sep Oct Nov Dec

Substance use _____

Health problems _____

Psychiatric symptoms _____

Legal problems _____

Work problems _____

Marital problems _____

FIGURE 4–3.   Sample parallel-timeline followback.

you #$%&*!!!"), it is much easier for the individual to become defensive and resist hearing anything that is said. Although it may be difficult to do, it is important for the individual providing the feedback to focus on the addicted individual, expressing concern. It is also important that feedback not be given while the individual is intoxicated because there is a good chance that the conversation will not be remembered. The clinician can help concerned family members by talking with them about some of the issues mentioned here. The clinician may also help to facilitate this process by having the significant other provide feedback in the relatively neutral setting of a health care facility. If initial attempts at providing feedback do not lead to immediate change, observations should be adjusted and repeated over time.

When the patient is in the contemplation stage regarding a particular behavior, the goal of the clinician is to assist the patient in moving from thoughts of changing the behavior to actual preparation for changing the behavior, the *preparation* stage (see Chapter 5, "Preparation"). Because of the great deal of ambivalence that often accompanies significant behavior change, a primary goal of the clinician is to help the patient recognize and examine factors on both sides of the argument, the pros and cons, benefits and costs, prospective gains and losses. Some individuals find it very useful to do this in a concrete way, with pen and paper. They may have thought about the various pros and cons but the act of committing them to paper and the visual confirmation provided by the list may be a very powerful motivator for some individuals. A *decisional balance sheet* (Figure 4–4) can be constructed and the patient can be assigned homework to complete the chart as honestly as possible. This can also be done in the office with the clinician. Either way, the chart should be reviewed with the clinician and patient (and significant others if possible) in order to clarify issues related to the various items listed. Just looking at the number of items in each column may not tell the whole story because certain factors may have significantly more importance or valence than others. It may help to assign a weighted value to each item before totaling the pros and cons.

Change behavior		Continue behavior	
Pros	Cons	Pros	Cons

FIGURE 4–4.   Sample decisional balance sheet.

Clinically, it is important to have the patient honestly and accurately look at the *positive* aspects of the substance use. Focusing only on the negative aspects often leads the individual to possess more knowledge about the problem but does not lead to further, long-lasting change. Disregarding the disease model of addiction and the changes in brain function that can accompany substance dependence and make change difficult, it may be helpful to point out to the patient that if there were no positive aspects to the behavior, then it would not make sense for the individual to continue the behavior. If efforts are not made to recognize, address, and compensate for the positive aspects of the substance use, the individual often reverts back to the more familiar behavior. Asking the patient to talk about the positives may also help reinforce the perception of the clinician as being nonjudgmental.

As a variation of the paper-and-pencil decisional balance sheet, an actual *balance scale* can be purchased and used as a visual aid in demonstrating the pros and cons of substance use. Coins, stones, weights, or marbles can be used and allow for relative values to be placed on certain factors (e.g., using two marbles for fighting with one's spouse vs. three marbles for incarceration, or using weights of different amounts for different factors). As the scale tips one way or the other, the clinician can ask for other factors to help weigh the scale in the desired direction. For clinicians with a flair for the dramatic, the scale can be suddenly upset as a limit of cons is reached, with marbles rolling all over the desk and floor. This visual display may help some individuals better appreciate the greater magnitude of negative effects of the problematic behavior.

Standardized scales have also been developed to assist clinicians in helping patients look at behaviors and contemplate change. Two examples of the more commonly used scales are the University of Rhode Island Change Assessment (URICA; DiClemente and Hughes 1990; McConnaughy et al. 1983) (Appendix A) and the Stages of Change Readiness and Treatment Eagerness Scale

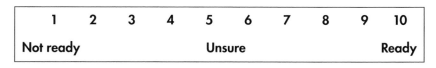

1	2	3	4	5	6	7	8	9	10
Not ready				**Unsure**					**Ready**

FIGURE 4–5.   The Readiness Ruler.
Source.   Adapted from Miller and Rollnick 2002.

(SOCRATES; Miller and Tonigan 1996) (Appendix B). More scales can be found in Treatment Improvement Protocol 35 of the Center for Substance Abuse Treatment (1999), which is part of the Substance Abuse and Mental Health Services Administration within the U.S. Department of Health and Human Services. All are in the public domain and can be used freely by clinicians. They are designed to be completed by the patient in a few minutes. Each measure has subscales that are designed to help the clinician and patient look at various domains like stages of change, ambivalence, and appreciation of pros and cons. Clinicians can use these scores to provide patients with feedback about their behavior. When the scales are readministered over time, changes in scores can help assess the impact of an intervention on problem recognition, ambivalence, and progress on making changes. A drawback to the use of some of these scales is that they require some amount of scoring by the clinician.

Briefer scales have also been used, including Rollnick's visual analogue *Readiness Ruler* (Figure 4–5; Miller and Rollnick 2002) and Sobell and Sobell's (1993) verbal *two questions* rated on a 100-point scale, as shown below:

1. "At this moment, how important is it that you change your current drinking?"

    Not important at all=0
    About as important as most of the other things I would like to achieve now=50
    Most important thing in my life now=100

2. "At this moment, how confident are you that you will change your current drinking?"

    I do not think I will achieve my goal=0
    I have a 50% chance of meeting my goal=50
    I think I will definitely achieve my goal=100

These brief scales can be used very quickly and changes in scores can be easily monitored over time. The clinician can also challenge the patient to consider change with questions such as, "Can you see yourself going from a 2 to a 4 [on the Readiness Ruler]?" or "What would it take to move from a 50 to a 60 [in ratings on Sobell and Sobell's questions]?"

Goal setting is another useful technique that can help an individual to recognize that he or she may have a problem with drugs or alcohol. The clinician can ask the patient to think of general life goals and things that prevent these goals from being realized. The clinician can help the patient recognize the role of substance use in setting goals by helping develop discrepancies between the past or current situations and the patient's goals for the future. For some patients, this exercise may help them to reevaluate behaviors and their effects on their life. A patient can then be asked to *envision* what his or her life would be like if the harmful behavior were changed. Specific, realistic, short-term goals can then be set as the patient moves into the preparation stage.

Ultimatums (rewards or punishments made contingent on a change in behavior) can be very powerful in assisting an individual to more closely contemplate his or her behavior. As with the process of providing feedback discussed above, it is important that ultimatums be presented out of care for the individual, not out of anger. In order for the contingency to be effective in promoting the individual's awareness of the problem, it is important that meaningful consequences be identified. Equally important is the identification of consequences that the concerned individual is willing and able to carry out. If threats are made and not followed through, the affected individual's rationalization and denial may become stronger. Some examples of consequences are not allowing a 15-year-old to take driving lessons until he or she stops smoking marijuana, not allowing a grandfather to visit with his grandchildren while consuming alcohol, not allowing an individual to remain in the home if he or she continues to use drugs, and marital separation if the spouse continues to drink alcohol. Obviously, many of these consequences are extremely difficult (emotionally and sometimes practically) for the significant other to enforce. The parent may have been waiting for years for a child to get a license so that the parent can stop being a taxi service. The grandfather may be a useful babysitter for busy parents. As mentioned above, it is very important for the concerned other to seriously consider the ultimatum and his or her ability to carry it out.

The clinician also may have control over certain reinforcers that are important to the patient (see Chapter 6, "Action," for a discussion of positive and negative reinforcement). The use of certain medications may be relatively or absolutely contraindicated with concomitant alcohol use. The physician may tell the patient that the physician is not able to prescribe the medication if the patient continues to drink alcohol. As with all ultimatums, it is important that an ultimatum be conveyed as being given out of concern for the patient, not as punishment. Reframing a patient's complaints about being coerced can be difficult but is important in order to help the patient understand the reasons for the ultimatum.

Suggestions for Teaching and Supervision

Teachers and supervisors can have trainees pick a behavior that they would like to change and have them construct a decisional balance sheet, encouraging them to pay attention to the positive aspects of the behavior to be changed. Trainees can also use a simple rating scale to evaluate the behavior and follow their ratings over time.

Trainees can also learn from role-playing, with one trainee (or the supervisor) acting as the clinician and the other acting as the patient. This can be done in a group with other trainees watching and providing constructive feedback.

Another useful technique is the audio or video recording of actual patient encounters with subsequent reviewing of the encounter with a supervisor. Obviously, this requires consent from the patient as well as a greater deal of planning and work related to the recording equipment, but the benefit of reviewing a session with a supervisor can be invaluable.

There are also useful videos (DiClemente 2004; D'Onofrio et al. 1997; Miller et al. 1998; Winters 2004) and Web sites with excellent educational material on Motivational Interviewing. Many of these show practitioners interacting with real or simulated patients and can be very useful in showing trainees many of the principles and techniques discussed in this chapter.

Movie: *Days of Wine and Roses*

Excellent examples of the stage of contemplation can be found in the film *Days of Wine and Roses*. Not only does the movie have individual scenes that depict the contemplation stage, the entire movie is an excellent depiction of the fluid, dynamic process of change. It also shows many of the concepts discussed in this chapter including ambivalence, provision of information, testimony from role models, feedback, self-observation, and the use of ultimatums. It shows how one individual's attempts to change are significantly affected by and have effects on those around him.

This 1962 movie, directed by Blake Edwards, was nominated for several Academy Awards and Golden Globe awards including Best Actor in a Leading Role (Jack Lemmon), Best Actress in a Leading Role (Lee Remick), Best Motion Picture—Drama, and Best Motion Picture Director. (The movie is based on a 1958 Emmy award–nominated teleplay for the series *Playhouse 90* that was directed by John Frankenheimer and starred Cliff Robertson and Piper Laurie.) It is about an alcoholic man, Joe Clay, who meets a relatively naive woman, Kirsten Arnesen, who prefers chocolate to alcohol.

The first half of the 117-minute movie shows Joe's increasing loss of control and the consequences of his drinking. It also shows how Kirsten, as a result of Joe's continual encouragement (and chocolate-flavored brandy alexanders), begins to drink and develops alcohol dependence herself.

The second half of the movie focuses on the couple's efforts to change their behavior. The first glimpses of contemplation occur about two-fifths of the way into the movie when Joe, while very intoxicated and fighting with his wife, slams a door, awakening their baby. After taking another drink, Joe becomes thoughtful and says, "How could I do a thing like that…to a child?…What's the matter with me?" He proceeds to look at their sleeping daughter and, crying, proceeds to apologize profusely to his wife for his behavior: "I'm sorry…I'm sorry…I'm sorry."

The next morning, late for work, Joe seems to no longer be contemplating the consequences of his drinking as he shaves in the office and jokes with his boss about his hangover. He proceeds to be demoted and sarcastically states, "I understand," to which his boss replies, "I hope you do." Later that day, while talking to his wife about the demotion (while drinking), Joe says, "I tried to be honest with myself…asked myself if it's my fault." Again, he seems to be only vaguely contemplating the effects of his drinking as he is more preoccupied with a missing bottle of liquor than with recognizing his role in the events.

Later in the movie, after he has been fired from his job, Joe is walking by his favorite bar and stops to look at his reflection in the window. On returning home, he says to his wife, "I walked by Union Square Bar. I was going to go in…Then I saw myself…my reflection in the window…and I thought, 'I wonder who that bum is?' And then I saw it was me. Now look at me. I'm a bum. Look at me! Look at you. You're a bum. Look at you. And look at us. Look at us. C'mon, look at us! See? A couple of bums." He then proceeds to describe the beginnings of his contemplation phase: "It came to me all of a sudden…. I saw the whole thing. You know why I've been fired from five jobs in 4 years?…and it's not politics like we always say, it's not office politics or jealousy or any of that stuff…it's booze…it's booze." Kirsten, now drinking heavily herself and clearly in the precontemplation stage, protests, "A couple of drinks." Joe responds, "We have more than a couple of drinks; we get drunk, then we stay drunk most of the time…Look at that dump that we live in…and the clothes that we wear…We send that child off to school like she's…looking like…I'm a drunk and I don't do my job and that's it…I'm a drunk and I don't do my job and I got fired and I can't get a job now and I…We should have done this a long time ago…taken a look at ourselves and realized we've just turned into a couple of bums." He proceeds with the preparation stage, devising a plan for himself and his wife to stop drinking alcohol.

After several months of sobriety, the couple relapses and Joe ends up in a straitjacket and padded room in the violent ward of a hospital. After he calms down, he begins to contemplate changing his behavior again. A man from Alcoholics Anonymous comes to visit him in the hospital, saying, "The nurse says you want some help..." to which Joe nods his head. The next scene shows Joe, clearly now contemplating his behavior and the need for assistance in maintaining abstinence, telling Kirsten about the help that was offered to him. "I asked for it...I must've needed help, I was in the hospital." For the first time, Kirsten appears to be contemplating that she also has a problem with alcohol, but she does not feel that she needs help. "I know I can't drink because it gets the best of me so I...I...I will just use my willpower and not drink and that's the end of it."

Following this, Joe stops drinking as Kirsten progresses to heavy daily drinking, disappearing from home for days at a time. Joe finds her in a motel and attempts to convince her to stop drinking. She, in turn, uses guilt to try to convince him to resume drinking with her, "I'm lonely, Joe...have a drink with me...Too good to have a drink with me?...I don't want any more of your mealy mouthed, holier-than-thou, do-gooder Boy Scouts with their hot coffee and cold feet...I don't want anybody that doesn't have the guts to take a drink...Now go away...I'm not coming back, Joe...you're too good." With that, because of his ambivalence and love for her, he contemplates for a few moments and then pours himself a drink. The binge rapidly escalates and he ends up in a psychiatric ward. Even then, after apparently experiencing delirium tremens, Joe continues to display ambivalence in his decision to change, crying, "I want her with me...I love her."

In the final scene of the movie, Kirsten returns home to talk with Joe, who has been sober for almost a year. Although she has not had a drink for 2 days, she is clearly continuing to contemplate her drinking and the purpose that she feels it serves in her life. Joe says to her, "You don't look so...," at which point she cuts him off and says, "So bad?...Not as bad as you'd imagined I would... Thanks for trying, but I know how I look. This is the way I look when I'm sober. It's enough to make a person drink, wouldn't you say? You see, the world looks so dirty to me when I'm not drinking...Joe, remember Fisherman's Wharf? The water when you looked too close? That's the way the world looks to me when I'm not drinking." She continues, "I don't think I could ever stop drinking completely, not like you...I couldn't...If I wanted to...really wanted to...well, I don't...I know that now...I want things to look prettier than they are."

She again tries to appeal to Joe to allow her to return home. "I know I could be alright if you'd help me...I need to be loved." He responds, "I love you...but I'm afraid of you." She then says, "If we only had it back...like it was." To which he replies, "You remember how it really was? You and me and booze...a threesome...You and I were a couple of drunks on the sea of booze, and the boat sank...I got hold of something that kept me from going under, and I'm not going to let go of it...Not for you. Not for anyone. If you want to grab on, grab on. But there's just room for you and me...no threesome." Kirsten looks at him, clearly contemplating. She walks to the window and looks out, "I can't get over how dirty everything looks." She then walks to the bedroom door to look at their daughter whom she has not seen for a year. "I can't...I can't... Better give up on me." Joe calmly replies, "Not yet." Kirsten smiles and responds, "Thanks...Goodnight." as she walks to the door and proceeds to leave. Joe, again ambivalent, calls for her and goes to open the door but stops himself and watches her through the window as she walks down the street.

Key Clinical Points

- The stage of contemplation may last a long time.

- Ambivalence is often present as an individual begins to contemplate changing behavior.

- In order for an individual to comprehensively consider the consequences of a behavior, it is important that he or she consider the positive aspects of the behavior as well as the negative.

- Even once an individual is able to recognize that he or she does have a problem, it is often difficult to move toward preparing to change because the individual feels that he or she is unable to make the change. However, with the help of an understanding and hopeful clinician, patients are more likely to feel empowered to change.

Multiple-Choice Questions

For the correct answers to these questions, including explanations of answers, please see the Answer Guide at the end of this book.

1. All of the following are true about the contemplation stage, EXCEPT:
   A. Ambivalence is very common.
   B. Most people move into the preparation stage within days of beginning to contemplate.
   C. Most people have many more pros for changing than cons against.
   D. Health care practitioners can often help patients contemplate behavior change.

2. Which of the following is NOT generally an effective technique used by clinicians to help a patient contemplate behavior change?

A. Provision of feedback.

B. Inducing guilt.

C. Use of a decisional balance sheet.

D. Provision of factual information.

3. Which is NOT a scale used to help assess an individual's readiness to change a behavior?

A. The University of Rhode Island Change Assessment (URICA).

B. The Readiness Ruler.

C. The Stages of Change Readiness and Treatment Eagerness Scale (SOCRATES).

D. The Princeton Level of Attention to Treatment Obstacles (PLATO).

4. All of the following are generally seen as primary goals of the clinician working with a patient in the contemplation stage, EXCEPT:

A. Helping the patient to recognize and work through ambivalence.

B. Helping the patient to recognize the benefits of change.

C. Helping the patient to achieve a sense of self-efficacy.

D. Helping the patient to regain things he or she has lost as a result of the addiction.

5. All of the following are typical phenomena seen in individuals in the contemplation stage, EXCEPT:

A. Rationalization.

B. Procrastination.

C. Dissociation.

D. Ambivalence.

References

Baumeister RF: The crystallization of discontent in the process of major life change, in Can Personality Change? Edited by Heatherton TF, Weinberger JL. Washington, DC, American Psychological Association, 1994, pp 281–294

Center for Substance Abuse Treatment: Enhancing Motivation for Change in Substance Abuse Treatment (Treatment Improvement Protocol Series, No 35; DHHS Publ No [SMA] 05–4081; publication reprinted as [SMA] 08–4212). Rockville, MD, Substance Abuse and Mental Health Services Administration, 1999

DiClemente C: Addiction and Change: How Addictions Develop and Addicted People Recover. New York, Guilford, 2003

DiClemente C: Stages of Change and Addiction. Hazelden Clinical Innovators Series (video and clinician's manual). Center City, MN, Hazelden, 2004

DiClemente CC, Hughes SO: Stages of change profiles in alcoholism treatment. J Subst Abuse 2:217–235, 1990

D'Onofrio G, Bernstein E, Bernstein J: The Emergency Physician and the Problem Drinker: Motivating Patients for Change. Boston, MA, Join Together, 1997

Janis IL, Mann L: Decision Making: A Psychological Analysis of Conflict, Choice, and Commitment. London, Cassel and Collier Macmillan, 1977

McConnaughy EA, Prochaska JO, Velicer WF: Stages of change in psychotherapy: measurement and sample profiles. Psychotherapy: Theory, Research and Practice 20:368–375, 1983

The Merriam-Webster Dictionary, New Edition. Springfield, MA, Merriam-Webster, 2005

Miller WR, Rollnick S: Motivational Interviewing: Preparing People for Change, 2nd Edition. New York, Guilford, 2002

Miller WR, Tonigan JS: Assessing drinkers' motivation for change: the Stages of Change Readiness and Treatment Eagerness Scale (SOCRATES). Psychol Addict Behav 10:81–89, 1996

Miller WR, Rollnick S, Moyers TB: Motivational Interviewing. Professional Training Videotape Series. Albuquerque, NM, Center on Alcoholism, Substance Abuse and Addictions, University of New Mexico, 1998

National Institute on Alcohol Abuse and Alcoholism: Helping Patients Who Drink Too Much: A Clinician's Guide (NIH Publ No 05–3769). Rockville, MD, National Institute on Alcohol Abuse and Alcoholism, 2005

Prochaska JO, DiClemente C: Stages and processes of self change of smoking: toward an integrative model of change. J Consult Clin Psychol 51:390–395, 1983

Prochaska JO, DiClemente CC: The Transtheoretical Approach: Crossing Traditional Boundaries of Therapy. Homewood, IL, Dow Jones-Irwin, 1984

Sobell M, Sobell L: Problem Drinkers: Guided Self-Change Treatment. New York, Guilford, 1993

Sobell LC, Sobell MB: Timeline FollowBack (TLFB) – User's Guide: A Calendar Method for Assessing Alcohol and Drug Use. Toronto, ON, Canada, Centre for Addiction and Mental Health, 1996

Winters K: Brief Intervention. Hazelden Clinical Innovators Series (video and clinician's manual). Center City, MN, Hazelden, 2004

Appendix A:
University of Rhode Island Change Assessment (URICA)[a]

Each statement below describes how a person might feel when starting therapy or approaching problems in his or her life. Please indicate the extent to which you tend to agree or disagree with each statement. In each case, make your choice in terms of how you feel right now, not what you have felt in the past or would like to feel. For all the statements that refer to your "problem," answer in terms of problems related to your drinking (or illegal drug use).

There are five possible responses to each of the items in the questionnaire:
1 = Strongly disagree; 2 = Disagree; 3 = Undecided; 4 = Agree; 5 = Strongly agree

Circle the number that best describes how much you agree or disagree with each statement.

	Strongly disagree	Disagree	Undecided	Agree	Strongly agree
1. As far as I'm concerned, I don't have any problems that need changing.	1	2	3	4	5
2. I think I might be ready for some self-improvement.	1	2	3	4	5
3. I am doing something about the problems that had been bothering me.	1	2	3	4	5
4. It might be worthwhile to work on my problem.	1	2	3	4	5
5. I'm not the problem one. It doesn't make much sense for me to consider changing.	1	2	3	4	5
6. It worries me that I might slip back on a problem I have already changed, so I am looking for help.	1	2	3	4	5

Appendix A:
University of Rhode Island Change Assessment (URICA)[a] *(continued)*

	Strongly disagree	Disagree	Undecided	Agree	Strongly agree
7. I am finally doing some work on my problem.	1	2	3	4	5
8. I've been thinking that I might want to change something about myself.	1	2	3	4	5
9. I have been successful in working on my problem, but I'm not sure I can keep up the effort on my own.	1	2	3	4	5
10. At times my problem is difficult, but I'm working on it.	1	2	3	4	5
11. Trying to change is pretty much a waste of time for me because the problem doesn't have to do with me.	1	2	3	4	5
12. I'm hoping that I will be able to understand myself better.	1	2	3	4	5
13. I guess I have faults, but there's nothing that I really need to change.	1	2	3	4	5
14. I am really working hard to change.	1	2	3	4	5
15. I have a problem, and I really think I should work on it.	1	2	3	4	5
16. I'm not following through with what I had already changed as well as I had hoped, and I want to prevent a relapse of the problem.	1	2	3	4	5
17. Even though I'm not always successful in changing, I am at least working on my problem.	1	2	3	4	5

Appendix A:
University of Rhode Island Change Assessment (URICA)[a] *(continued)*

	Strongly disagree	Disagree	Undecided	Agree	Strongly agree
18. I thought once I had resolved the problem I would be free of it, but sometimes I still find myself struggling with it.	1	2	3	4	5
19. I wish I had more ideas on how to solve my problem.	1	2	3	4	5
20. I have started working on my problem, but I would like help.	1	2	3	4	5
21. Maybe someone or something will be able to help me.	1	2	3	4	5
22. I may need a boost right now to help me maintain the changes I've already made.	1	2	3	4	5
23. I may be part of the problem, but I don't really think I am.	1	2	3	4	5
24. I hope that someone will have some good advice for me.	1	2	3	4	5
25. Anyone can talk about changing; I'm actually doing something about it.	1	2	3	4	5
26. All this talk about psychology is boring. Why can't people just forget about their problems?	1	2	3	4	5
27. I'm struggling to prevent myself from having a relapse of my problem.	1	2	3	4	5
28. It is frustrating, but I feel I might be having a recurrence of a problem I thought I had resolved.	1	2	3	4	5

Appendix A:
University of Rhode Island Change Assessment (URICA)[a] *(continued)*

	Strongly disagree	Disagree	Undecided	Agree	Strongly agree
29. I have worries, but so does the next guy. Why spend time thinking about them?	1	2	3	4	5
30. I am actively working on my problem.	1	2	3	4	5
31. I would rather cope with my faults than try to change them.	1	2	3	4	5
32. After all I have done to try to change my problem, every now and again it comes back to haunt me.	1	2	3	4	5

[a]URICA is in the public domain.
Source. McConnaughy EN, Prochaska JO, Velicer WF: Stages of change in psychotherapy: measurement and sample profiles. *Psychotherapy: Theory, Research and Practice* 20:368–375, 1983.

Scoring

Precontemplation items (PC)	1, 5, 11, 13, 23, 26, 29, 31
Contemplation items (C)	2, 4, 8, 12, 15, 19, 21, 24
Action items (A)	3, 7, 10, 14, 17, 20, 25, 30
Maintenance items (M)	6, 9, 16, 18, 22, 27, 28, 32

Note. The subscales can be combined arithmetically (C + A + M – PC) to yield a second-order continuous Readiness to Change score.

Appendix B: Stages of Change Readiness and Treatment Eagerness Scale (SOCRATES 8A)[a]

Instructions: Please read the following statements carefully. Each one describes a way that you might (or might not) feel *about your drinking*. For each statement, circle one number from 1 to 5, to indicate how much you agree or disagree with it *right now*. Please circle one and only one number for every statement.

	NO! Strongly disagree	No, disagree	? Undecided or unsure	Yes, agree	YES! Strongly agree
1. I really want to make changes in my drinking.	1	2	3	4	5
2. Sometimes I wonder if I am an alcoholic.	1	2	3	4	5
3. If I don't change my drinking soon, my problems are going to get worse.	1	2	3	4	5
4. I have already started making some changes in my drinking.	1	2	3	4	5
5. I was drinking too much at one time, but I've managed to change my drinking.	1	2	3	4	5
6. Sometimes I wonder if my drinking is hurting other people.	1	2	3	4	5
7. I am a problem drinker.	1	2	3	4	5
8. I'm not just thinking about changing my drinking, I'm already doing something about it.	1	2	3	4	5
9. I have already changed my drinking, and I am looking for ways to keep from slipping back to my old pattern.	1	2	3	4	5

Appendix B: Stages of Change Readiness and Treatment Eagerness Scale (SOCRATES 8A)[a] (continued)

	NO! Strongly disagree	No, disagree	? Undecided or unsure	Yes, agree	YES! Strongly agree
10. I have serious problems with drinking.	1	2	3	4	5
11. Sometimes I wonder if I am in control of my drinking.	1	2	3	4	5
12. My drinking is causing a lot of harm.	1	2	3	4	5
13. I am actively doing things now to cut down or stop drinking.	1	2	3	4	5
14. I want help to keep from going back to the drinking problems that I had before.	1	2	3	4	5
15. I know that I have a drinking problem.	1	2	3	4	5
16. There are times when I wonder if I drink too much.	1	2	3	4	5
17. I am an alcoholic.	1	2	3	4	5
18. I am working hard to change my drinking.	1	2	3	4	5
19. I have made some changes in my drinking, and I want some help to keep from going back to the way I used to drink.	1	2	3	4	5

[a]SOCRATES is in the public domain.
Source. Miller WR, Tonigan JS: Assessing drinkers' motivation for change: the Stages of Change Readiness and Treatment Eagerness Scale (SOCRATES). *Psychology of Addictive Behaviors* 10:81–89, 1996.

SOCRATES 8A Scoring Sheet

Transfer the patient's answers from questionnaire:

Recognition (Re)	Ambivalence (Am)	Taking steps (Ts)
1 _____	2 _____	
3 _____		4 _____
		5 _____
	6 _____	
7 _____		8 _____
		9 _____
10 _____	11 _____	
12 _____		13 _____
		14 _____
15 _____	16 _____	
17 _____		18 _____
		19 _____

Totals: Re: _____   Am: _____   Ts: _____

SOCRATES 8A Profile Sheet

Decile scores	Recognition (Re)	Ambivalence (Am)	Taking steps (Ts)
90 (very high)		19–20	39–40
80		18	37–38
70 (high)	35	17	36
60	34	16	34–35
50 (medium)	32–33	15	33
40	31	14	31–32
30 (low)	29–30	12–13	30
20	27–28	9–11	26–29
10 (very low)	7–26	4–8	8–25

Raw scores   Re = _____   Am = _____   Ts = _____
(from Scoring Sheet)

Guidelines for Interpretation of SOCRATES 8A Scores:

Using the SOCRATES Profile Sheet, circle the client's raw score within each of the three scale columns. This provides information as to whether the client's scores are low, average, or high *relative to the scores of people already seeking treatment for alcohol problems.* The following are provided as general guidelines for interpretation of scores, but it is wise in each individual case also to examine individual item responses for additional information.

Recognition

HIGH scorers directly acknowledge that they are having problems related to their drinking, tending to express a desire for change and to perceive that harm will continue if they do not change.

LOW scorers deny that alcohol is causing them serious problems, reject diagnostic labels such as "problem drinker" and "alcoholic," and do not express a desire for change.

Ambivalence

HIGH scorers say that they sometimes *wonder* if they are in control of their drinking, are drinking too much, are hurting other people, and/or are alcoholic. Thus a high score reflects ambivalence or uncertainty. A high score here reflects some openness to reflection, as might be particularly expected in the contemplation stage of change.

LOW scorers say that they *do not wonder* whether they drink too much, are in control, are hurting others, or are alcoholic. Note that a person may score low on ambivalence *either* because they "know" their drinking is causing problems (high Recognition), *or* because they "know" that they do not have drinking problems (low Recognition). Thus a low Ambivalence score should be interpreted in relation to the Recognition score.

Taking Steps

HIGH scorers report that they are already doing things to make a positive change in their drinking, and may have experienced some success in this regard. Change is underway, and they may want help to persist or to prevent backsliding. A high score on this scale has been found to be predictive of successful change.

LOW scorers report that they are not currently doing things to change their drinking, and have not made such changes recently.

CHAPTER 5

Preparation

Jose P. Vito, M.D.

In this chapter, I discuss the preparation stage (experimenting with small changes), which is before the action stage (taking a definitive action to change) and after the contemplation stage (weighing benefits and costs of behavior and the proposed change). Note that the preparation stage was not an original part of the Stages of Change. Precontemplation, contemplation, action, and maintenance were in the early version of the Stages of Change model, whereas the preparation stage was added later (DiClemente 1991).

Early on, the investigative actions that were used to assess information collected on the Stages of Change model recommended a four-step standard (precontemplation, contemplation, action, and maintenance) (McConnaughy et al. 1983, 1989). Soon after, using a different statistical investigative tactic was deemed more appropriate. This presented a better endorsement for the significance and the importance of the preparation stage (DiClemente 1991; Prochaska et al. 1992). As a result, precontemplation, contemplation, preparation, action, and maintenance are now the five basic stages of change within the model.

In the preparation stage, patients are planning to initiate change in both their attitude and their behavior. In most instances, they have learned important lessons from previous failed attempts to change (Prochaska and DiClemente 1992). In this stage, patients are planning a specific change, and they secure their planning and commitment to make that change. Their determination to change will intensify as they try to make minor modifications (e.g., a patient who chooses to lose weight may try low-fat food as a start).

When patients try to alter their behavior, such as trying to decrease smoking, they are moving into a more significant plan. It is critical for the clinician to support the patient and to help the patient deal with difficulties in achieving the plan, while persisting to investigate the patient's ambivalence toward change. Then tactics should shift from motivational technique to action.

In the preparation stage, patients feel an increasing sense of the need to change (Zimmerman et al. 2000). Here, patients talk about their decision to change, whereas in the contemplation stage patients still merely desire or hope for change. In the preparation stage, a patient selects a well-defined goal, such as "I will smoke 18 cigarettes instead of a pack a day." The patient may also declare an exact time period to start the goal (e.g., "Next week I will...."). After having chosen a specific course of action, the patient now asks for a potential health treatment plan. The patient anticipates and weighs the costs, the time required, potential physical discomfort, and embarrassment. Patients often think about the response of family members or others who may be threatened or refuse to go along with the change, such as a spouse or partner who smokes. Sometimes this occurs because individuals anticipate pressure from their own problems. In some cases, family members or others may oppose the patient's choice to change due to some concern about being inconvenienced (e.g., the wife who must leave work early to take care of the children while the husband attends a Sex Addicts Anonymous meeting). There is also the risk of humiliation if family members or others discover the addiction (e.g., the husband being seen entering the building where a sex addiction program takes place).

In addition, preparation is a watershed stage. Miller and Rollnick (2002) divide Motivational Interviewing into phase 1 and phase 2. Phase 1 involves building motivation, whereas phase 2 involves strengthening motivation and developing a plan of action. Phase 1 corresponds to the early stages, namely precontemplation and contemplation, and phase 2 corresponds to action and maintenance. Work during the preparation phase includes both phase 1 and phase 2 issues; therefore, it is a pivotal stage of transition toward establishing desired change.

Clinical Case

Tiffany is a 40-year-old divorced mother who works as an emergency room nurse. She was self-referred for intake in an outpatient drug treatment program. She has been abusing prescription drugs. As an emergency room nurse, she has easy access to painkillers, stimulants (such as amphetamines), and benzodiazepines. Her work shifts change from time to time with some mandated overtime work. Because money is always a challenge, Tiffany jumps at every opportunity to work for 16 hours straight. Tiffany has three children: a 5-year-old boy, an 8-year-old girl, and a 13-year-old girl, all from different fathers who are not involved in raising the children. She is in the process of taking legal action against her first ex-husband, who has stopped paying child support. Tiffany's mother occasionally babysits the children. However, Tiffany does not have a good support system and wishes that she had more time with the kids. In order to be alert at work she takes amphetamines, and later she takes benzodiazepines to calm down and fall sleep. She believes that these behaviors are helping her cope; however, she is irritable, screams at the children, has difficulty focusing on tasks, and is jittery and lethargic. Tiffany denies any other drug use but occasionally has one glass of wine at night before bedtime. She has been smoking cigarettes, one pack daily, for almost 20 years.

Tiffany has realized that she is overwhelmed with the kids and work. She is aware that while under the influence of drugs, she is more likely to make errors at work that could have dire consequences for her patients and could result in losing her children. She believes that one of her coworkers suspects that she is stealing and taking prescription medications. This coworker confidentially confronted her to seek help. Tiffany confided that she made numerous attempts in the past to stop "cold turkey" by herself but has been unsuccessful. Although she has tried reducing her drug usage, she finds she only craves more. This is where Tiffany has decided to initiate change (the preparation stage). Tiffany's plan is to utilize all her paid vacation days to seek outpatient care and assistance from her second ex-husband. She plans to make the first appointment next week.

Discussion of the Clinical Case

Tiffany's choice to seek outpatient drug treatment was a difficult decision because it may she jeopardize her job. She is emotionally ready for change in both attitude and behavior. She is now in the preparation stage. She has made the decision and is planning on making changes. Her determination is demonstrated by several planned behavior changes, such as making an appointment for outpatient care and seeking assistance from the second husband. Tiffany shows a firm commitment and has engaged herself in the process of change. She had set the specific date, that is, next week.

Suggestions for Treatment

Patients in the preparation stage have determined, during the contemplation stage, the difficulties they will encounter and have committed to a plan soon to be put into practice. However, ambivalence on the part of the patient can continue and must be addressed (Carroll 1996). The idea behind the suggestions for treatment that things flow perfectly in the preparation stage is not reality. The patient can move forward and be on the verge of action and still fall back on old ways or have residual negative thoughts. The clinician needs to be alert to these possibilities. The primary question that the clinician needs to assess is, does the patient want to change? How much the patient wants to commit to change in the preparation phase is in no small measure dependent on how much input the patient has in this stage; therefore, preparation can contain alternatives and additions to the plan, especially changes initiated by the patient. This is important because patient-initiated adjustments to the plan will increase patients' feelings of empowerment and will help them assume more ownership of their treatment. With further considerations of treatment, clinicians need to think outside the box. For example, if the patient verbalizes strong spiritual and religious feelings or beliefs, participation in a faith-based community support system can be included as a component of the treatment plan (rabbis and priests often offer substance abuse counseling). Patients who like to gather information in order to know their options may be directed to Hazelden Publishing (www.hazelden.org), a company with a long history of publishing literature dealing with substance use and abuse tailored to a broad range of readers.

Another important aspect of this stage is the difference between short- and long-term preparation for the action stage. What could be more important than getting through the first day of treatment and then the next couple of days? Building on small initial accomplishments is essential. The clinician should consider increasing interaction with patients during this stage. As the preparation stage moves forward, having the patients take ownership will increase the commitment. The characteristics of patients in this stage are shown in Table 5–1.

A significant yet incorrect belief held by some clinicians is that as soon as a choice has been made, patients move into the action stage. This is not always the case. The goal of the clinician for patients in the preparation stage is the development of planning and commitment. It is the effectiveness of the plan and the depth of the commitment that will allow patients to choose the right actions and to pledge to pursue them.

In the preparation stage, the clinician helps patients by enhancing motivation to build their action plans (DiClemente 1991). The clinician needs to work decisively regarding any unwillingness to change and to clearly distinguish the benefit of sobriety versus abuse. Planning must consist of the tactics to progress effectively and the abilities required to put them into practice. A significant contribution from the clinician is to offer an assessment of the skills required to execute the patient's plan and to avoid any shortfalls.

Furthermore, it is important to identify the lack of proper support that impacts the actions of the patients. The clinician needs to set definite planning goals with specific recommendations for patients, which can include joining a support group for substance abusers.

Evidence from smoking cessation literature supports there being a greater probability of moving into the action stage when the action plan is specific,

---

TABLE 5–1. **Common characteristics of individuals in the preparation stage**

A. Planning to alter their behavior

B. Willing to change in terms of both outlook and behavior

C. Being on the verge of taking action

D. Making a commitment to follow through

E. Deciding to change

Source. Adapted from Connors et al. 2001, p. 22.

---

such as setting a date (The Agency for Health Care Policy and Research Smoking Cessation Clinical Practice Guideline 1996). The action plan should anticipate different scenarios and contain specific patient behaviors and actions about how to handle them. The plan also should 1) identify a support structure, 2) identify a worst-case scenario, and 3) offer a contingency plan. The level of detail depends on the patient's need, terms of treatment, setting, and intensity.

Prior efforts to change behavior can be very helpful and can give insight. Some of the necessary questions to ask patients include the following: what were the previous plans, how long did the patient remain abstinent (e.g., abstaining from drug use), and what were the conditions of relapse? The feedback can give an overall analysis of the tough conditions and challenges that a patient finds difficult to overcome. In the clinical case presented earlier, Tiffany's failed prior efforts contained elements of accomplishments. The clinician should include those examples in the current planning. The skills and tactics to deal with these challenges must be addressed in the current change plan.

With the clinician's support, the next critical task in the preparation stage is development of the patient's commitment:

- Having choices increases commitment (Prochaska and DiClemente 1984).
- Offering patients alternative elements in their action plan can increase the level of commitment.
- Encouraging and positive words reinforce the patient's ability to change, which may recall past efforts that were successful.
- Positive images of success, such as visualization, can enhance commitment.
- Eliminating the last vestiges of the patients' ambivalence can be viewed as enhancing commitment.

Once the action plan is designed and the commitment confirmed, the patient enters the action stage.

During the preparation stage in a group setting, the key objective with patients is to give the encouragement and the validation needed to move the plan forward. This helps patients pursue their goal to change. In other words, the group functions such that patients support each other in initiating change. Keep in mind that in the preparation stage, there is a reduced level of denial and ambivalence. But until commitment and planning are set, patients may revert to the precontemplation or contemplation stage. Therefore, the group can assist by supporting the commitment to continue the change in behavior. A patient's efforts need to be acknowledged by the group because this will enhance the individual's confidence and commitment. The patient will start to feel competent to face all the obstacles and challenges that he or she might encounter in moving forward.

The group can also be helpful by observing and witnessing any relapse in behavior and confronting the patient about this issue. The group can give recommendations on ways to avoid hazardous behaviors and avoid trigger situations that can cause a patient to relapse.

Suggestions for Teaching and Supervision

In supervising junior therapists, keep in mind that moving from contemplation to the preparation stage involves a change in patients' thinking—for example, a shift in their attitude and perceptions that have continued from substance use. However, the negative consequences of substance abuse now clearly outweigh the positive effects of continued alcohol and/or drug use. Patients in the preparation stage are ready for change, and they seek out information about their problems. They are determined to initiate new patterns of daily living habits and behaviors. They are more likely to seek new activities—activities other than substance use—and are more likely to rearrange their lives and avoid high-risk situations. They are more likely to develop new support systems.

Psychotherapy trainees may find it helpful to match specific patient characteristics with clinician strategies to enhance patients' motivation in the preparation stage (Table 5-2). For example, patients who begin to express commitment to specific goals will likely benefit from a negotiation of a specific timetable. Such patients choose a time to begin their course of change and the steps necessary to carry them out. Clinicians should record data (e.g., start date), provide encouragement, and help patients select an explicit tactic that may consist of planned actions or recommendations.

For reinforcement of motivation to change, open-ended discussions can be effective. The clinician expresses support by participating in ongoing conversations and reassures patients that initiating action to change is always a positive step. Even when patients' attempts to change are not successful, the experience

TABLE 5–2. **Strategies to enhance patients' motivation in the preparation stage**

Patient characteristics	Clinician strategies
Understands that change is needed	Summarize patient's reasons for change
Begins to form commitment to specific goals, methods, and timetables	Negotiate a start date to begin some or all change activities
Can picture overcoming obstacles	Encourage patient to announce plans publicly
May procrastinate about setting start date for change	Arrange a follow-up contact with patient and clinician for shortly after the plan start date

Source. O'Connell 2003.

yields helpful information and lessons learned. Encourage patients to tell their support group and others about their plans to change their behavior so that they can maintain their promises. Arranging follow-up with patients, such as scheduling an appointment for a date after their action plan has started, is helpful before patients reach their proposed start date. Reinforcement by clinicians is important for change to continue. The clinician helps patients fortify their goals with specific, detailed actions that must be carried out. After that, the clinician needs to support patients to strengthen their commitment by setting an exact time for an exact route of action. Junior therapists must note that change is natural and intrinsic. In addition, they should retain the belief that people are capable of planning and that this capability can be facilitated in a supportive environment.

Movie: *28 Days*

The movie *28 Days* (released by Columbia Pictures in 2000) portrays the different stages of change, in particular, the preparation stage. The main character, Gwen Cummings, was arrested for driving while intoxicated. She was given a choice between going to prison or checking into a drug rehabilitation facility for a 28-day program. She chooses the latter. At first, she is in denial and unwilling to take part in any of the treatments. She does not accept or recognize her addiction. She continues her drug, nicotine, and alcohol use—sneaking in drugs and running out of the center, to return drunk hours later and past curfew. There are moments in the movie when she is aware of her substance dependency: after witnessing the suicide of her 17-year-old heroin addict roommate, after enabling her boyfriend to supply her with drugs, and when her sister confronts her about her behavior during her sibling's wedding. She recognizes that the path to successful recovery is not guaranteed after she observes the relapse of a surgeon who had completed the same 28-day program.

A critical scene in the movie is when Gwen eventually comes to terms with her alcoholism and substance abuse. Her counselor threatens to throw Gwen out of the program and into jail after she returns drunk past curfew. Gwen is angry and throws her recreational drugs (pills) out the window in her room. Not being able to deal with her current emotions and the thought of going to jail, Gwen later tries to climb down the building from her window to obtain the drugs she had thrown out earlier. She falls and breaks her leg and is brought to the facility's medical clinic. The medical doctor tells her that she will not be given any painkillers because of her addiction. Gwen then catches sight of her reflection in a glass door. She does not like what she sees. She immediately seeks help from her counselor, letting him know how much she needs rehab treatment instead of going to prison. At that moment, she enters the preparation stage.

Gwen finally understands the need for change in her behavior and her commitment to being drug and alcohol free. She negotiates her plans of behavior change with the counselor, but she is very specific about her start date for change as she wants to complete the 28-day program. To start her smoking cessation, she begins to chew gum. She also begins to distance herself from her drug-dependent boyfriend.

Key Clinical Points

- The preparation stage is when a patient plans to begin change with a set date in the future.

- In the preparation stage, the clinician's primary focus is planning and commitment enhancement.

- Patients in this stage have made the choice to change their behavior but may have some resistance about their decision.

- The patient's willpower to change is evidenced by making small incremental changes. Patients occupy this stage for a short period of time. However, this does not guarantee that they will move into the action stage. There is the possibility that patients will revert back to contemplation when hit with frustrating obstacles.

- A realistic action plan is critical and anticipates barriers, identifies solutions, and provides concrete recommendations.

Multiple-Choice Questions

For the correct answers to these questions, including explanations of answers, please see the Answer Guide at the end of this book.

1. Rashad is a 40-year-old male with a history of heavy nicotine addiction for over 20 years. His lover, who has been a smoker for over 35 years, was recently rushed to the emergency room and was diagnosed with emphysema. Rashad is aware of his nicotine dependence and has tried numerous times to quit. He attributes this addiction to his partner. After hearing the emphysema diagnosis, Rashad immediately went on the Internet to research nicotine cessation. He scheduled an appointment with his doctor to discuss his nicotine dependence. Rashad is also searching for a support group. Rashad is in what stage of change?

    A. Precontemplation.
    B. Contemplation.
    C. Preparation.
    D. Action.

2. Charles is a 40-year-old married male with a 9-year-old daughter. He works as an executive in a busy, high-pressure accounting firm. He denies any alcohol or drug use. He verbalized being sexually dissatisfied with his wife. He spends much time searching pornographic Web sites on his laptop. In fear of being discovered by his wife, he started using his laptop in the basement. At first, he would spend an hour after work surfing the Internet, then it grew to 4 hours. Now, it has consumed him so that he is surfing the Internet for porn during business hours. Two weeks ago, his assistant walked in on Charles sniffing a thong while watching pornographic material during lunch. Embarrassed, Charles quickly turned off his computer and hid the thong in his desk drawer and threatened to fire the assistant if she were to mention this to anyone. The assistant promises to keep his secret in confidence. In order for Charles to be in the preparation stage, which of the following statements is correct?

    A. "Who, me? I have no problem. I can stop surfing the Internet for pornographic Web sites whenever I want to. Besides, I am a top executive in this company. Anyway, nobody monitors my computer because I am the boss."

B. "I think I might have a problem controlling my urges and surfing the Internet for pornographic Web sites. It was really embarrassing that my assistant caught me in the act. What if my wife knew?"

C. "I have a problem controlling my urges and surfing the Internet for porn. I could lose my job if my assistant reports me to human resources. My wife will find out, divorce me, and not let me see my daughter. Tomorrow, I will take a day off from work and will seek professional help."

D. "It was really embarrassing that my assistant caught me. Since then, my wife and I have attended couples counseling and I see a psychiatrist who has prescribed medication for me."

3. What is the most important component in moving a patient from contemplation into the preparation stage so that the patient can be successful in dealing with his or her problem?

A. The patient believes and understands that he or she has a problem and plans to do something about it in the future.

B. The patient identifies the pros and cons of change.

C. The patient describes a plan in detail and follows it as part of his or her regular activity.

D. The patient expresses feelings about how much the change has actually improved the patient's life and reflects on the long-term goal.

4. How can a clinician know if the patient is ready to move from the preparation stage to the action stage and be successful?

A. Feedback from the patient regarding the treatment plan and whether he or she is ready to move from the preparation state to the action stage is the best indicator.

B. Using urine toxicology is the best way to assess the stage of change and readiness to move forward.

C. The scope of the treatment plan determines the appropriate time to move to the next stage.

D. The preparation stage typically lasts for 6 months, after which the patient transits to the action stage.

5. Which patient characteristic best increase the chances of success when entering the preparation stage?

A. The patient realizes that he or she is substance dependent and is aware of the negative consequences of his or her behavior. Therefore, the patient plans to set a date in the future to change the behavior.

B. The patient believes that there are fewer opportunities when he or she stops using drugs and thinks, for example, "We are all going to die anyway, might as well die high."

C. Younger substance abusers have fewer established negative behavioral patterns than older users; they are better candidates for substance use cessation.

D. The patient is being forced by society to change his or her behavior; for example, a heroin-dependent teenager is mandated by the court to attend a drug treatment program.

References

The Agency for Health Care Policy and Research Smoking Cessation Clinical Practice Guideline. JAMA 275:1270–1280, 1996

Carroll KM: Integrating psychotherapy and pharmacotherapy in substance abuse treatment, in Treating Substance Abuse: Theory and Technique. Edited by Rotgers F, Keller DS, Morgenstern J. New York, Guilford, 1996, pp 286–318

Connors GJ, Donovan DM, DiClemente CC: Substance Abuse Treatment and the Stages of Change: Selecting and Planning Interventions. New York, Guilford, 2001

DiClemente CC: Motivational interviewing and the stages of change, in Motivational Interviewing: Preparing People to Change Addictive Behavior. Edited by Miller WR, Rollnick S. New York, Guilford, 1991, pp 191–202

DiClemente CC, Prochaska JO: Toward a comprehensive, transtheoretical model of change: stages of change and addictive behaviors, in Treating Addictive Behaviors, 2nd Edition. Edited by Miller WR, Heather N. New York, Plenum, 1998, pp 3–24

McConnaughy EA, Prochaska JO, Velicer WF: Stages of change in psychotherapy: measurement and sample profiles. Psychotherapy Theory, Research, Practice, Training 20:368–375, 1983

McConnaughy EA, DiClemente CC, Prochaska JO, et al: Stages of change in psychotherapy: a follow-up report. Psychotherapy Theory, Research, Practice, Training 26:494–503, 1989

Miller WR, Rollnick S: Motivational Interviewing: Preparing People for Change, 2nd Edition. New York, Guilford, 2002

O'Connell D: Behavior change, in Behavioral Medicine in Primary Care: A Practical Guide, 2nd Edition. Edited by Feldman MD, Christensen JF. New York, Lange Medical Books/McGraw Hill, 2003, pp 135–149

Prochaska JO, DiClemente CC: Stages of change in the modification of problem behaviors, in Progress in Behavior Modification, Vol 28. Edited by Hersen M, Eisler RM, Miller PM. Sycamore, IL, Sycamore Publishing, 1992, pp 183–218

Prochaska JO, DiClemente CC: Self-change processes, self-efficacy and decisional balance across five stages of smoking cessation, in Advances in Cancer Control. Edited by Epstein PF, Anderson PN, Mortenson LE. New York, Alan R. Liss, 1984, pp 131–151

Prochaska JO, DiClemente CC, Norcross JC: In search of how people change: applications to addictive behaviors. Am Psychol 47:1102–1114, 1992

Zimmerman GL, Olsen CG, Bosworth MF: A 'stages of change' approach to helping patients change behavior. Am Fam Physician 61:1409–1416, 2000

Action

Gary P. Katzman, M.D.

Maintenance of abstinence is a highly active process. It is not simply the cessation of using a substance. Helping patients develop lifestyles that support abstinence and that are less compatible with substance use is the major goal of treatment during the transition between the action and maintenance phases. Cognitive-Behavior Therapy (CBT), based on principles of learning, is one type of psychotherapy that is effective for developing healthy lifestyles that support abstinence. CBT rests on the assumption that symptoms are related to the interaction of thoughts, behaviors, and emotions. It is intensely active and collaborative, albeit prescriptive, and focuses on identifying and directly changing thoughts and behaviors that may be maintaining symptoms. Using specific approaches discussed in this chapter, patients can learn and practice alternative, healthier, non-substance-using patterns of living.

Although there is a strong technical base to CBT, one of the most powerful factors in the motivation for change is the therapeutic relationship. Greatly influenced by Carl Rogers's Client-Centered Therapy (Rogers 1951), Motivational Interviewing is a method for enhancing a person's intrinsic motivation to change by exploring and resolving ambivalence about behavior change. Its main goal is to identify and amplify discrepancies between a person's present behavior and the person's broader goals. The two phases of Motivational Interviewing are 1) building motivation and 2) strengthening the commitment to change. Motivational Interviewing emphasizes the therapeutic alliance and is nonjudgmental. It attempts to create an environment that feels safe and comfortable, so that patients can be more disclosing and trustful. The assumption is made that people generally know what they need to do. Instead of pedantically providing instruction such as "You need to have more structure in your day," Motivational Interviewing supports a more collaborative approach: "What do you need to do to be less bored and lonely during the day?" In many ways, we try to help patients become cotherapists. They actively participate in the design of their treatment and engage in the treatment work between therapy sessions (Kadden et al. 1992). CBT involves a lot of planning, and when done in a style consistent with Motivational Interviewing, ambivalence can be addressed and motivation can be maintained and enhanced, improving the likelihood that patients will establish the new habits that lead to the maintenance of abstinence (Foote 2006).

Below is a brief vignette that illustrates how substance use affects multiple areas in the patient's life. In this chapter, several approaches are discussed, some applicable to helping this patient, Joe, assess his problem areas, identify his strengths and weaknesses in dealing with stressors, and evaluate and change some of his patterns of thinking and behaving to manage the identified problem areas.

Clinical Case

Joe is a 34-year-old man who has been in ongoing therapy with a psychiatrist for alcohol dependence. He started drinking heavily for the first time while in his school fraternity and over the past 8 years has increased his consumption to five drinks of vodka per day, four to five times per week. He would occasionally experience morning shakes, relieved by drinking alcohol. He reports using cocaine once to twice per month. He last used alcohol and cocaine 2 weeks ago, at which time he decided to abstain from all substance use.

Currently, he is having difficulty sleeping, feels anxious, and is frequently irritable. He has been arguing more than usual with his live-in girlfriend of 3 years. She is dependent on alcohol, sells and uses cocaine on the weekends, and becomes verbally abusive when he suggests that she has a problem with substances.

He has attended Alcoholics Anonymous (AA) meetings in the past, but very sporadically. He reports good compliance with his drug therapy, taking a selective serotonin reuptake inhibitor for anxiety and naltrexone to decrease alcohol cravings. He has never tried to hurt or kill himself and his most angry outburst resulted in punching a door.

Both of his parents were "heavy drinkers, but functional." He always struggled in school and was often the class clown. Joe is currently employed as a salesman and enjoys his work, although he dreams of a career in politics. He does not have any hobbies, does not engage in any recreational or physical activities, and is overweight. He is very close with his two sisters, although they are wary of getting too involved in his care, having felt manipulated in the past. Joe has a few acquaintances from work with whom he used to get drunk, but "no real friends." He experiences a great deal of shame and embarrassment when he thinks about the pain he has inflicted on his family and friends over the years. He views himself as "messed up" and thinks he has very limited dating options. He worries that he won't be able to socialize without the help of alcohol.

Discussion of the Clinical Case

The case suggests a family history of alcohol dependence, a likely biological or hereditary contribution to his substance use. Another possible predisposing factor is attention-deficit/hyperactivity disorder, as deduced from his history of poor classroom performance and class-clown behavior, which is highly comorbid with alcohol dependence. Joe's college fraternity drinking days and possible social anxiety disorder may have precipitated his long history of binge alcohol use. His tumultuous relationship with his drug-using girlfriend and his anxiety, insomnia, and unfulfilled dream of a life in politics may all have contributed to the perpetuation of his substance use. Joe is currently in the action phase of the stages of change described in the Transtheoretical Model of Change (Prochaska et al. 1994). He not only has the desire to abstain from the maladaptive pattern of substance use, he actually stopped using drugs 2 weeks ago. Given the natural course of substance dependence (considered a relapsing and remitting illness), his continued relationship with his drug-abusing girlfriend, his lack of involvement in alternative interests and activities, and his limited social network, the risk for imminent resumption of substance use remains high. Joe has a diagnosis of alcohol dependence and cocaine abuse, both in early remission. The remainder of this chapter focuses on how to help Joe consolidate his gains and minimize the risk of relapse.

Suggestions for Treatment

As seen in the vignette, Joe's history reveals a number of behaviors and thoughts that are associated with risk for relapse. To sustain abstinence, patients develop alternative behaviors and thought patterns that not only are healthy and satisfying, but also can compete with the allure of substance use. These new behaviors and thoughts often coalesce to become a new lifestyle, replacing the former one that was narrowly focused on acquiring and using substances. In CBT, the patient and therapist work together to introduce new, healthier behaviors and cognitions, ones that are incompatible with substance use. This collaboration optimally leads to the development and practice of new behaviors and thoughts until they become the default patterns.

Behavioral Component of CBT

Behavior Therapy, which developed before the advent of Cognitive Therapy, rests on the notion that both healthy and maladaptive (unhealthy) behaviors are governed by the same principles of learning. Specific, maladaptive behaviors can be modified by learning new, more appropriate behaviors. The first step toward making change is helping patients become nonjudgmental observers of their own behaviors and patterns of thinking. Most of our patterns of interacting, thinking, and reacting are somewhat automatic processes that have been learned over time and reinforced.

Through monitoring, patients can become more aware of these processes. Patients are encouraged to keep a dedicated notebook in which they make an entry each time they notice a behavior or thought they want to change. People often say, "I'm aware of what I do; I'll just pay more attention to it." Although it is true that people are aware of many of their patterns, writing things down makes the process of change much more active and purposeful and tends to lead to much more change than merely making a mental note (Kadden et al. 1992).

One of the cornerstones of Behavior Therapy is that behavior is a function of its consequences. If the consequence is favorable, then the behavior is more likely to be repeated. We refer to this type of consequence as a *reinforcer* (further discussed later in this chapter, in the section "Self-Efficacy and Locus of Control"). When something is done or added to provide reinforcement, it is called *positive reinforcement* (this includes social reinforcers such as praise and affection, and material reinforcers such as gifts and money). When a stimulus is removed (typically something aversive) in order to provide reinforcement, it is called *negative reinforcement*. This term is often confused with punishment. Whereas both positive and negative reinforcement strengthen behaviors, punishment is intended to weaken a behavior. *Extinction* refers to the weakening of a behavior by the attenuation of positive or negative reinforcement (Carroll 1998).

The following is an example that highlights the above principles, referred to as *operant conditioning*. Hypothetically, let's assume the case of Joe is different than detailed earlier. If Joe wants a drink of alcohol and his girlfriend attempts to thwart him from drinking, he may start screaming and cursing. Joe's girlfriend at first may hold her ground and tell him he cannot have the alcohol. Joe may escalate his screaming. The girlfriend, head throbbing in pain, finally relents, letting Joe have the drink. As soon as Joe gets the alcohol, he stops screaming. Everyone is now at least partially relieved…until the next time. Joe negatively reinforces the girlfriend's capitulatory behavior by removing the aversive stimulus of screaming. The girlfriend positively reinforces Joe's demanding behavior whenever he wants something he doesn't get right away by giving in to his demand for alcohol. If the girlfriend did not positively reinforce the screaming behavior, the screaming and cursing would eventually diminish or be extinguished. The same would be true if Joe did not stop the screaming when the girlfriend finally gives in: in the future, the girlfriend would not give in as a way to quiet screaming Joe.

Many patterns of substance use are maintained through positive and negative reinforcement. Often, these patterns are shaped by operant conditioning in a somewhat haphazard and even random fashion. Behavior Therapy attempts to use operant conditioning, systematically, to strengthen adaptive patterns of living and to weaken maladaptive ones.

When helping patients develop behaviors and thoughts that are incompatible with substance use, it is important to remember that not everyone perceives the same things as reinforcing. Some people may like being told they have done a good job and may enjoy the taste of chocolate; they therefore find these reinforcing. Someone else, however, may find it embarrassing to be complimented and may be allergic to chocolate or not care for it, making these behaviors nonreinforcing or even punishing. We say that reinforcers need to be in the currency of the recipient.

Assertiveness

One of the most important aspects of the behavioral management of substance use is the ability to stand up for oneself in the face of discomfort. The alternative response, passivity, usually leads to anger and frustration: at the person for the offense and at oneself for not speaking up. This in turn may be a trigger for substance use. *Assertiveness*, the preferred adaptive response, is the capacity to ask for what one wants, without undue guilt or anxiety, in a manner that projects confidence but does not trample on the rights of others. The important thing to remember is that assertiveness is more about the belief that one has the capacity to manage an adversarial situation than actually acting on it. For example, if an infirm elderly person cuts in to the front of a line of people, one may choose to say nothing because it may have little practical significance. If this is not the case, one might say, with good eye contact and voice projection, "Excuse me, I need to dash out and am on line here." Very few people are adept at this vital skill, and most of us have contextual deficits. For example, some people are assertive at work but nonassertive at home. Unfortunately, assertiveness is often misunderstood and confused with aggressiveness. Aggressiveness is also a way of getting what one wants, but this tends to offend—such as saying "Hey, you &!?@, get to the back of the line like everybody else!" in the situation above—and promotes more distance in a relationship.

Assertive refusal is an essential skill to delay or avoid substance use when the substance or trigger is present. It is important for patients to avoid using excuses such as "I'm on antibiotics" or vague refusals such as "I'm OK for now." Statements need to be clear, firm, and nonapologetic: "I have stopped drinking alcohol" or "No, thank you, I won't be drinking." Justifying substance refusal with excuses perpetuates the belief there is something wrong with disclosing abstinence or a substance use problem. The therapist might role-play, pressuring the patient to have a drink. The patient can then practice assertive refusal. The therapist may reinforce assertive behaviors while prompting for alternatives to be practiced. The therapist and patient may then switch roles so the therapist can model assertive refusal. Patients can also practice assertive refusal using imagery: patients picture walking into a trigger-rich environment, and in a confident manner either avoid the trigger or refuse an offer to use a substance. The patient can imagine feeling proud and determined. Imaginal exposure is often a safer way to practice the desired responses and can help a patient become desensitized to triggers (Kadden et al. 1992).

Patients are encouraged to have a checklist of behaviors that are part of the new behavioral lifestyle. Patients can carry this checklist and refer to it each morning and bring it to each therapy session to increase the likelihood that these behaviors and activities won't be forgotten.

Problem Solving

Problem solving is a collection of techniques that help a patient identify the current circumstances, the desired goals, and possible ways to accomplish the goals—and then weigh the pros and cons of the generated options and choose the optimal one. Often, the first recognizable sign of a problem is a negative emotion. Patients may first notice feelings of anger, sadness, anxiety, and so forth. These feelings may even be preceded by physiological responses such as sweaty palms, indigestion, or feeling hot. Other clues indicating that there is a problem may be behavioral responses such as impulsivity, overworking, or isolation. After potential goals are explored, an exhaustive list of possible solutions is generated. Patients can then do a cost-benefit analysis. It is important to generate a cost-benefit analysis for each option as well as a cost-benefit analysis for not choosing that option. Once a solution is chosen and implemented, the patient's progress needs to be evaluated, with attention paid to any difficulties encountered and the degree of effectiveness.

Patients are encouraged to list a hierarchy of the triggers that were most associated with their substance use and another hierarchy of the triggers that are the most difficult to avoid. For each trigger, the patient might generate multiple strategies to avoid the trigger or alter the trigger if it occurs. Prompting and suggesting ideas to manage triggers can be saved until after the patient first tries. As patients practice problem solving, they get better at it and develop a sense of increased self-efficacy (Kadden et al. 1992).

Self-Efficacy and Locus of Control

Self-efficacy refers to the individual's belief that he or she has the capacity to effect change. Motivational Interviewing techniques are designed to enhance patients' confidence in their ability to change. For example, on hearing Joe report initiating a conversation at a party, the therapist might ask, "How did it feel to do what is usually uncomfortable for you?" or "Did you expect it to work out the way it did?" (Miller and Rollnick 1991). The therapist's positive reinforcement of the more adaptive behavior is important, such as "You did a great job approaching that woman at the party." Clinicians also want to promote self-reinforcement, such as by asking, "What do you think about the change you made?" This relates to another concept called locus of control.

Locus of control refers to the source of patients' reinforcement. Reinforcers can be external, such as praise and gifts, or internal, such as self-affirmations and self-praise. Although both can be therapeutic, often it is the capacity to generate strong internal reinforcers that leads to the greatest motivation to sustain change. When patients recognize a disproportionate desire for external reinforcers, they can practice refraining from behaviors designed to elicit those responses. For example, if someone routinely seeks external reinforcement (e.g., "Tell me I'm beautiful"; "Am I smart?"; "Tell me again that you love me"), he or she may monitor this behavior and practice refraining from the habit. Patients could monitor their cognitions that are associated with concern for their looks or other qualities and use cognitive restructuring exercises, discussed later in this chapter (see "Cognitive Restructuring"), to challenge maladaptive thought patterns that may be perpetuating the desire to seek self-reassurance. It can also be helpful to coach members of the patient's network to avoid engaging in the reinforcing behaviors that the patient is seeking. To generate more internal reinforcers, patients can repeat daily affirmations, practice replacing self-deprecating comments with more descriptive ones, and evaluate and change unrealistic expectations of themselves and others (Fay 1998).

Behavioral Activation

One of the commonly used techniques for dealing with a sense of emptiness, often present during early abstinence, is *behavioral activation,* which involves programming daily activities that the patient finds reinforcing. Substance-related behaviors and thoughts can occupy large portions of the day. When drug usage stops, many patients feel a large void characterized by boredom, loneliness, and despair. Behavioral activation attempts to fill the abyss with naturally reinforcing activities such as exercise, socializing, eating, hobbies and interests, chores, work, reading, and other activities. In addition, when patients have minimal social supports, exposing them to new and interesting activities and pursuits can expand their network. Given that Joe lacks interests and hobbies and has a limited social network, behavioral activation can play an important role in reducing his risk for relapse (American Psychiatric Association 2006).

Cognitive Component of CBT

When we refer to the Cognitive Therapy portion of CBT, the term *cognition* encompasses a variety of thoughts, assumptions, expectations, beliefs, values, attributions, predictions, standards, and rules. Cognitions often intersect with behaviors and emotions, which may impact the course of substance use or abstinence. One of the fundamental principles of Cognitive Therapy is that situations or stimuli are often the triggers of, but do not directly cause, emotional reactions. It is the interpretation and assessment of situations, or cognitions, that lead to our feelings about them. It was the Greek Stoic philosopher Epictetus who said 2,000 years ago, "We are disturbed not by events, but by the views which we take of them." Many of our cognitions are habitual patterns of thinking that are automatic and outside of conscious awareness. Carefully observing and evaluating cognitions associated with negative emotions—and replacing irrational or inaccurate ones—often lead to improved mood, decreased anxiety, and generally greater life satisfaction (Beck 1976).

Cognitive Restructuring

One way to help patients change their patterns of thinking is through a process known as *cognitive restructuring*. This involves examining the link between an emotion and an underlying cognition, sometimes referred to as an *automatic thought*, evaluating the veracity of that thought, and replacing inaccurate or irrational thoughts with more balanced and healthy ones. With practice and repetition, the new, more adaptive thoughts become the default cognitions. For example, if Joe feels anxious in anticipation of meeting friends in a setting that may involve alcohol use, he may identify the underlying cognition: "My friends will think I am weak if I tell them I've stopped drinking." Joe is then asked to examine the evidence that supports this assertion. Evidence for the assertion might be, "My friends have always teased someone who doesn't drink," or "My friends seemed to enjoy my silliness when I drank." Joe then examines the evidence that does not support the underlying cognition. Evidence against it might be, "My close friends are generally supportive and would like to see me happy," or "During times when I haven't been drunk, my friends seemed to enjoy my company." If Joe determines that his initial assessment was not quite on the mark, he comes up with alternative cognitions, such as "Although my friends may have to get used to me not drinking, we'll all still have a good time. If they reject or ridicule me for not drinking, maybe they aren't really my friends." The positive alternative is certainly associated with less anxiety and is actually an invitation to venture out, not to avoid contact. Joe is also asked to rate the levels of anxiety he experienced before evaluating the automatic thought and after generating the alternative cognition. The patient can learn how different thoughts lead to different intensities of emotions—or different emotions altogether.

Although alternative cognitions may seem obvious, it usually is essential for patients to go through this process, especially early on in their treatment. With practice, patients learn to become observers of their underlying thoughts and get faster at replacing harmful ones with more accurate and healthier ones. The patient must internalize this new way of thinking. The therapist simply calling attention to and correcting maladaptive cognitions does not usually lead to change. It just leads to responses such as, "Yeah, I know that. I just can't stop thinking this way." The idea is to teach patients to evaluate their thoughts critically and rationally, not to tell patients the "correct" way to think. If Joe, during his evaluation, actually discovers that there is indeed a high likelihood that he will be ridiculed for refusing to drink, then this is helpful information. Joe can then think about the following questions: What is the worst that will happen if this is true? Will it destroy his evening or his friendships? Does it mean he just needs to educate his friends, or will it be desirable to find more supportive friends? Such follow-up questions often challenge the underlying belief that it is catastrophic if the initial automatic thought is accurate. As we can see, this process creates options and brings greater control over the patient's thoughts, feelings, and responses (Carroll 1998).

It is sometimes useful to help patients label the specific errors involved in their thought patterns. For this purpose, clinicians can give patients a list of the most common cognitive errors or distortions to make it easier for patients to monitor them. Some common cognitive errors are included in Table 6–1.

Cognitive Dissonance

It is recommended that the therapist explore client expectancies and determine discrepancies. *Cognitive dissonance* is the tension associated with incompatible ideas or information that contradicts closely held beliefs. In Motivational Interviewing, we encourage patients to amplify dissonance to create the initial drive for change. Once a change has occurred, we might help patients to decrease the cognitive dissonance associated with any discomforting thoughts, especially if they may interfere with more adaptive behaviors. For example, if Joe decides to end his relationship with his girlfriend, he can decrease dissonance by focusing on the reasons her influence was toxic for him. When he finds himself brooding, he can replace longing thoughts of cute dimples and wonderful sex with images of her being vindictive and irascible. People have more life

---

TABLE 6–1.   Common cognitive distortions

Overgeneralization—evidence is drawn from one experience or a small set of experiences to form an unwarranted conclusion with far-reaching implications

Magnification—exaggeration of the meaning of an event

Catastrophic thinking—thinking in which the impact of a clearly negative event or experience is amplified to extreme proportions (e.g., "If I am rejected, it will be disastrous.")

All-or-none, dichotomous thinking—an unnecessary separation of complex or continuous outcomes into polarized extremes (e.g., "Either I am a success at this job or I am a total failure.")

Confusing the person with the behavior—a negative characteristic of a person or an event defines that person or event. Failure at something is translated to, "I am a failure." Losing a job means, "I am a loser."

Negative predictions—the application of a pessimistic bias to undetermined future events so that failure or harm is inappropriately predicted

Mind reading—negative inferences about the thoughts, intentions, or motives of others

Personalization—interpretation of an event, situation, or behavior as indicative of a negative aspect of self

Selective abstraction—selectively seizing on negative events from a field of many events that may have variable positive and negative valences, and responding only to the ones that are selected

Should, ought, and must—imperative statements about the self or others involving the application of rigid standards

---

satisfaction and tend to make healthier decisions when they feel that they can exert some control over their thoughts and feelings. Decreasing cognitive dissonance is one technique to effect that change (Fay 1998).

Functional Analysis: Identifying and Working With Triggers and Consequences

A *functional analysis* is an assessment of the chain of events that precedes and the events that follow the use of a substance. Helping patients to understand the antecedents, or the potential triggers, and the consequences of their substance use are important steps toward effective behavior change. Then stimulus control techniques (changing the determinative effect that environment has on a behavior by directly modulating the environment) and the avoidance and alteration of cues can be employed to decrease the likelihood of engaging in the problem behavior. If triggers cannot be avoided or altered, techniques to manage them are used. The following three skill sets broadly outline how to help patients avoid substance use:

1. Identify high-risk situations (triggers and cues).
2. Avoid triggers.
3. Cope and manage high-risk situations and triggers when present.

Patients are encouraged to label two columns on a sheet of paper as "Triggers" and "Effects." It is useful to explain the reason for doing this by saying, "I'd like to understand how substance use fits into your life." Help patients identify antecedents to their past substance use. Asking patients to recall specific examples helps them identify the chain of events that preceded their substance use as well as the consequences. Connecting the consequences of the behavior to the triggers helps clarify the triggers' contributions to the behavior (Kadden et al. 1992).

The goal is to help patients discover the links among triggers, their substance use, and the consequences—not to convince or pressure the patient who is considering change. The spirit of Motivational Interviewing is evocation, not education (Miller and Rollnick 1991). It is important for the patient to explore and acknowledge the positive consequences of a behavior as well as the negative ones. As mentioned earlier (in the section "Problem Solving"), helping patients perform a balanced cost-benefit analysis that compares using versus not using is an important tool for patients to have. The final step is to generate additional options to avoid triggers and to manage discomfort if the triggers are unavoidable.

One benefit of having patients identify the positive consequences of their substance use is that they can then be asked to identify alternatives that may satisfy the same goal. For example, Joe reported a beneficial effect from alcohol during social situations. Assertiveness training and exercises in exposure and response prevention (refraining from avoiding the anxiety associated with the exposure) will help Joe manage his social anxiety without the use of drugs.

It is a common myth that triggers cause substance use. In reality, they merely increase the likelihood of use due to the desire to decrease discomfort. This subtle distinction helps patients learn that substance use is a result of choosing to use, regardless of psychological or physiological discomfort. Although there may be biological determinants, patients can learn that they are ultimately responsible for their behaviors. The enhanced awareness can result in a powerful cognitive shift that empowers the person to change (Center for Substance Abuse Treatment 1999).

External Versus Internal Triggers

Triggers can be externally derived from the environment or come from within the patient. It is important to help patients distinguish between external and internal triggers, or cues, that may precede substance use. Patients often like the pithy phrase "people, places, and things" (as coined by Alcoholics Anonymous) to help them identify and categorize potential external triggers or cues.

Whereas external triggers are often easier to identify, internal triggers can be quite powerful but easily overlooked. Internal triggers may be sensory, such as pain and muscle stiffness; emotions, such as anger, sadness, and shame; or thoughts, memories, and images. Internal triggers vary from person to person, with sadness, boredom, and shame being some of the more common ones. Although depression or sadness may have been present before abstinence, sadness often develops as patients learn that many of their difficulties related to substance abuse do not disappear once the substance use has stopped. The loss of friends, family, and lifestyle during the period of substance use—as well as losses due to the new, alternative pattern of living—often create a sense of sadness. Helping patients cope with sadness and loss while engaging in problem solving to create positive feelings associated with their abstinence, and restructuring sad thoughts to better reflect the new lifestyle modifications that were chosen, are necessary (Foote 2006).

Loneliness, boredom, and shame as triggers.   Loneliness and boredom may be consequences of abandoning maladaptive patterns and relationships. Often, someone's social network is intertwined with individuals with whom the patient used substances. These could have been friends, family members, or intimate partners. Unless these interactions are replaced with ones that do not reinforce substance use, patients are likely to be lonely or bored.

Shame and embarrassment are common as patients assess the damage they have inflicted on themselves and others. Although sadness and regret about the hurt caused to others is an appropriate emotion, shame conveys a moral judgment and is often associated with feelings of inferiority and worthlessness and even the belief that one should be punished. These thoughts only weaken a person's sense of confidence and can lead to isolation, sadness, and even anger, generating even more potential triggers. Helping patients distinguish between sadness and shame is important. When feelings of shame and its associated thoughts are recognized, patients can then challenge some of the negative self-talk and focus on behaviors that will help maintain their abstinence, increase their sense of self-efficacy, repair damaged relationships, and have other positive effects (Foote 2006).

Anger as a trigger.   When patients are facile at expressing their feelings and getting their needs met, they tend to more easily resist substance use. When they have difficulties with assertiveness, anger is often a resulting emotion that can be a strong internal trigger for substance use. The popular conceptualization of anger is that if it is not let out, it will become pent up until it erupts like a volcano. However, many experts now regard anger as a potentially maladaptive emotion based on faulty assumptions that reflect grandiose and self-righteous thinking, and some believe that anger often leads to maladaptive behaviors. Although this view may be somewhat reductionistic—as everyone experiences this emotion—anger can be associated with preoccupations of revenge, an antagonistic attitude, and a predisposition to violence, and it often provides only momentary relief. An extreme example of unchecked anger is road rage, which is often based on the assumption that an offending act was intentional, prompting the urge to get even or right the perceived injustice.

Often, anger is actually a reflection of other emotions such as fear, hurt, shame, or sadness. When a parent yells at a child for running into the street, it is in response to fear. Although it is rational to feel fear for a child's safety, it is quite irrational to be angry at a child for simply running into the street. After all, it is normal for young kids to run into the street; the activity just happens to be unsafe. Both the behavioral response and the emotion can be altered. Although the behavior of yelling may be an attempt to punish the child so that in the future the behavior won't be repeated, there are usually more effective ways to teach a child. Hence, cognitive restructuring can be used with patients to manage their distortions in thinking that may lead to anger—and substance use.

In addition, people who are better at getting what they want also tend to feel less angry. Assertiveness is the quintessential anger management skill. A CBT therapist may teach patients how to express emotions assertively rather than aggressively—which tends to be blaming and punitive. Helping patients shift the responsibility of their emotions to themselves is an important way to regain control over how they feel (Foote 2006).

Craving as a trigger.   Craving, which is generally defined as a strong desire to use a substance, and may even include physical or sensory experiences associated with using, such as sweating or tightness in the stomach, is one type of potential internal trigger that deserves special mention. Cravings are often associated with other cues or triggers. They are often accompanied by strong imagery, symbolic of the romance of the substance. For example, patients may imagine sensually caressing the stem of a wine glass, gently swirling the liquid, sitting back in a seductive pose, and letting the warm liquid glide down their throat. During these moments, after much practice, patients can learn to, as the AA saying goes, "Play the tape forward." Patients can then carry the reverie further, imagining slurring their words, saying embarrassing things they will later regret, and culminating in vomiting on someone's shoes. The idea is to think of the negative consequences of drinking and to stop idealizing the drink.

This exercise helps patients to gain control over their thoughts, and to un-couple positively associated thoughts from the substance. It is important to re-member that cravings usually peak after a few minutes and then abate. Rarely do they last more than a few hours. Stimulus control techniques (discussed ear-lier; see "Functional Analysis: Identifying and Working With Triggers and Consequences"), distraction, and reframing the cognitions and imagery associ-ated with the craving can all be useful to get people out of a high-risk situation (Foote 2006).

Attributional styles.   Another factor that can influence internal triggers is a patient's attributional style. In other words, it would be helpful to know whether Joe would attribute a good conversation with someone at a party to some external factor, with thoughts such as "She must have been drunk"; "She just broke up with someone and was lonely"; or "I was just lucky." Or would he attribute the positive outcome to something that he did? "I took a few deep breaths, sweated a little, but started talking to her anyway and I enjoyed it." With monitoring and awareness, patients can modify their attributional styles, which can lead to a greater sense of self-efficacy.

When asking patients what they like about using a substance or what the positive consequences are of using a substance, clinicians also elicit a patient's perceptions or expectations about the substance use. Distinguishing actual con-sequences from desired or expected consequences can help patients evaluate the costs and benefits of using a substance. Patients are encouraged to identify both external consequences of their use (such as effects on their relationships, fi-nances, and health) and internal consequences (such as shame, depression, anx-iety, and loneliness) (Miller and Rollnick 1991).

When people stop using a substance they feel much better about them-selves and often receive a lot of positive reinforcement for their abstinence. Pa-tients often expect that all the other areas of their lives will subsequently improve. Disappointment may lead to negatively laden emotions, which may in turn be a risk factor for relapse. Analysis of expectations related to abstinence may prepare the patient for more realistic outcomes.

Avoiding relapse justifications.   Learning to cope with triggers requires a cognitive shift as well. It is not willpower that prevents substance use. It is a set of skills that enables the patient to replace older, maladaptive habits with a lifestyle less associated with substance. As the patient progresses from ac-tion to maintenance, it is generally thought that maintenance is sustained through consistent use of new behaviors and cognitions. It is actually rare that relapse happens at the drop of a dime. What is more likely is that the patient will drift away from the behaviors that maintain abstinence. Patients may start skipping AA meetings or be inconsistent about taking their medications. They may start spending time in high-trigger places or with high-trigger

---

TABLE 6–2. **Common relapse justifications**

Other people made me do it.

    My husband brought it home....

    I was in a bar and someone offered me some....

I was testing myself.

    I wanted to see if I could be around it and say no....

    I needed some money and thought I would sell a little without using....

    I'm stronger now....

It was an accident.

    I was in a bar and someone offered me....

    I found some in my car....

I was celebrating.

    I've done great, so one time won't be a problem....

    This occasion deserves a reward....

I felt depressed, angry, and bored.

    Things are not going to get better. I may as well use....

    Things are too overwhelming for me....

There was a specific purpose.

    I was gaining weight and needed to control it by using....

    I needed to do something to relieve my social anxiety....

There was a catastrophic event.

    My wife left me. I may as well use....

    I got fired, so I may as well just use....

---

people. Often, the insidious slide is easily rationalized as a response to their environment. This rationalization is aptly referred to as *relapse justification*. Frequently, relapse justifications are shaped by the belief that external forces drive the patients' behaviors and that the patients have limited control over these influences. Some common justifications are listed in Table 6–2. Patients often benefit from monitoring their patterns of thinking and recording what they say to themselves when they are in environments that have been conducive to substance use in the past. An example might be, "I'll just have one drink since I made it 90 days without drinking; I'm strong enough now" (Center for Substance Abuse Treatment 1999). Patients can then challenge these self-statements to stop the slide.

Developing coping strategies.   In the spirit of Motivational Interviewing, it is best to collaborate with the patient to develop situation-specific options and alternatives to cope with triggers and stress. The goals are 1) to help the patient build an armamentarium for managing stress, anxiety, and triggers; and 2) to strengthen the patient's capacity and confidence to generate new coping skills without the help of the therapist. Positive reinforcement of the successful application of coping strategies is essential, even if the outcome is suboptimal. Future modifications can be explored to work toward the desired goal. If a coping strategy has failed, it is important to help the patient analyze the process dispassionately and look for ways of modifying the approach. Patients can make a detailed plan of what they may do in response to each one of their triggers and carry index cards with the planned responses. These cards can be reviewed daily and also when a trigger arises. Some common coping mechanisms include calling a sponsor, therapist, or other support person; jogging or doing push-ups; using breathing or progressive muscle relaxation exercises; or listening to music (Miller et al. 1992).

Importance of Social Supports

Involving the patient's support network is an invaluable part of treatment. A patient's network may include, but certainly is not limited to, a spouse or other family members, friends, a sponsor, neighbors, and members of a support group (Fay 1998).

Substance abuse almost always affects a patient's interpersonal relationships. Although patterns that develop between patients and their network members can be supportive, they are often reinforcing of the substance use. For example, Joe's girlfriend tends to be generally vindictive but is usually only emotionally and physically present when they use drugs together. The shame and anger that Joe likely feels may be a trigger for further substance use. Both the patient's network members and the patient can learn to be more effective partners, manage each other's negative contributions, and be more positively reinforcing of adaptive patterns. Network members can provide help by monitoring the patient's behaviors, modeling and reinforcing new and more adaptive behaviors, providing accurate feedback to the patient and to the therapist, involving the patient in new social and recreational activities, and providing emotional and even logistical support.

It can be helpful to understand how members of the network feel about a patient's substance use. A very different dynamic exists when a family member is also using. Table 6–3 lists some relevant questions to consider about the patient's support system. People in the patient's network may benefit from correction of misconceptions regarding substance use. The network is encouraged

TABLE 6–3.   Important questions regarding a patient's social support network

Does the support network member:

Know that the patient uses?

Know of the use but not say anything about it?

See the use as a problem?

Want the patient to stop using?

Try to actually stop the patient from using?

Get involved in the patient's life or treatment?

Refuse to get involved in the patient's life because of the use?

Get angry or punitive?

Drink or use as well?

Mistrust the patient?

to eschew judgments and instead focus on the practical sequelae of substance use. However, issues of mistrust often exist. Discussions about the terms of any relationship must incorporate these sensitive but understandable elements.

Even after patients have made real changes consistent with sobriety, those in their network may continue to behave in the same way to which they are accustomed. The support system members will benefit from guidance to adjust to new roles and patterns of relating. Some of their established roles will need to be reevaluated and changed. Individuals in the patient's network are often invited into therapy meetings, as well as being offered outside group and individual counseling.

It is crucial to help patients evaluate their potential supports and decide when and how to best incorporate them into their treatment. Ceasing to view a drug supplier as a friend may help loosen the grip of the supplier. Sometimes patients need to distance themselves from an abusive relationship. This may be necessary for Joe with his girlfriend if she continues not to support him in his abstinence (Carroll 1998).

Self-Help and Support Programs

Ongoing support from self-help programs can be an important part of a patient's treatment. (See also Chapter 12, "Engaging in Self-Help Groups.") The most widely known and attended are the 12-step programs, the best known of which is AA. Many similar programs have grown from the same model, such as Al-Anon (support for family and friends), Alateen (support for teenagers), Cocaine Anonymous, Sexual Compulsives Anonymous, Gamblers Anonymous, Narcotics Anonymous, Overeaters Anonymous, Debtors Anonymous, Co-Dependents Anonymous, and so forth. These groups are composed of members who support each other in their quest to maintain abstinence from a substance or from a set of maladaptive behaviors. The only requirement for attendance at their meetings is the desire for change. The meetings are free, are available throughout the United States 7 days a week, day and evening, and are run by the members. No outside financial support or other kind of sponsorship is allowed. AA meetings in hotels or cruise ships are often inconspicuously advertised as "Friends of Bill W.," aptly honoring Bill Wilson, a New York stockbroker, and cofounder of AA along with Bob Smith, a surgeon in Akron, Ohio ("Dr. Bob"), in 1935. Meeting locations and times can be found on the Internet or by contacting local centers listed in telephone directories or regional intergroup offices, such as those of AA.

Anonymity has been paramount in fostering an atmosphere of trust and openness. While members may choose to attend different group meetings, a *home group*—the group whose meetings a member preferentially and routinely attends—also serves to promote a familiar, safe, and comfortable environment.

The 12 steps and traditions in AA and other 12-step programs provide structure for introspection and maintaining sobriety. "Trust God, clean house, help others," courtesy of Dr. Bob, nicely encapsulates the 12-step process (Anonymous 1980). Admitting lack of control over the use of a substance (or other behavior) and recognizing the presence of a higher power to give strength are cornerstones of the first three steps. Recognizing one's fallibilities, striving to improve shortcomings, and apologizing and making amends for harm done to others when possible reflect the next steps. The final, twelfth step is the evangelical spreading of the good word.

Participants are encouraged to find a sponsor, usually a member who has been sober for more than 1 year, who helps guide the patient through the 12 steps and offers support and education. Most members are familiar with the tome *Alcoholics Anonymous: Big Book* (Alcoholics Anonymous World Services 2001), colloquially referred to as "The Big Book." This is a compilation of inspirational and moving testimonials written by the founders of AA, their wives, and many who have come after them. Patients and therapists alike can learn much from this book. In addition, many patients benefit from supplementary or even stand-alone bibliotherapy, an essential intervention in CBT. There is a plethora of self-help books that may appeal to patients, such as *Overcoming Your Alcohol or Drug Problem: Effective Recovery Strategies,* 2nd Edition (Daley and Marlatt 2006), which I use in my practice. Given the critical importance of social skills and networks in the cultivation and maintenance of abstinence, I also recommend *Making It as a Couple: Prescription for a Quality Relationship* (Fay

1998), which is applicable to all types of relationships. Patients have found these and other books useful for home study in conjunction with formal therapy.

Some people are deterred by the emphasis on accepting a higher power within the framework of the 12 steps. Increasingly, for some individuals, the "higher power" is a belief in something other than a deity, such as an abstract belief in something greater than themselves—e.g., nature, the group, or their community. Because not all meetings are alike, patients can be encouraged to go to a few different ones to see whether any resonate with them.

Twelve-step meetings may not be for everyone. Recently, a number of alternatives to AA have sprung up around the country. SMART Recovery (an acronym for Self-Management and Recovery Training) and Rational Recovery are both CBT-oriented organizations. SMART Recovery offers group meetings throughout the country, in addition to publications and an Internet Listserv discussion group; Rational Recovery offers educational workshops and publications. Secular Organizations for Sobriety (SOS; also known as Save Our Selves), with hundreds of groups around the country, offers a nonreligious perspective. Women for Sobriety, Inc., emphasizes that women have distinct emotional needs to be addressed during their recovery (Foote 2006).

Contingent Reinforcement

Contingent reinforcement rewards people only if certain behavioral milestones have been met. It has been studied in a variety of therapeutic settings. While patients work to develop alternative and more adaptive behaviors and lifestyles, they can be rewarded for abstinent behaviors or milestones. For example, negative urine toxicologies can be reinforced by giving the patient money at each testing. Vouchers or points may be redeemed at a later time for cash or prizes, such as electronic items. These programs offer a high level of structure, with clear expectations for parameters that are specific, measurable, and time limited. There is some debate regarding the effectiveness of cash versus vouchers as incentives. Cash may be a stronger reinforcer because it may be more desirable and is usually given close to the time that the desired change has occurred. It does carry some risk, though, if having available cash is a cue or trigger to acquire and use a substance. If this is the case or the concern, a nonusing support member can hold the awarded money until the patient has chosen something to purchase. Vouchers or points allow for patients to select for themselves the rewards they receive and may lead to more internal reinforcement. It may also teach patients to delay gratification while their points accumulate (American Psychiatric Association 2006).

The *community reinforcement approach* (CRA) is a multifaceted program designed to make abstinence more reinforcing than the patterns associated with substance use. It attempts to use external reinforcers that are directly related to previously delineated goals. For example, 90 days of abstinence, as assessed by some predetermined measure, might be reinforced by the patient's children coming over for dinner. The reinforcer in this case is one that is directly related to the patient's previously stated goal of being closer to his or her family. Creative ways to make naturally occurring reinforcements contingent on abstinence can be useful, such as family visits, financial support, or other rewards (American Psychiatric Association 2006).

CRA also builds coping skills through the use of functional analysis. Social skills and job training, if necessary, and self-management skills, such as assertiveness training and time management, are all incorporated into the program. Some CRA programs include a highly structured program called The Job Club. It offers skills training in making telephone contact, job application and résumé preparation, interviewing, and assertiveness. Even though the data strongly support its use, CRA is rarely utilized, likely due to logistic and economic constraints.

Another approach, computer-assisted training based on principles of CBT, has yet to be incorporated into mainstream treatment for substance use disorders, but research suggests that it provides better outcomes than therapy sessions alone. Virtual reality sessions in high-risk places such as virtual bars offer realistic sights and sounds that help patients become desensitized to certain triggers and give them opportunities to practice their skills managing high-risk situations.

Summary

Clearly, there is an abundance of available techniques, both behavioral and cognitive, to initiate and strengthen more adaptive patterns of living. When combined with a Motivational Interviewing approach, treatment is greatly enhanced. This work, done during the action phase, greatly contributes to the continuation of abstinence and to greater life satisfaction.

Suggestions for Teaching and Supervision

- Listen with a keen ear. What people say is often a window into their underlying cognitions. Semantic restructuring often leads to a change in feelings. For example, if a patient consistently replaces "I am so lazy" with "I procrastinate a lot," the person tends to feel less hopeless and down. It also challenges the cognitive error of confusing the person with the behavior, by relabeling a judgment of the self with a description of a specific behavioral pattern.

- Challenge patients to actually test their assumptions. Often we take at face value our assumptions and regard them as fact. Patients can learn that an initial assumption may have been off the mark.

- The more actively patients monitor a behavior or thought that they want to change, the more likely they are to be able to make a change. Suggest that patients keep a log of their behaviors and thoughts that are earmarked for change. Review the notes with them. If they are reluctant, explore the rationalizations as to why.

- Teach through modeling. Be a nonjudgmental, assertive, inquisitive, active, and experimental therapist and the patient will be more apt to follow suit.

- It is better to positively reinforce actual behavior changes, not plans. Otherwise we risk simply strengthening planning and promises, and not an actual change in behavior. Reinforce specific behaviors, not general behavioral patterns. "It means a great deal to me when you sit and engage me in conversation" is much more effective than "I enjoy when you pay attention to me." Although external reinforcers can be potent motivators for change, teach the patient to generate his or her own internal reinforcers.

- Be collaborative. The goal is to teach patients how to be active agents of change, not to tell them what they should be doing.

- Bring in the patient's network. Make it a habit at some point in the treatment to meet with the patient's friends and family members. It can make the difference between change and stagnation.

- Focus on developing a strong relationship. Allen Fay, my mentor, once told me, "If you have a great relationship with a patient, you can ask them to try almost anything."

- Have fun. Therapy, like life, is serious business but the process can be enjoyable and even fun. Use humor when appropriate. Smile at the beginning, middle, and end of each session, if appropriate.

Movie: *Ray*

The 2004 movie *Ray* charts some of the more poignant moments in the life of Ray Charles, one of the great American musicians and entertainers of the twentieth century. From the struggles of being born the son of a sharecropper in the South, becoming blind as a child, overcoming his opiate addiction, and experiencing marital distress to navigating the vicissitudes of the entertainment world, we see a man who learned how to cope with adversity.

In one scene, Ray is caught with illicit substances at the airport by federal agents while disembarking the plane. He then faces possible prison time, and his wife threatens to leave him. His wife asks, "Is that poison worth losing everything?" Ray decides to stop using opiates entirely. He is then seen writhing in pain and agony while going through opiate withdrawal. He is offered, but refuses, agonist therapy. He even refuses intravenous fluid hydration, stating, "No more needles for me."

After his period of withdrawal, we see Ray playing chess with his physician. His doctor informs him that to obtain a positive report to keep him out of prison, he will have to attend a therapy program and receive periodic drug testing. We can infer that he complies with the treatment recommendations, as he manages to avoid incarceration. We also see him spending more time with people who do not use substances, and dedicating himself to his career and to philanthropic endeavors.

Besides highlighting the transition from the action phase to the maintenance phase, these scenes demonstrate the complicated interplay between internal and external motivators for change. While we try to help patients increase their internal motivation to change, we cannot ignore the often useful leverage that some external factors can offer. Sometimes threats of abandonment or legal or penal consequences can lead to substance abstinence. Regardless of how someone gets to the action phase, we can still help them strengthen the behaviors and cognitions that might result in continued abstinence.

Key Clinical Points

- The action phase of the Transtheoretical Model of Change is a very active process, whereby a patient ceases to engage in a maladaptive behavior or set of behaviors.

- Motivational Interviewing is a style of therapy that helps to clarify and resolve ambivalence, build motivation, and strengthen patients' commitment to change.

- CBT, based on principles of learning, helps patients replace maladaptive or unhealthy patterns of behaving and thinking.

- Although CBT is often a prescriptive and directive approach, it can work well with the evocative style of Motivational Interviewing to increase the motivation for change.

Multiple-Choice Questions

For the correct answers to these questions, including explanations of answers, please see the Answer Guide at the end of this book.

1. A patient's wife giving a warm embrace and encouragement when her partner comes home from an AA meeting is an example of:

   A. Positive reinforcement.
   B. Negative reinforcement.
   C. Community reinforcement.
   D. Contingency management.

2. When a person says, "I can't have fun at a party without alcohol":

   A. This is a cognition that needs to be accepted.
   B. This indicates that parties always need to be avoided.
   C. This is an assumption that is testable.
   D. All of the above.

3. If a trigger cannot be avoided, some useful techniques to cope or manage
   the person's response to triggers include:

   A. Assertive refusal.
   B. Imaginal flooding with negative consequences, such as vomiting.
   C. Contacting a healthy social support.
   D. All of the above.

4. When someone stops using a substance, which of the following is most
   likely to occur?

   A. Most areas in the person's life now become stable and fulfilling.
   B. Many people, at least temporarily, have difficulty adjusting to life
      without substance use.
   C. Most relationships, damaged as a result of substance abuse, are re-
      paired.
   D. Patients have a new clarity and realize that the substance was the cause
      of most of their difficulties.

5. With regard to a patient's social network:

   A. Only family members should be included in the treatment.
   B. The individual being treated is the patient, and he or she needs to re-
      cover without interference from network members.

C. Often, network members have negatively contributed to a patient's substance use or to the dysfunctional relationship. Involving such a person is a risk for relapse.

D. Substance use usually involves interpersonal issues. Involving the network can greatly enhance the treatment.

References

Alcoholics Anonymous World Services: Alcoholics Anonymous: Big Book, 4th Edition. New York, Alcoholics Anonymous World Services, 2001. Available at: http://www.aa.org/bigbookonline. Accessed February 12, 2010.

American Psychiatric Association: Treatment of patients with substance use disorders, 2nd edition. Am J Psychiatry 163(8 Suppl):5–82, 2006

Anonymous: Dr. Bob and the Good Oldtimers (2nd printing edition). New York, Alcoholics Anonymous World Services, 1980

Beck AT: Cognitive Therapy and the Emotional Disorders. New York, International Universities Press, 1976

Carroll KM: National Institute on Drug Abuse Therapy Manuals for Drug Addiction: A Cognitive-Behavioral Approach: Treating Cocaine Addiction (NIH Publ No 98–4308). Rockville, MD, National Institute on Drug Abuse, 1998

Center for Substance Abuse Treatment: Enhancing Motivation for Change in Substance Abuse Treatment (Treatment Improvement Protocol Series, No 35; DHHS Publ No [SMA] 05–4081; publication reprinted as [SMA] 08–4212). Rockville, MD, Substance Abuse and Mental Health Services Administration, 1999

Daley DC, Marlatt GA: Overcoming Your Alcohol or Drug Problem: Effective Recovery Strategies, 2nd Edition. New York, Oxford University Press, 2006

Fay A: Making it as a Couple: Prescription for a Quality Relationship. Essex, CT, FMC Books, 1998

Foote J: Group Motivational Intervention (GMI-20) Manual: A Cognitive-Behavioral-Motivational Treatment Approach. New York, National Development and Research Institutes, 2006

Kadden R, Carroll KM, Donovan D, et al: Cognitive-Behavioral Coping Skills Therapy Manual: A Clinical Research Guide for Therapists Treating Individuals With Alcohol Abuse and Dependence (Project MATCH Monograph Series, Vol 3; DHHS Publ No [ADM] 92–1895). Rockville, MD, National Institute on Alcohol Abuse and Alcoholism, 1992

Miller WR, Rollnick S: Motivational Interviewing: Preparing People to Change Addictive Behavior. New York, Guilford, 1991

Miller WR, Zweben A, DiClemente CC, et al: Motivational Enhancement Therapy Manual: A Clinical Research Guide for Therapists Treating Individuals With Alcohol Abuse and Dependence (Project MATCH Monograph Series, Vol 2; DHHS Publ No [ADM] 92–1894). Rockville, MD, National Institute on Alcohol Abuse and Alcoholism, 1992

Prochaska JO, Norcross JC, DiClemente CC: Changing for Good: A Revolutionary Six-Stage Program for Overcoming Bad Habits and Moving Your Life Positively Forward. New York, W Morrow, 1994

Rogers CR: Client-Centered Therapy. Boston, MA, Houghton Mifflin, 1951

CHAPTER 7

Maintenance

Jennifer Hanner, M.D., M.P.H.

Mark Twain is quoted as having said, "Quitting smoking is easy. I've done it hundreds of times." His statement describes what many patients struggle with in addictive disorders—that it is easier to stop an addictive behavior than to remain that way—that is, to achieve sustained abstinence. Substance use disorders are common and may manifest as a substantial factor in the medical histories of patients treated in all areas of medicine. Yet only a small percentage of patients who need help with these disorders seek treatment. Some seek help through their primary care physician whereas others need treatment from psychiatrists for co-occurring mental health disorders. Some become involved in self-help groups such as Alcoholics Anonymous (AA) or Narcotics Anonymous.

Because patients can present at both low and high levels of motivation for making changes in behavior, it is important for clinicians to be able to recognize a patient's level of readiness in order to provide the most appropriate response and treatment. In this chapter, I discuss Prochaska and DiClemente's maintenance stage of change, in which the patient has accomplished the desired change and now seeks to sustain the change for the long term (Prochaska and DiClemente 1984), as well as its ties to Miller and Rollnick's Motivational Interviewing (Miller and Rollnick 2002). Patients may enter this phase with confidence in having achieved their goal but may find themselves surprisingly challenged or even struggling to maintain the change for which they have worked so hard. This is where the clinician's support of the patient's motivation is vital to continued success and stability in behavior change.

Clinical Case

Jim is a 35-year-old patient who has been sober for 11 months with active involvement in AA after completing a 28-day rehabilitation program. He had a
prior history of drinking up to a quart of vodka daily and required multiple
detoxification admissions. He presents to a psychiatrist at the recommendation
of the group counselor in his substance abuse program with complaints of low
mood and increased anxiety.

He has been dating a woman for the past few months and has felt some increased uneasiness in social situations. His new girlfriend is a socialite, with a
full schedule of events planned for the winter holidays. She is aware of his
drinking history but seems not to be particularly sensitive to his vulnerability.
He recalls that last year he was in rehab treatment during the holidays. Though
he has been through much hardship because of his alcoholism—losing his
driver's license, jeopardizing his job, and dealing with estrangement from his
family—he acknowledges still having nostalgia at moments when recalling the
euphoric relationship he once had with drinking during the winter holidays. He
admits that he has had a passing thought or two about having just one cup of
eggnog or a glass of champagne to partake in the festivities and to alleviate his
feelings of tension. At other times, he is acutely aware of a feeling of being outside looking in at others who are "normal" drinkers. And everywhere, everyone
is drinking in the name of good holiday cheer. He has also been thinking a great
deal about his mother, who died 5 years ago from cancer around this time of the
year. She had always been a big part of his family's holiday celebrations. He
wishes she could see him now, with several months of sobriety. His drinking
had cast a pall over many family get-togethers in years past. The patient reports
that he has not been sleeping well, but his energy during the day is still adequate. He feels distracted during the day with worries about his new girlfriend
when trying to concentrate at his job in an advertising agency.

Discussion of the Clinical Case

In the above case, the patient is in remission from his alcohol dependence. Jim
has remained in a treatment program following his completion of a rehab program, as well as continuing 12-step work with AA. But he now faces challenges
in living life without alcohol. He describes the common experience of patients
who are at this point in their recovery. On first impression, it might seem hard
to believe that a patient could describe nostalgia for experiences with substance
dependence, because there has typically been a great deal of turmoil and loss
before arriving at treatment. Jim has had hospitalizations and many negative
consequences as a result of his drinking. Yet those memories are not always salient when in a crowd during the holidays, when drinking is equated with the
enjoyment of the season. He is also faced with the social pressure to engage in
what would be considered "normal" behavior among his peers—brought to
heightened attention by his new dating situation. In addition, he is dealing

with the challenge of having a new romantic partner who does not seem to grasp or appreciate his vulnerability to alcohol. AA typically recommends no new relationships in the first year of sobriety so that the focus remains on an individual's recovery. This patient's dilemma demonstrates the complications that can arise.

It might be tempting for a clinician to rush to confront the patient about his misguided thoughts, perhaps even to be critical of the patient's flawed judgment in considering having a drink. But this would only risk alienating the patient who has come seeking help. It would be more helpful to take a curious and interested position—to consider the patient's perspective on the positives and negatives of his recent thoughts about using alcohol and the consequences of either outcome.

The patient describes recent symptoms suggesting a possible co-occurring affective disorder, with mood changes, anxiety, and some neurovegetative symptoms. Because patients with substance use disorders often also have other psychiatric disorders, it is important for clinicians to be thorough in evaluating for them, though a complicated substance use history can confound diagnostic clarity. The patient is additionally dealing with grief related to the anniversary of his mother's death during the holidays, as well as feelings of guilt that have arisen when recollecting the negative impact of his drinking on past family gatherings. These types of stressors are common to patients in substance abuse treatment and may create substantial challenges to recovery. In the present case, it is important for the clinician to screen further for a co-occurring mood or anxiety disorder, as the patient may require management with medication in addition to psychotherapy. His symptoms may also be related to his adjustment to a new relationship and sobriety during an emotion-laden time of the year. The clinician will be challenged to support the patient's level of motivation for sobriety in the face of these other stressors.

Suggestions for Treatment

Maintenance Stage

In the Prochaska and DiClemente (1984) Stages of Change model, maintenance involves a period of sustained behavior, with a patient typically having taken action to change behavior more than 6 months prior (though in some cases it may require much longer) and involves a process just as in other stages of change (DiClemente and Velasquez 2002). The patient in this stage has had a successful period in which his or her efforts in the action stage have become consistent and sustained. There may be a lessening of the intensity and tenacity with which the patient approaches the change in behavior. In the case of alcoholism, for example, he or she may now go to AA meetings a few times a week rather than every day. The fact that behavior change is not necessarily fixed is important for clinicians to recognize, for it will then not be a surprise to see patients struggling at times to maintain abstinence. Some will have a brief return to drinking or drug use after a period of abstinence, referred to by clinicians as a *lapse* (Daley and Marlatt 2005) or a *slip*. Some lapses may lead to a full relapse to the previous behavior and the patient then cycles again through the stages of change, though with improved chances for sustained abstinence the next time through (DiClemente and Velasquez 2002). In AA literature and meetings, the phrase "progress, not perfection" describes this expectation associated with maintenance. Recognizing these normal aspects of the maintenance stage, clinicians are better able to support patients by providing techniques to avoid lapses or interrupt them if they should occur.

Maintenance and Motivational Interviewing

The integration of the Stages of Change model with Motivational Interviewing techniques (Rollnick et al. 2008) is accomplished in the maintenance stage by first recognizing the continued role of motivation (DiClemente and Velasquez 2002). Patients need continued support and fostering of their efforts to remain with their choice of change and to manage challenges that may impede or deter their progress (Center for Substance Abuse Treatment 1999). The maintenance stage is characterized by active effort on the part of the patient rather than passivity or complacency, which both may create vulnerability to relapse. Motivational Interviewing techniques during this stage can be used to bolster the patient's sense of self-efficacy in maintaining the desired change. Multiple studies have also shown that Motivational Interviewing helps to increase patients' involvement with and adherence to substance abuse treatment, which is associated with improved outcomes (Zweben and Zuckoff 2002). Miller and Rollnick (2002) describe two phases of Motivational Interviewing, with phase 1 applying to the building of motivation in the early stages of change and phase 2 being the reinforcing of the commitment to the change once action has begun. In phase 2, the importance of motivational style on the part of the clinician remains paramount, as patients may still have ambivalence about their decision or insecurity about their ability to continue following through. The clinician's efforts are collaborative with the patient's efforts in forming plans, drawing on the patient's responsibility to make the choices but also providing some direction for the patient's consideration.

For patients in the maintenance stage, sustained change requires continued self-assessment and preparation for anticipated stresses or situations that may threaten their stability. The clinician is in the role of supporter, commending the patient on his or her continued efforts, and asking questions out of interest and curiosity, rather than suspicion or distrust. The clinician also remains the empathic responder to all reactions and experiences the patient may have while maintaining the change in behavior, offering advice or reflective feedback when needed. The patient is encouraged to have a vigilant attitude, though not overtly fearful or overwhelmingly anxious, to safeguard against threats to sobriety. The maintenance stage is a team effort between the patient and clinician, but may also require and benefit from other sources of support, such as self-help support groups, sponsors, and family members (Center for Substance Abuse Treatment 1999). When patients have a lapse or even a full relapse, the motivational style is still maintained 1) to reassure patients that their crisis is not a failure but something that can be used as a chance to learn more about what continued abstinence will require, and 2) as a means of encouraging them to renew their motivation to take up the early stages of change again (DiClemente and Velasquez 2002).

Clinical Interventions Using Motivational Style

The Substance Abuse and Mental Health Services Administration's Treatment Improvement Protocol No. 35 (Center for Substance Abuse Treatment 1999) provides a useful guide for utilizing a motivational style in starting treatment with patients. The following is a summary of several of those steps, with the underlying goal of retaining the patient in treatment:

1. The first goal is to establish a therapeutic connection with the patient based on trust and good rapport. Patients need a level of comfort and feelings of safety and security while participating in treatment. They should be approached in a way that is respectful and culturally sensitive.
2. Provide the patient with explicit and clear information about the goals and expectations of treatment. This also allows the patient a chance to clarify any points of confusion and ask questions.
3. Ask the patient about his or her expectations of treatment. For example, he or she may have had negative treatment experiences previously, with residual fears that can be assuaged before delving into the work of treatment. Bring up other patients' past comments so that this patient feels comfortable to speak freely. Be sure the patient has realistic goals for treatment and understands its limitations as well as its potential to help.
4. Anticipate and discuss common stumbling blocks, such as feelings of embarrassment or strong emotions that may come up during treatment. Being

made aware of the likelihood of stumbling blocks, patients can prepare themselves and perhaps then be less likely to have abrupt reactions such as terminating treatment.

5. Explore possible obstacles to treatment such as language or reading skill level. Address possible transportation or child care constraints, as well as financial issues that may hinder compliance with treatment attendance.

6. Every patient has unique triggers, what AA calls the "people, places, and things" that increase the risk of substance use. Explore the triggers preceding the patient's substance use as well as the consequences. The discussion should be specific and detailed, drawing on actual episodes of use. Kadden and Cooney (2005) also recommend the use of assessment instruments to help with identifying triggers.

7. Design a plan of coping strategies for individual situations and triggers. The plan may need to be adjusted over time to accommodate needs that arise as the patient continues working to sustain change.

8. Enlist the help of family members and other supportive people if possible. Discuss with the patient which family members or friends could be resources to help reinforce the desired change. Support can be given in many ways, whether keeping patients accountable in meeting their responsibilities, providing assistance with child care or transportation, or planning for emergencies and ways the support person could help if the patient encounters a high-risk situation. For patients with few emotional supports, the fellowship of a 12-step group and the help of a sponsor can sometimes fulfill these needs.

In ongoing visits, the clinician continues to check in with the patient about how well he or she is maintaining the desired change and asks directly about slips or recent cravings. Below are some examples of questions for clinicians to use during treatment sessions:

1. "How have you been doing without drinking/using drugs? Any recent slips? If so, how did you deal with them?" Be prepared that the patient may feel defensive in reaction to these questions.

2. "Any recent cravings? Tell me more about them." "How are your meetings going? What has your sponsor been talking with you about lately?"

3. "Have you noticed changes in friends or family in reaction to your efforts to stay sober?"

4. "Do you anticipate any upcoming situations that might tempt you to drink/use drugs?"

It is important to convey to the patient that the questions are meant to be supportive rather than mistrustful or accusatory. Reassure patients that cravings are a normal part of the recovery process and that lapses can be opportunities for learning rather than being viewed as failings to be criticized or condemned (Daley and Marlatt 2005).

Relapse Prevention

Relapse prevention is a treatment approach that has the goal of preventing lapses or relapse by providing coping skills and alternatives to repeating previous unwanted behaviors (Marlatt and Witkiewitz 2005). It has the secondary goal of managing lapses if they do occur, in order to prevent a total relapse. The approach is based in a cognitive-behavioral framework drawing from the earlier work of Marlatt and Witkiewitz (2005), who developed a classification of high-risk circumstances and relapse determinants from the patterns of male chronic alcoholic patients. These determinants encompass both aspects of the individual and his or her environmental interactions in predicting responses to high-risk situations, described in two categories—intrapersonal and interpersonal (Daley and Marlatt 2005). The intrapersonal category includes negative and positive emotional states, urges, and temptations, whereas the latter includes conflicts in relationships and social pressure to drink or use. The role of self-efficacy is also noted to be an important individual component, in that a person needs not only the skills to cope with situations but also the confidence that he or she is able to carry them out (Marlatt and Witkiewitz 2005).

Kadden and Cooney (2005) describe elements of coping skills training employed by relapse prevention as including 1) anticipation of decisional patterns that have a high likelihood of subsequently leading to risky situations, 2) exploration of activities that create higher possibilities for substance use, and 3) early recognition of high-risk situations if they occur so that they can be addressed and managed. Patients benefit from the utilization of coping skills and alternative activities to avoid lapses, as well as the simple realization that they have other choices besides using drugs or drinking to meet their needs. Before the training, patients may describe feeling that there is no other choice than to use once a strong craving has been triggered. The skills provided by relapse prevention work interrupt that pattern of thinking. Relapse prevention models may vary somewhat based on the drug of choice and context, but all provide multiple tools to help sustain patients in the maintenance stage by using various coping skills.

Suggestions for Teaching and Supervision

Students will benefit from an early introduction to the concepts of the Stages of Change model and Motivational Interviewing. Understanding the process of change will help them to develop therapeutic skills to target the patient's current stage. Students often make the early mistake, for example, of not fully assessing in what stage the patient is presenting before delving into therapy that assumes a certain level of motivation. Case vignettes can be a helpful way of differentiating the stages and how patients may present. Understanding and utilizing Motivational Interviewing approaches will also help students to have better experiences and outcomes with patients. Learning about how to address resistance from a Motivational Interviewing perspective, for example, will help students avoid the pitfalls and resulting frustrations of an overly confrontational approach.

Movie: *SherryBaby*

In the movie *SherryBaby* (2006), the actress Maggie Gyllenhaal portrays a young woman named Sherry who has just completed a prison sentence for drug-related crimes. She has a history of heroin addiction. She has been abstinent from heroin for 2½ years while incarcerated but now struggles to maintain her sobriety in the face of the daunting challenge of reassimilation to normal life. Her character is involved in 12-step work, though not formal substance abuse treatment. Sherry is motivated to maintain abstinence mainly by her desire to reclaim her young daughter, who has been raised by her brother in her absence. We see the character triggered to use drugs by intolerable negative emotions—frustration with her family situation, dissatisfaction with the housing situation she finds herself in, and the pain of rejection by her daughter. Were she a patient in treatment, Sherry's situation would present multiple opportunities for intervention. She has a level of motivation that can be harnessed and reinforced, but she needs to learn further coping skills in dealing with the triggers that precede her cravings for heroin.

Key Clinical Points

- The maintenance stage as described by Prochaska and DiClemente (1984) involves a process in which, despite achieving success in sustaining abstinence from drinking or drug use, patients may struggle with temptation, disappointment, and doubts about their decision.

- Motivational Interviewing can be used to help sustain the positive and desired change patients have made by reinforcing their confidence and supporting their efforts to stay the course, and helping them confront remaining obstacles to their goals.

- Relapse prevention is a treatment that employs a cognitive-behavioral model of approach to help patients avoid lapses and relapses by using coping skills and alternative behaviors.

- Active involvement in self-help work through AA, Narcotics Anonymous, or other 12-step-based organizations can provide additional supports for patients' efforts to sustain desired change in the maintenance phase.

Multiple-Choice Questions

For the correct answers to these questions, including explanations of answers, please see the Answer Guide at the end of this book.

1. Which of the following correctly describes the maintenance stage of change?
   A. A period during which patients are unaware of having a problem behavior.
   B. A period of abstinence in which the desired behavior change has become sustained.
   C. A period during which patients consider changing their behavior.
   D. A period during which patients take concrete steps to change their behavior.

2. Which of the following is NOT a Motivational Interviewing style of response to a patient who has acknowledged a lapse into drinking?
   A. "You should have known better than to make a mistake like that."
   B. "Can you tell me more about what thoughts and emotions you were having before you took the drink?"
   C. "What can we learn from the episode of drinking that will help you in the future?"
   D. "Having a slip is a common setback that patients experience, but it is not a failure."

3. Which of the following is NOT a recommended coping skill in relapse prevention?

   A. A patient attends anger management classes to learn how to deal with this emotion.
   B. An alcoholic patient repeatedly returns to a bar where he or she used to drink to desensitize himself or herself to cravings.
   C. A patient carries around an index card with a list of reminders about the negative consequences of drinking.
   D. A patient decides to begin a new hobby that he or she enjoys.

4. In beginning treatment with patients, it is recommended that therapists do all of the following EXCEPT:

   A. Provide the patient with a clear explanation of the goals of treatment.
   B. Establish a therapeutic connection.
   C. Make clear to the patient that any deviation from therapy goals could be grounds for termination.
   D. Explore the patient's expectations from treatment.

5. A *lapse* is defined as:

   A. A strong craving to use alcohol or drugs.
   B. A period of time between the action and maintenance stages of change.
   C. A full-blown return to the previous pattern of behavior.
   D. A brief return to drinking or drug use after a period of abstinence.

References

Center for Substance Abuse Treatment: Enhancing Motivation for Change in Substance Abuse Treatment (Treatment Improvement Protocol Series, No 35; DHHS Publ No [SMA] 05–4081; publication reprinted as [SMA] 08–4212). Rockville, MD, Substance Abuse and Mental Health Services Administration, 1999

Daley DC, Marlatt GA: Relapse prevention, in Substance Abuse: A Comprehensive Textbook, 4th Edition. Edited by Lowinson JH, Ruiz P, Millman RB, et al. Philadelphia, PA, Lippincott Williams & Wilkins, 2005, pp 772–785

DiClemente CC, Velasquez MM: Motivational interviewing and the stages of change, in Motivational Interviewing: Preparing People for Change, 2nd Edition. Edited by Miller WR, Rollnick S. New York, Guilford, 2002, pp 201–216

Kadden RM, Cooney NL: Treating alcohol problems, in Relapse Prevention: Maintenance Strategies in the Treatment of Addictive Behaviors, 2nd Edition. Edited by Marlatt GA, Donovan DM. New York, Guilford, 2005, pp 65–91

Marlatt GA, Witkiewitz K: Relapse prevention for alcohol and drug problems, in Relapse Prevention: Maintenance Strategies in the Treatment of Addictive Behaviors, 2nd Edition. Edited by Marlatt GA, Donovan DM. New York, Guilford, 2005, pp 1–44

Miller WR, Rollnick S: Motivational Interviewing: Preparing People for Change, 2nd Edition. New York, Guilford, 2002

Prochaska JO, DiClemente CC: The Transtheoretical Approach: Crossing Traditional Boundaries of Therapy. Homewood, IL, Dow Jones-Irwin, 1984

Rollnick S, Miller WR, Butler CC: Motivational Interviewing in Health Care: Helping Patients Change Behavior. New York, Guilford, 2008

Zweben A, Zuckoff A: Motivational interviewing and treatment adherence, in Motivational Interviewing: Preparing People for Change, 2nd Edition. Edited by Miller WR, Rollnick S. New York, Guilford, 2002, pp 299–319

CHAPTER 8

Relapse

Benjamin Cheney, M.D.
Daniel McMenamin, M.D.
Daryl I. Shorter, M.D.

Relapse or recycling (i.e., reentering the cycle of the stages of change) comes about frequently in working with patients who have a history of substance abuse and can be challenging for both patient and clinician. Although many patients graduate from the maintenance stage of change to termination (i.e., remain symptom-free without any further professional help), a significant number of our patients relapse. When a patient resumes substance use after a period of sobriety, treatment can be interrupted and the patient may not return. In many cases, however, he or she does return for help and the opportunity emerges to restart treatment work together.

The relapse state can lead patients to reassess the reasons why they do or do not use, and following the relapse a patient may enter a stage of change other than maintenance, ranging from precontemplation, to contemplation, to preparation or action (Figure 8–1). The change in motivation can be influenced by the relapse, in that the patient often feels discouraged by the return to use and believes that it is not possible for him or her to stay sober. The clinician working with the patient can also feel discouraged if the clinician views the relapse as a sign of failure on the clinician's part or as somehow undoing the work that previously led the patient to the maintenance stage. It is important to be aware of this tendency in both patient and clinician and to not be judgmental about relapse. In fact, relapse is considered a normal part of the passage through the different stages of motivation.

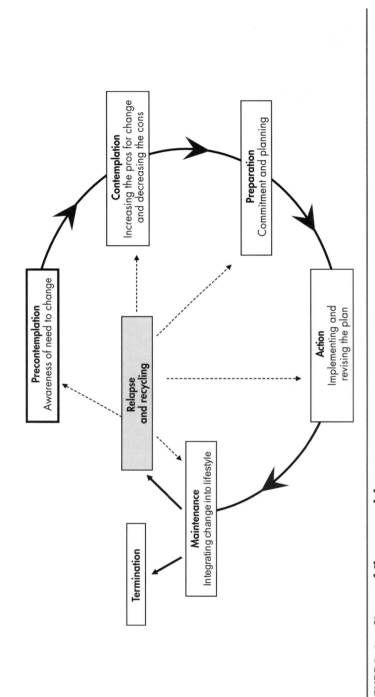

FIGURE 8–1. Stages of Change model.
Source. Adapted from DiClemente 2003.

When a patient relapses, the clinician should try to ascertain what led to the relapse as well as to determine what the patient would like to do following the relapse. The patient may require a different treatment, such as a detoxification process or a stay in a rehabilitation facility. The clinician should understand that the patient is likely to be in a different stage than the patient was before the relapse and should tailor the approach to the patient's current stage of change.

In this chapter, we discuss the case of a patient who stops smoking and then relapses several times to cigarette use before achieving a sustained state of abstinence. Our discussion focuses on how the clinician identifies the patient's motivational stage during each relapse and works with the patient using techniques appropriate to that stage. We also highlight and discuss an example of relapse taken from the movie *The War of the Roses*.

Clinical Case

Josh, a 21-year-old male college student with no history of medical or psychiatric illness, made an appointment with his internist, Dr. X, for a routine physical and checkup. At his appointment, Josh discussed his social alcohol use of two drinks a few times per month, past experimentation with marijuana, and cigarette use of approximately 1½ packs per day. Josh began smoking at age 15, with occasional use that increased to a half pack per day by age 17, then to 1½ packs daily after entering college. Josh would smoke his first cigarette shortly after waking up and smoked during class breaks. He smoked the most at night, when studying.

Dr. X, who had recently attended a continuing medical education course on brief interventions in the primary care setting, asked Josh how he felt about his tobacco use. Josh quickly told his doctor that he was aware that it is an unhealthy habit that he needed to quit because of its potential to cause lung cancer.

Sensing that Josh might be telling him what he wanted to hear, but not having time to further explore Josh's reaction, Dr. X told Josh that he was right that smoking can substantially increase someone's risk of developing lung cancer. "Unfortunately," Dr. X continued, "smoking also increases the risk of several other medical problems, including heart disease, stroke, and emphysema." Dr. X also told Josh that quitting is difficult but that there are medications that can help reduce use and cravings.

Josh thanked Dr. X for his advice and said that he would think about what he had told him and try to cut down after the semester ended, when he wouldn't be feeling so much pressure from his coursework.

Josh returned a year later for another checkup and to inquire about treatment recommendation for headaches he had when he felt stressed with work. Dr. X reviewed his previous notes and recalled his discussion with Josh about his smoking. In reviewing Josh's substance use, Dr. X learned that Josh had increased his smoking to 2 packs of cigarettes daily. Josh somewhat sheepishly told Dr. X that he remembered saying he'd intended to cut down but never made the effort. Given that he was in his senior year of college and applying to

Decisional matrix

	+	**−**
Continuing to smoke	*Helps concentrate on work* *Alleviates anxiety* *Improves mood* *Provides temporary relief from schoolwork* *Something to do when bored*	*Health concerns* *Harder to exercise* *Yellow teeth* *Smelly breath and clothing* *Expensive* *Unappealing to his girlfriend*
Giving up smoking	*Better health* *Extra money* *Will probably eventually feel better* *Independence from a drug*	*Will feel crummy* *Harder to focus on work, particularly in the beginning* *Worried it might affect relationships with friends who smoke (don't want to be one of those "obnoxious" quitters who can't be around other people who smoke)* *May not concentrate as well when studying*

law school, he figured he would try to quit once he had completed his exams and law school applications.

Dr. X decided at this point to complete a decisional matrix with Josh, reviewing the benefits and disadvantages of quitting tobacco use and continuing smoking, as shown above.

Dr. X gave Josh a copy of the decisional matrix and suggested he take it with him to review at his leisure, reminding him that if he decides to quit and finds it difficult, there are medications that may help him.

Josh returned for a follow-up appointment for his headaches 6 months later, at which time he informed Dr. X that he had managed to quit smoking on his own after taking the Law School Admission Test and reported being abstinent for the past 3 months. Josh reported that he had felt irritable, restless, and "a bit cloudy" at first but had been able to push through it, and now felt "much better" and had also discovered that he had better performance and endurance when he played basketball with friends. Josh said he felt confident that he'd never pick up a "cancer stick" again.

Two years later, however, Josh returned and told Dr. X that since starting law school he had fallen back into his habit and was now smoking 2 packs of cigarettes daily. He said that he'd tried to quit a few times, but that he found it difficult to deal with the stresses of law school while simultaneously dealing with nicotine withdrawal symptoms and cravings, which seemed more pronounced than they did the first time he quit. In addition, he felt more stressed in law school than he did in college. Cigarettes helped him concentrate better and deal with his stress, and thinking back to his decisional matrix (which he said he had kept), he wondered if he could quit given the benefits cigarettes conferred. He reiterated his concern that he might just be "a smoker for life," noting that his 56-year-old father started smoking in his teens and has never been able to quit.

Dr. X considered a trial of varenicline for Josh. Varenicline is a medication that works as a nicotine receptor partial agonist and is used to treat tobacco addiction. Varenicline acts by reducing cravings for cigarettes as well as decreasing the pleasurable aspects of smoking (Jorenby et al. 2006). Dr. X wrote Josh a prescription for varenicline, which Josh agreed to try. Josh returned to his follow-up appointment reporting that the medication helped reduce his cravings but made him feel sad and more anxious. Concerned about these side effects and recognizing that Josh could benefit from more extensive counseling, Dr. X decided to discontinue varenicline and refer Josh to a psychiatrist, Dr. Y. Josh initially refused to see Dr. Y because he didn't think he had enough time in his schedule. A year later, however, after learning that his father had been diagnosed with emphysema, Josh decided to contact Dr. Y.

Dr. Y asked Josh about the process by which he had resumed smoking. Josh recalled that he first relapsed during final exams in his first year of law school, when in the midst of a stressful study session, he decided to take a break; as he stood outside the library, he watched a classmate smoke a cigarette. He recalled how cigarette breaks had made him feel a sense of relief from anxiety and broke up the monotony of studying. After "bumming" a cigarette from his friend, he recalled feeling simultaneously calmed and energized. He subsequently decided to buy a pack of cigarettes to help get him through the remainder of the semester and went through the pack in less than a day. He recalled feeling discouraged by resuming smoking and feeling resigned to the fact that he had to "use a crutch" to get through his exams. In the following weeks, he continued smoking.

Working with Dr. Y, Josh learned that he held two incorrect and maladaptive beliefs about his relapse. The first was that his relapse was inevitable because "cigarette smoking is in my genes." The second was that he had no other way to deal with the demands and lifestyle of a law career than by smoking. In addition, Josh expressed the belief that his relapse and subsequent inability to quit proved he lacked the capacity to quit and remain abstinent.

As they explored the circumstances that led to Josh's relapse, Dr. Y noted that Josh had restarted smoking at a particularly stressful time and that it seemed Josh had come to conclusions about himself as a person based on this one event. He suggested to Josh that by making broad assumptions about himself from the event, he seemed to be selling himself short, and that this distorted way of viewing himself might be preventing him from quitting. On reflection, Josh agreed to make another attempt at quitting. Dr. Y prescribed a nicotine nasal spray to help with craving and withdrawal symptoms.

Two years later, Josh called Dr. Y to check in with him. In their phone conversation, Josh told Dr. Y that he "fell off the wagon again with the cigarettes a few days ago" and was hoping to come in to discuss how to proceed "before things get out of hand again." In the session, Josh told Dr. Y that he started smoking again after meeting up with an old college friend (who smoked) for a drink after work. He had since smoked 4 packs of cigarettes. Dr. Y also learned that Josh's father's emphysema had worsened due to his inability to stop smoking. Josh appeared anxious as he spoke of his concerns about relapsing. Dr. Y commended Josh for seeking help in what was clearly a difficult moment in maintaining his abstinence. He reminded Josh that slips do not necessarily lead to full-blown relapses but instead may provide an opportunity to learn about how to remain abstinent.

Dr. Y. also provided psychoeducation about the stages of change in addiction, and suggested that Josh think about his slip as a not entirely unexpected movement from the maintenance stage toward an earlier stage—from which he previously had been able to advance back into maintaining abstinence. Josh was able to identify the factors that led to his lapse (drinking alcohol in a bar, a stressful day at work, reuniting with an old smoking buddy) and decided to avoid these precipitants when possible (and find other ways to deal with the stress of work) while he continued to work on remaining abstinent.

Discussion of the Clinical Case

Josh's struggle with nicotine dependence illustrates the dynamic nature of the stages of change: Josh shifted from the precontemplation to contemplation to preparation to action to maintenance stages, after which stressful circumstances led to relapse and the precontemplation stage. The cycle occurred again until he had an additional lapse and then shifted back into the maintenance stage, where the case ends. An appreciation of the Transtheoretical Model of Change (Prochaska and DiClemente 1984) allowed Drs. X and Y to both avoid becoming overly discouraged by Josh's occasional movement backward and to provide the necessary interventions to prevent Josh from abandoning his efforts to become and remain abstinent from smoking.

In reviewing the techniques used in the treatment, note that Dr. X initially raised concerns in his brief intervention after first learning about Josh's nicotine use. It is important that Dr. X avoided reprimanding Josh, lecturing him, or commanding him to quit. Instead, by expressing empathy, providing necessary health information outlining the dangers of smoking, and allowing Josh to come to his own decision, Dr. X focused on building an alliance with him while providing information that could promote change in him and lead him to the contemplation stage. The decision matrix exercise helped Josh shift into the preparation and action stages.

When Josh relapsed, Dr. Y was able to recognize an important pattern that is common to people who shift out of the maintenance stage, which is that lapses frequently lead patients to feel a lowered sense of self-efficacy—attributing the shift (which often has specific transient or external contributing factors) to an inherent inability to stay abstinent. It is believed that such a tendency to attribute a lapse to internal, stable, and global factors (also known as the *abstinence violation effect*; see the following section "Suggestions for Treatment," item number 3) can play a role in turning a temporary lapse into a full-blown relapse. Dr. Y's intervention, which was repeated in Josh's subsequent lapse, was to help rebuild Josh's confidence in his ability to become abstinent again. Dr. Y restored Josh's faith in himself by addressing Josh's cognitive distortions (Josh's generalizations about himself based on a solitary event); by providing psychoeducation about the addiction and the Transtheoretical Model of Change—which helped Josh normalize his behavior; and by reframing the relapse so that Josh could see it as a learning experience rather than as a failure.

One final note should be made regarding this case: nicotine does not cause the same behavior changes or acute health risks as other addictive substances. This case, therefore, does not address the need for the treatment provider to consider more acute levels of care (e.g., inpatient rehabilitation or an intensive outpatient program) when a patient relapses—as should be considered for a patient who abuses substances like alcohol and opioids. With respect to this issue, the reader is asked to refer to the "Suggestions for Treatment" section below.

Suggestions for Treatment

A return to substance use can be disconcerting for both the patient and the clinician. The way a clinician should respond depends on numerous factors. The clinician's approach to treatment requires an assessment of the patient and the relapse event. To help organize the clinician's approach to this potentially chaotic event, we have divided this section into steps the clinician might take when faced with a relapsed patient:

1. *Don't forget to be nonjudgmental and empathic.* People become frustrated when they feel that their investment of time and effort has not yielded the intended results, so the clinician naturally and understandably can feel frustrated with a patient during relapse. This feeling of frustration frequently leads the clinician to respond in exactly the wrong way to a patient who feels shame and a loss of self-efficacy. It is important for clinicians to remind themselves to resist the urge to blame or judge but to instead make an effort to appreciate the patient's feelings of distress or self-blame. Remembering to be curious about how the patient is feeling and to make empathic statements (e.g., "This must be a very confusing time for you") will strengthen the clinician's alliance with the patient.
2. *Assess safety and appropriate level of care.* Before deciding on a means of intervention, it is important to first reassess the level of care that would be most beneficial or is medically necessary for the patient. Although the se-

lection of the appropriate level of care for a substance abuse patient remains a debated topic, the most commonly accepted means of determination is provided by the American Society of Addiction Medicine's Patient Placement Criteria (Mee-Lee et al. 2003). The society recommends assessing a patient's need for treatment along six dimensions (intoxication and withdrawal, biomedical conditions, emotional/behavioral conditions, treatment acceptance/resistance, relapse/continued use potential, and recovery environment), then using the assessment to recommend placement (level of treatment), which could range from continued outpatient services to partial hospitalization to medically managed inpatient treatment.

Although the treatment algorithm is beyond the scope of this chapter, it is worthwhile to consider the following questions when assessing whether a patient should receive a higher level of care:

- Does the patient have a history of serious withdrawal symptoms? Is he or she currently having withdrawal symptoms?
- Does the patient have any severe health problems?
- Is the patient in imminent danger of harming himself or herself or others? Is the patient unable to attend to activities of daily living?
- Are there components of the patient's environment that will threaten the patient's safety or prevent recovery?

3. *Determine whether the patient's return to use is an actual relapse—or just a lapse.* In their discussion of Relapse Prevention therapy, Marlatt and Donovan (2005) distinguish between a *lapse* (a singular, discrete episode of use) and a *relapse* (a full return to regular use). Marlatt and Donovan's research suggests that a patient's emotional response can affect the likelihood of proceeding to a full-blown relapse via a phenomenon they term the *abstinence violation effect*. With the abstinence violation effect, a lapse causes feelings of guilt, failure, or helplessness as patients attribute the lapse to factors that are "internal, global, and uncontrollable" (Marlatt and Donovan 2005, p. 3). These negative feelings lead patients to abandon the abstinence attempt, presumably because they lose faith in their sense of self-efficacy and because they know they can rely on the addictive substance or behavior to escape their feelings.

    Patients who manage to seek treatment following a lapse are considered to be in the maintenance stage of change, in which case a relapse prevention approach is indicated. On the other hand, patients who present after a full-blown relapse may have shifted from maintenance to any of the earlier motivational stages of change.

4. *If the patient has lapsed, then assess the patient's emotional reaction and sense of self-efficacy.* Self-efficacy is defined as a "personal perception of mastery over [a] risky situation" (Larimer et al. 1999, p. 153). Following a lapse, a pri-

mary role of the clinician is to help the patient maintain the belief that he or she has the power to overcome the forces of addiction and to stay abstinent. It is therefore helpful to identify negative cognitive distortions such as all-or-none thinking, overgeneralization, mental filters, disqualifying the positive, jumping to conclusions, catastrophization, emotional reasoning, *should* statements, labeling and mislabeling, and personalization—all of which may contribute to the patient's tendency to attribute his or her relapse to global factors, and in turn, decrease the patient's sense of self-efficacy. Pointing out the irrational nature of these distortions and helping the patient create rational responses will help increase the patient's sense of self-efficacy.

Other ways of enhancing self-efficacy as noted by Larimer et al. (1999; p. 156) include helping the patient "break down the overall task of behavior change into smaller, more manageable subtasks" and "providing patients with feedback concerning their performance on other new tasks, even those that appear unrelated to alcohol use [...] (e.g., showing up to appointments)."

5. *If the patient has relapsed, then assess the patient's motivational stage of change.* If a patient has experienced a full-blown relapse, he or she may present in any of the first four motivational stages of change (precontemplation, contemplation, preparation, or action). As with any other case, a therapeutic intervention is more likely to be effective if it is correctly matched to the appropriate motivational stage of change.

6. *Help the patient see the lapse or relapse as a learning experience.* This intervention is helpful in two ways: a) it reframes the event into an experience with a potentially positive outcome, thus helping the patient defend against catastrophization and other self-debasing cognitive distortions; and b) it serves to help the patient prevent future relapses. This is a particularly helpful intervention after a lapse or after the patient has progressed past the contemplation stage of change. Areas worthy of exploration include identification of high-risk situations and decisional patterns that have a high likelihood of subsequently leading to risky situations, both of which are discussed further in Chapter 7 ("Maintenance").

Suggestions for Teaching and Supervision

One useful exercise in teaching and supervising clinicians about the relapse state is to role-play a sample situation in which the supervised clinician can play both a clinician and a patient. In the exercise, the clinician should be encouraged to think creatively about possible factors that could lead a patient to relapse and also to envision additional supports to help a patient who has already relapsed. In the role-playing scenario, the clinician also can be asked to imagine the emotional states held by clinician and patient, in particular negative emotions that might frustrate treatment. In the supervision, the clinician can also practice using specific motivational techniques such as the decisional matrix or having the patient, as played by the supervisor, imagine how the patient would like his or her life to be different in the future.

In an actual situation involving a patient who relapses, it is important to ask the clinician about his or her own reaction to the relapse to ensure that the clinician has not taken it personally.

Movie: *The War of the Roses*

In the 1989 film *The War of the Roses*, Danny DeVito plays divorce attorney Gavin D'Amato, who narrates this tale of love, hate, and comic tragedy. He weaves the story of Barbara and Oliver Rose (played by Kathleen Turner and Michael Douglas): the couple who meet, fall madly in love, and get married, only to have their imperfect union devolve into petty squabbling, violence, and ultimately death. In his opening monologue, Gavin lights up a cigarette and states, "I gotta cut this out. It's gonna kill me," as he explains that he had not smoked for 13 years before relapsing. Gavin's thinking is reflective of the contemplation stage of motivation. Having achieved a significant amount of time abstinent from nicotine, he seems to have progressed back to an earlier stage of change, as can be the case for many patients who relapse. Although he recognizes and voices a clear need for change, he does not state any intention to make changes in the near future (e.g., the next 6 months), nor does he seem to be preparing to take some sort of action toward quitting smoking.

For some individuals struggling with addictive behavior following a relapse, a focus on the loss of sobriety may overshadow the successful recovery that preceded it, creating feelings of guilt and shame and an attitude that future efforts at abstinence are futile. In these cases, it is important to remind patients of their success and to help identify those factors that may have assisted in their ability to achieve and maintain sobriety. Interestingly, Gavin is able to identify an important factor that helped him to maintain abstinence from smoking. He says, "I kept the last cigarette from my last pack. I said if I never smoke this one cigarette, I'll never smoke again. Period. Thirteen years I kept that cigarette." By keeping a symbol or token, he held onto a physical representation of his abstinence, which ultimately assisted him in remembering his commitment to long-term abstinence. This type of psychological reinforcement may be important for many patients in recovery and is similar to the coins and/or chips used by members of 12-step groups like Alcoholics Anonymous. Rather than obtaining a reward from the pleasurable effects of smoking, Gavin receives powerful self-reinforcement of his decision to not smoke by viewing this symbol of his success. Working with patients to identify and practice such a relapse prevention technique represents a core component of treatment during the maintenance phase; at this stage, however, treatment for Gavin should focus on instilling a sense of hope in order to reduce negative feelings about himself and the relapse. Additionally, it would be appropriate to discuss, in an empathic and nonjudgmental fashion, any difficulties Gavin may have with reengaging in the recovery process. In this overall approach, the ultimate goal would be to assist Gavin in discovering his own level of desire to change and to assist him in transitioning from contemplation to preparation as he becomes ready to change.

Key Clinical Points

- Relapse is commonly encountered in work with people with substance use problems, and despite the temptation for clinician and patient to become demoralized, should be viewed as an opportunity to reengage in treatment.

- Once a patient relapses, it is important to be supportive, nonjudgmental, and empathic in your approach as a clinician.

- Following a relapse, the clinician should assess the patient's stage of motivation, tailor the treatment approach to the patient's particular stage of change, and determine what additional supports or strategies would be helpful to the patient to continue his or her progress.

Multiple-Choice Questions

For the correct answers to these questions, including explanations of answers, please see the Answer Guide at the end of this book.

1. A patient resumes drinking alcohol for a month after attaining 1 year of sobriety. He visits his therapist to discuss the relapse. The patient could be in which of the following stages of change as identified by Prochaska and DiClemente (1984)?

    A. Precontemplation.
    B. Contemplation.
    C. Action.
    D. Any of the above.

2. During a relapse, a patient tells the clinician who is working with her that "I should just keep on drinking. I've lost my sobriety now." This patient is most likely in which of the following stages of change?

    A. Precontemplation.
    B. Contemplation.
    C. Preparation.
    D. Maintenance.

3. With the abstinence violation effect:

    A. Patients attribute their loss of sobriety to factors beyond their control.
    B. Patients maintain their confidence that they can return to abstinence.
    C. Patients view their return to substance use as a learning experience.
    D. Patients remain in the maintenance stage of change.

4. Which of the following is NOT an example of a common pitfall for clinicians in working with patients who have relapsed?

    A. Having a judgmental attitude toward the patient.
    B. Having self-critical thoughts about how you, the clinician, could have prevented the relapse.
    C. Expressing your (the clinician's) desire for the patient's immediate return to a state of abstinence.
    D. Having an open-minded viewpoint about the patient's motivation to change his or her behavior.

5. Which of the following is NOT an example of a motivational approach for the clinician to take with patients who relapse?

   A. Identify the possible factors that may have led to the relapse.
   B. Use a decisional matrix to analyze the pros and cons of continuing to use the substance.
   C. Determine additional supports for patients to help them reestablish their abstinence.
   D. Tell patients that the relapse shows how powerful their disease is and that they will need to be stronger next time.

References

DiClemente C: Addiction and Change: How Addictions Develop and Addicted People Recover. New York, Guilford, 2003

Jorenby DE, Hays JT, Rigotti NA, et al: Efficacy of varenicline, an alpha4beta2 nicotinic acetylcholine receptor partial agonist, vs placebo or sustained-release bupropion for smoking cessation: a randomized controlled trial. JAMA 296:56–63, 2006

Larimer ME, Palmer RS, Marlatt GA: Relapse prevention: an overview of Marlatt's cognitive-behavioral model. Alcohol Res Health 23:151–160, 1999

Marlatt GA, Donovan DM (eds): Relapse Prevention: Maintenance Strategies in the Treatment of Addictive Behaviors, 2nd Edition. New York, Guilford, 2005

Mee-Lee D, Shulman GD: The ASAM placement criteria and matching patients to treatment, in Principles of Addiction Medicine, 3rd Edition. Edited by Graham AW, Schultz TK, Mayo-Smith MF, et al. Chevy Chase, MD, American Society of Addiction Medicine, 2003, pp. 453–465

Prochaska JO, DiClemente CC: The Transtheoretical Approach: Crossing Traditional Boundaries of Therapy. Homewood, IL, Dow Jones-Irwin, 1984

CHAPTER 9

Working With Dually Diagnosed Patients

Stephen Ross, M.D.

Motivation to change behavior in individuals with addictive disorders is a complex phenomenon that has multiple dimensions including neurobiological, cognitive, behavioral, psychodynamic, spiritual, and experiential dimensions. It can broadly be influenced by both intrinsic factors (those within the individual—such as internal, intentional states) and extrinsic factors (those outside the individual—such as external incentives and coercion). Alteration in motivational intent and behavior change represent a core, fundamental aim of psychotherapy for individuals with addictive disorders. This is particularly important for those with co-occurring disorders, who constitute the majority of our patients.

In the National Comorbidity Survey, 50.9% of individuals with a lifetime mental illness had a history of a substance use disorder (SUD), and conversely, 51.4% of those with a lifetime SUD met criteria for a lifetime mental disorder (Kessler et al. 1996). In addition, almost all psychiatric disorders have higher rates of co-occurrence of SUDs compared with the rate at which SUDs occur in people without mental illness, but rates are particularly high in people with affective disorders (especially bipolar spectrum disorders), psychotic disorders, anxiety spectrum disorders (especially posttraumatic stress disorder and panic disorder), attention-deficit/hyperactivity disorder (ADHD), eating disorders (mostly bulimia nervosa), and personality disorders (especially antisocial and borderline personality disorders) (Ross 2008). The prevalence of individuals with co-occurring disorders is dramatically elevated from a baseline of 3%–4% of people living in the community to 40%–60% of those in mental health treatment settings and 50%–60% of those in substance abuse treatment settings (Hendrickson 2006). Of patients with co-occurring disorders, those with severe and persistent mental illness, such as schizophrenia or bipolar spectrum disorders, have a particularly high co-occurrence of SUDs, estimated to be as many as 4 million adults in the United States (Substance Abuse and Mental Health Services Administration 2004).

From a treatment delivery system perspective, integrated treatment for patients with co-occurring disorders has generally been associated with better outcomes than treatment in either serial or parallel treatment paradigms, especially with an increased duration/intensity of treatment and added ancillary services (Drake et al. 2004). Moreover, it has been well established that addiction treatment is effective across the spectrum of SUDs in multiple types of treatment settings—as well as being cost-effective and providing savings to patients, their employers, and society in general—with the following variables predicting better response to treatment (McLellan and McKay 2003):

- **Pretreatment:** Increased motivation beyond the precontemplation stage; active employment; low severity of psychiatric symptoms or addictive disorder; having a supportive social network
- **Intratreatment:** Longer length of time spent in treatment; having an individual therapist as part of treatment; receiving proper psychotropic interventions for both psychiatric and addictive disorders; reduction of psychiatric symptomatology; participation in voucher-incentivized behavioral reinforcement programs; having added ancillary services to treat ongoing psychiatric, medical, and/or family problems
- **Posttreatment:** Participation in mutual-help programs such as Alcoholics Anonymous (AA) and Narcotics Anonymous (NA) has been associated with improved treatment outcomes such as increased abstinence rates.

Individuals with co-occurring disorders, in particular those with severe and persistent mental illness, face unique challenges regarding their ability to engage in an intentional process of change, whether it relates to the initiation, commitment, or maintenance of positive changes. As such, they pose a heightened problem regarding their relation to treatment engagement, motivation for change, sustained change, relapse rates, and overall treatment outcomes (DiClemente et al. 2008). Compared with patients with only one mental disorder, patients with co-occurring disorders across a broad spectrum of diagnostic types and combinations have greater severity of illness and a worse longitudinal course of illness in multiple domains, including the following (Hser et al. 2006; Mueser et al. 1998; Ziedonis 2004):

- Increased risk for psychiatric and substance use relapses
- Higher rates of recidivism
- Higher levels of psychological distress
- Poorer quality of social networks
- Worse overall psychosocial functioning
- Poorer treatment engagement
- Worse treatment retention
- Poorer medication compliance
- Higher rates of violence, suicide, legal difficulties, medical problems, and family stress
- Higher utilization of health care services such as emergency room and in-patient services.

In addition, irrespective of the etiology of co-occurring illness, there is a bi-directional effect whereby failure to treat one disorder (either the mental illness or the SUD) negatively affects the severity of illness and longitudinal course of the other (Hser et al. 2006). Along with all the above items, this makes the success of engagement and motivational change that much more imperative in this patient population. Moreover, the process of initiating and maintaining positive change relates to dimensions of both the mental illness and the SUD, and the process of changing one needs to occur independently and in parallel with the process of changing the other. In this chapter, I review the core evidence-based motivational approaches used to initiate change in patients with co-occurring mental illness and SUDs. I focus on treatments commonly used to leverage change in all addictive disorders and in particular highlight approaches that are unique in being able to engage and motivate individuals with co-occurring disorders, especially those with severe and persistent mental illness. A large spectrum of approaches is discussed, ranging from intrinsically oriented treatments, such as Motivational Interviewing, to extrinsically oriented ones, such as contingency management and coercion. I also discuss motivational augmentation strategies such as pharmacotherapy and the use of creative arts therapies and paradigms for how to combine various modalities. A clinical case provides a vehicle to introduce each of these techniques and to illustrate a methodology of how and when to apply different types of motivational approaches, and how co-occurring mental illness and SUDs necessitate a uniquely tailored approach to influence the intentional and nonintentional processes of change.

Clinical Case

Joan is a 21-year-old unemployed single woman, living with her parents, who first presented for treatment complaining of mood swings and stating that she has to stop using heroin because "my parents say I have to." She was using eight bags of heroin intravenously per day for the year before presentation and had never been to an inpatient detoxification program or a rehabilitation program. Her parents had become fed up with her "lying and stealing addict behavior." They suspected that she had started to sell heroin and wanted her out of the house. Joan was described as a sweet and sensitive child who did well academically but had difficulty socializing; she had always been the "special" one in the family. She described herself as awkward and felt ostracized at school. She started smoking cigarettes and drinking alcohol at age 16 and began to experiment recreationally with cocaine and heroin at age 19, despite being warned of their dangers in health education classes throughout middle and high school. She found that heroin was effective at diminishing the anxiety and depression that she had experienced on and off since age 12. She had been in therapy but stated that her drug use had never been addressed. Joan made it to her senior year of college before her use of heroin dramatically escalated in the setting of a breakup with a boyfriend. She went from weekend intranasal use to daily intravenous use. She took a leave of absence from school after being arrested for heroin possession. She came home to live with her parents, who were furious at her and scared that their daughter had become a "junkie."

At the initial evaluation, Joan did not acknowledge the severity of the problems she faced and felt that her parents were overreacting. The parents appeared to be scared and exasperated. They could not understand how their daughter had become addicted but wanted to do everything they could to help her. After an assessment, Joan was diagnosed with bipolar II disorder, ADHD, and heroin dependence. Given that she was in the precontemplation stage, Motivational Interviewing was begun to increase her intention to change. After completing a decisional matrix that highlighted the risk–benefit ratio of her continued use, Joan displayed greater cognitive dissonance toward her heroin use and began to contemplate change. However, on a fundamental level, she still viewed the risk of use as being less than the risk of change. A family component was added to the treatment to improve her motivational state. Although Joan continued to become more contemplative over time regarding her motivation to change her relationship with heroin, her stated goal became that of moderation management. Angry, her family insisted that she get inpatient treatment. She was admitted to an inpatient detoxification unit, underwent a methadone taper, and transitioned to a 1-month rehabilitation program. Following this, she attended an intensive outpatient program for addiction for several months. She remained abstinent for 3 months taking naltrexone, valproic acid, and bupropion, with thrice-weekly addiction psychotherapy including relapse prevention and family therapy, but then became nonadherent with her medications and relapsed to heroin use. The family was furious at her for "not trying harder." Buprenorphine was offered to the patient, but the family was invested in a sober outcome and the patient felt she could be abstinent if she just tried harder. After several months of increased heroin use and mood lability, the patient and the family agreed on rehospitalization to an inpatient detoxification unit. Here, the patient and family agreed to buprenorphine induction, and Joan resumed taking her psychotropic medications. A residential program was offered, but Joan refused and she went back to living with her parents and attending an intensive outpatient program.

Again, she was stable and sober for several months before sequentially becoming more nonadherent with therapy, the intensive outpatient program, and her medications. She returned to using heroin and began to sell it as well. After being arrested again for heroin possession, she was offered court-monitored treatment as an alternative to incarceration. Joan said that this "woke me up," and she began attending a treatment program in conjunction with a drug court. She remained sober for 4 months and began to feel that the drug court, and in particular, the benevolent but firm judge, was helping her stay sober. However, in the setting of increased stress from being unemployed and fighting with her parents, she slipped back into using heroin. Her parents stated that they "couldn't do this anymore," decided on a path of tough love, and proceeded to tell Joan to leave their house and that she would have to hit rock bottom and really want to get better for herself before they would help her further. Joan became panicked after hearing this because she felt as if her parents were withdrawing "their love for me." She became acutely suicidal and stated she would kill herself by purchasing a gun. She refused to go to a psychiatric emergency room, so her treating psychiatrist called 911 and hospitalized Joan involuntarily on a dual-diagnosis inpatient unit. Joan was furious at her treating psychiatrist for doing this and said, "I never want to see you again." She was hospitalized for 2 weeks and agreed to a 30-day rehabilitation program. On getting to the program, she immediately left against medical advice. The treating psychiatrist received a frantic call from the family saying that Joan had come home and that she said she was leaving to kill herself. The psychiatrist immediately called 911, and luckily, the police found her in a nearby alley, passed out but alive after injecting heroin and with a gun nearby. She was rehospitalized involuntarily in the same dual-diagnosis inpatient unit. This time she was even angrier than before. She attempted to spit on her treating psychiatrist when the psychiatrist came to visit her and said, "I hope you die." Her family called to say that they were "done" with Joan and did not want any further contact and felt there was no more hope of saving her.

On admission to the unit, Joan was in a mixed manic state and was acutely suicidal. She was placed on a one-to-one observation that lasted for approximately 2 weeks. For the first 2 weeks on the unit, Joan went to court several times to be released but was retained by court order. She refused all psychotropic medication until a court order mandated that she begin taking medication over her objection. Electroconvulsive therapy was considered, but after restarting her psychotropic medications, her mood lability and suicidal ideation began to improve. However, she continued to refuse to meet with her treatment providers or family and would simply not leave her room. She went to no group meetings and in particular cursed the existence of spiritual-type treatments on the unit, such as daily AA and NA groups, because she was an avowed atheist and felt that "God must be dead if this is happening to me."

Finally, after 3 weeks on the unit and through persistent coaxing by the unit's charismatic and tirelessly optimistic music therapist, Joan agreed to come to a music therapy group but agreed to do so only if the group agreed to play one of Joan's favorite songs, "Don't Stop Believing" by Journey. Joan played guitar and sang passionately in the group as the other patients joined in. It was a dramatic and symbolic moment that would translate into an even more surprising series of transformational events. Joan began to participate actively in her treatment and discharge planning over the next several weeks of her inpatient stay. She participated in individual and group Motivational Interviewing, relapse prevention, and all of the creative arts therapy activities including music, art, dance, and yoga therapy. She also enthusiastically participated in the peer-led token economy contingency management program on the unit, earning enough points to be elevated to level 3, which allowed her to go to the roof and attend the semiweekly rewards meeting where prizes such as food and clothing items were awarded. Even more surprising, she began to religiously attend all of the AA and NA group meetings and found them to be very useful. She particularly liked reciting the serenity prayer and found meaning and hope in the words. The concept of recovery through connection with a transcendent "higher power," which she came to conceptualize as the sum of the care of her fellow patients and treatment providers, appealed to her and provided a great sense of comfort and ongoing motivation. She agreed to a long-term residential program and was discharged to an 18-month modified therapeutic community for dually diagnosed individuals.

Despite the fact that Joan was one of the youngest patients and despite reports of others abusing drugs during their stay in the facility, she completed the 18-month program, being abstinent the whole time. She served as chief expeditor of the therapeutic community for the last 6 months of her treatment stay. After completing the program, she obtained employment at a Starbucks coffee store and moved into her own apartment. Over the next year, she remained psychologically stable, sober, and engaged in treatment, and she talked about plans for her future. She continued to go to AA and NA meetings up to five times a week, connected with a sponsor, worked through all 12 steps, and eventually became a sponsor herself, which she took great pride in. Vocationally, she decided she wanted to be an emergency medical technician and eventually obtained her license despite numerous regulatory hurdles and setbacks in training. It was remarkable to see her change from her previous mode of impulsivity and need for instant gratification to her increased tolerance of delayed gratification and the acquisition of the ability to self-soothe and self-regulate. In addition, she met a man, fell in love, and moved in with him.

Discussion of the Clinical Case and Suggestions for Treatment

Start With Noncoercive, Intrinsically Oriented Treatments: Psychoeducation and Motivational Interviewing

The first motivational techniques used with Joan were two types of brief interventions: 1) psychoeducation delivered in health classes at various points of her schooling and 2) Motivational Interviewing delivered early on in her treatment course. Brief interventions are time-limited, client-centered therapeutic techniques, easily administered and cost-effective, in which the goal is a specific behavior change and improved medication adherence (Graham and Fleming 2003). Broadly, three main types of brief interventions are psychoeducation, Motivational Interviewing, and Screening, Brief Intervention, and Referral to Treatment (SBIRT; discussed further later in this chapter). Both psychoeducation and Motivational Interviewing are techniques that lack any coercive measures. With psychoeducation, straightforward facts about drug use and addiction are presented and often include the harmful effects of compulsive drug use, such as psychiatric and medical sequelae, but can also include positive properties of certain drugs (e.g., cardioprotective effects of low-dose alcohol consumption). No attempt is necessarily made to change behavior, although the hope is that increased knowledge about the harm of drugs will prompt the individual to change his or her behavior. On the other hand, Motivational Interviewing is a technique drawing on the principles of motivational psychology and Rogerian therapy (Martino et al. 2002) and is designed to help individuals resolve ambivalence inherent in the precontemplation and contemplation stages of change, thereby moving the individual along the motivational continuum. It is a nonconfrontational cognitive and experiential method whereby the therapist helps the patient explore and resolve ambivalence in order to increase motivation for behavior change. Rather than being confrontational, the therapist employs the principles of expressing empathy, developing discrepancy, rolling with resistance, and supporting self-efficacy to help individuals become better risk managers for themselves by weighing the relative pros and cons of continued substance use; it is hoped that increased cognitive dissonance will create a discordant internal state that will increase the intentional motivation to either reduce use or aim for abstinence.

It is valuable to start with a type of intervention like Motivational Interviewing that is nonconfrontational in nature. Addicted individuals tend to have a poor history of interacting with medical providers and too often are treated with disrespect, made to feel ashamed of their behavior, and told to simply stop behaving in such self-destructive ways. Such moralistic, heavy-handed, and at times mean-spirited approaches often adversely polarize the treatment relationship from the beginning and hamper crucial rapport building. Initially, it is best to take a supportive, curious stance and to assume that addicts do not start using drugs with the intention of eventually ruining their lives. Addiction often starts as a rational attempt at self-psychopharmacology to alleviate psychic distress. As we know, it eventually ends up in a deeply irrational, destructive process. However, it is always better to positively build rapport by expressing empathy and curiosity as a means to initially engage patients in treatment by assuming their use has or had a logical rationale. Such an approach is often disarming to addicted individuals and allows them to not hold on as tightly to denial and resistance. It further builds confidence by tapping into a patient's inner resources and sense of self-efficacy and aims to treat the executive and cognitive dysfunction seen in addiction by establishing or strengthening cognitive processes, such as weighing the pros and cons of behaviors, delaying gratification, diminishing impulsivity, and weighing the relative saliency of drug-oriented versus biologically oriented cues and rewards.

Although both psychoeducation and Motivational Interviewing were initially tried with Joan, they were clearly not sufficient to get her to significantly change her addictive and harmful behavior. The evidence for the efficacy of Motivational Interviewing has been well established across multiple drugs of abuse and in multiple treatment settings (Martino et al. 2002). Its use has been extended to include medical (Brodie et al. 2008) and psychiatric illnesses. Furthermore, recent work has looked at its applicability in patients with co-occurring disorders, with some positive preliminary findings (DiClemente et al. 2008; Drake et al. 2004). However, treatments such as Motivational Interviewing are not always useful or even possible in patients with co-occurring disorders. Motivational Interviewing presupposes sufficient intact cognitive substrates to be able to engage in the treatment. Patients such as those with mental retardation (e.g., fetal alcohol syndrome), neurological damage (e.g., strokes or dementing syndromes), advanced or refractory addictive disorders, or severe mental illness (e.g., avolition associated with major depression or positive and negative symptoms associated with schizophrenia) may simply not have the capacity to engage in Motivational Interviewing. Therefore, some investigators have suggested that extrinsic or external forces may be more salient to effect behavior change in patients with co-occurring disorders, especially those with severe and persistent mental illness (Bellack and DiClemente 1999).

Use Extrinsically Oriented Treatments Next

Screening, Brief Intervention, and Referral to Treatment

If initial noncoercive attempts at behavior change that affirm a patient's autonomy and try to tap into inner sources of self-efficacy and enhanced executive functioning fail, extrinsically oriented approaches are necessary. SBIRT, another brief intervention, is an example of one such approach. (See also Chapter 11, "Integrating Screening, Brief Intervention, and Referral to Treatment With Motivational Work.") Like Motivational Interviewing, SBIRT emphasizes empathic resonance, reviews the pros and cons of use behavior, and supports self-efficacy. However, unlike the less directive Motivational Interviewing, SBIRT approaches include overt and explicit treatment recommendations from the external treatment provider, such as advice to effect a change in drug or alcohol use behavior (either reduction of use or abstinence) using goal setting, behavior contracting, behavior modification planning, and referrals to specific treatment programs. This type of brief intervention has reliably been shown to reduce alcohol and other drug use behavior; the number and length of the intervention sessions can vary but typically involve 5- to 10-minute sessions repeated one to three times over a 6- to 8-week period (Graham and Fleming 2003). This type of intervention is well suited to and tends to work optimally in primary care or emergency room settings. In Joan's case, it had little impact. Simply being told that she had a problem, even repeatedly, and receiving advice to make a change were not enough. She needed a different type of external approach—coercion.

Coercion (Legal, Familial, Peer)

Coercive interventions are an integral part of treatment to effect changes in behavior in individuals with addictive disorders and co-occurring disorders. They include the following types: legal, familial, and peer. The majority of patients with addictive disorders alone (without comorbid mental illness) who present for treatment are in either the precontemplation stage (approximately 40%) or the contemplation stage (approximately 40%), both of which are marked by denial, ambivalence, and resistance to change (Velicer et al. 1995). In addition, individuals with co-occurring disorders may have even less volition and cognitive capacity to engage in internally oriented motivational treatments and their risk liability for bad outcomes (including self-harm, violence, and poor medical outcomes) is enhanced. The practice of total disengagement from the patient by the family and hoping the individual will hit rock bottom, allowing for transformative change, does not apply because the risk is too high and rock bottom for some of these individuals is the irreversible state of death.

Legal coercion. Legal interventions include diversion from jail or release from jail to participate in court-mandated drug treatment programs. Although these types of intervention are in their infancy, preliminary outcome data, including data on individuals with co-occurring disorders, suggest good outcomes including enhanced treatment utilization, enhanced motivation for change, decreased recidivism, and reduced overall cost (Drake et al. 2008; Gregoire and Burke 2004). Other legal coercive measures specific to those with co-occurring illness include involuntary psychiatric hospitalization and other court-mandated inpatient treatments for psychiatric patients who have demonstrated a history of repeated danger to themselves or others, such as New York State's Assisted Outpatient Treatment program; such programs also exist in some form in many other states (Kallert 2008). For Joan, being offered court-mandated treatment as an alternative to incarceration helped her engage in treatment and remain abstinent for 4 months. Also, she was involuntarily committed twice to an inpatient dual-diagnosis locked unit. At the time, Joan had particularly hated this approach and felt it violated her rights and volitional capacity. The reality is that this intervention, used sparingly and carefully, is necessary when risk liability for danger to oneself or others increases to unacceptable and dangerous levels. Looking back on her involuntary psychiatric hospitalizations, Joan remarked that "this is what saved my life." She reported being grateful that someone "cared" enough to do something so drastic because she lacked the volition and autonomy in her state of consciousness at the time.

Family coercion.   Family-oriented treatments are an integral part of addiction psychotherapy. In addition to providing support for sobriety, they can serve as a force to change the addicted individual's behavior. They can range from noncoercive interventions such as Community Reinforcement and Family Training (Meyers and Smith 1997; Miller et al. 1999) or Al-Anon and Alateen, to those with some degree of coercion such as network therapy (Galanter 1993; Galanter et al. 2002), to the most coercive—such as the original Johnson (1998) method of *intervention*, popularized in movies and television, with the goal of leveraging extensive family pressure and confrontation to break down denial and lead to treatment acceptance. Family interventions played a prominent role in Joan's treatment in both positive and negative ways. Joan's motivation initially improved after family therapy began, although not enough to move toward abstinence. Her family then demanded that she go into an inpatient setting, and without the intervention, she would likely not have made this decision.

Addiction causes immense strain on a family system, and the family does not always respond in optimal ways. In fact, one of the dark sides of addiction is that it can lead families to want to rid themselves of the addicted family member out of extreme states of fear and frustration. Worse, addiction can sometimes lead to total disintegration of family units. Joan's addiction pushed her family to the limit, and they responded at times in nonconstructive ways, such as refusing buprenorphine treatment out of a misguided but understandable desire for total abstinence. Even worse, out of desperation, they tried to disengage from her by throwing her out of the house after a relapse. This caused her to become acutely suicidal and necessitated an inpatient admission. Optimal engagement with addicted family members is a very tricky and difficult feat to accomplish; it is important to act in ways that reduce addictive behaviors through a combination of rewarding nonaddictive behaviors and providing coercion and even punishment when necessary, but to do so in an empathic and connected manner. Of course, this task is easier said than done, and in reality it is hard to finesse. Skilled treatment providers can help families navigate these difficult waters. A core aspect of recovery from addiction is reintegration back into the rewarding social network of the family. Ultimately, Joan returned to her family unit with a highly valued status as someone who had overcome enormous difficulties and odds to recover and become a productive member of the family and her community.

Peer coercion.   Often, the most patient-accepted form of coercive intervention takes place from patient to patient. In adolescents, just as peer pressure to use drugs is one of the most potent risks for drug initiation and use syndromes, positive peer influences can be protective (Brook et al. 1990, 2002). Two examples of coercive-type peer interventions that have an evidentiary base are 12-step-oriented treatments (e.g., AA, NA; Ferri et al. 2006) and therapeutic communities (Sacks et al. 2008). In 12-step mutual-help recovery movements, immersion, indoctrination, cohesion, and coercion are combined as part of a spiritually oriented yet medical model of recovery. To be part of the group, the individual has to relinquish his or her relation with drugs of abuse, although nicotine and caffeine are often absented from this requirement. There is group pressure to do this and any deviation from an abstinence model (i.e., a goal of moderation management) is not part of the treatment philosophy. Anyone is allowed to be part of the group as long as the person has a desire for abstinence. Although Joan at first vehemently resisted 12-step-oriented treatments, they became a very useful treatment modality both during her transformative hospital stay and afterward, as a cornerstone for maintaining her sobriety.

As in 12-step recovery programs, therapeutic communities employ aspects of peer coercion to promote behavior change and recovery. The core therapeutic principles of therapeutic communities lie in the "community as method" approach where the main treatment effect comes from the members of the group rather than from formal treatment providers. In the early and traditional therapeutic community models, coercive measures were often employed in ways that were overly harsh and even sadistic. Over time, modified therapeutic communities have incorporated the special needs of particular populations including adolescents, women with children, incarcerated individuals, and those with co-occurring disorders. Several studies have demonstrated the efficacy of modified therapeutic communities for dually diagnosed patients (including those with severe and persistent mental illness) in terms of improved motivation and overall positive treatment outcomes (Sacks et al. 2008). As mentioned in the clinical case, Joan completed 18 months of treatment in a modified therapeutic community for dually diagnosed patients. She credits this as being the treatment that really allowed her recovery to take hold and become long lasting.

Contingency Management

Contingency management is a type of behavioral treatment for addictive disorders predicated on the systematic application of external incentives and disincentives to optimally modify certain behaviors (Petry 2000). Based on behavioral theory, it uses positive reinforcement to reward proabstinent behaviors (e.g., vouchers for positive treatment engagement) and uses punishment (coercion) or the threat of punishment (e.g., loss of privileges for positive urine toxicology screening results) as a means to promote negative reinforcement. It is often administered in a community milieu, combined with principles of community reinforcement approaches. In fact, therapeutic communities in addition to the above-mentioned aspect of peer coercion are essentially predicated on a contingency management plus community reinforcement approach. Contingency management is one of the best-validated psychosocial treatment modalities in addiction treatment, and research includes positive findings in several studies of patients with co-occurring disorders (Drake et al. 2008). In addition to the positive influence that therapeutic community treatment had on Joan, she responded well to contingency management, which she first encountered during her last hospital stay; she successfully utilized the token economy system in the program to gain biologically oriented rewards (i.e., food, social affiliation) and to decrease the length of her hospital stay.

Augmentation Strategies

Pharmacotherapies

Although critical by themselves as a standard component of successful addiction treatment (with U.S. Food and Drug Administration–approved treatments for alcohol, nicotine, and opioid use disorders), pharmacotherapies are necessary to augment psychosocially based motivational approaches in patients with co-occurring disorders. For one thing, they can increase motivation for use reduction or abstinence through a variety of mechanisms, such as the following (Ross and Peselow 2009):

- Treating acute withdrawal states
- Interrupting the primary reinforcing and conditioning properties of drugs of abuse (i.e., agonist substitution, receptor antagonism, aversive conditioning)
- Compensating for neuroplastic brain changes related to chronic drug abuse (i.e., interrupting conditioned memories, strengthening the saliency of natural rewards, and interrupting the stress response system).

Moreover, as noted earlier, failure to adequately treat either mental illness or an SUD (using pharmacological and/or psychosocial approaches) in patients with co-occurring disorders adversely affects illness severity and longitudinal course of illness (Hser et al. 2006). Also, there is evidence that treating dually diagnosed patients with medication for their mental illness, such as mood disorders (Khantzian et al. 2005) or ADHD (Wilens et al. 2003), is associated with a trend toward a decreased use of substances of abuse. This indirectly suggests that some part of the association between a particular mental illness and an SUD is due to the mental illness causing or exacerbating the substance abuse problem. Given the high rate of medication nonadherence in patients with co-occurring disorders, especially those with severe and persistent mental illness, it is vital to monitor treatment compliance in this patient population (DiClemente et al. 2008). Joan clearly was more motivated and stable when compliant with her pharmacological treatments for her mental illness and addictive disorder and reliably decompensated during periods of medication nonadherence.

Alternative Therapies (Creative Arts)

Despite the successes of traditional motivational techniques such as the ones mentioned above for addictive disorders, their efficacy in individuals with co-occurring disorders still has not been definitively as well established as their efficacy in individuals who are singly diagnosed. Much more research is still necessary. Also, as previously discussed, traditional motivational treatment approaches usually need some modifications to address the special needs of dually diagnosed patients—or the approaches simply do not work. Thus, there continues to be a great need for novel motivational approaches to better engage, motivate, and retain in treatment those patients with co-occurring disorders. *Integrated treatment* is the buzzword for better treatment of co-occurring disorders; however, there is a range of possibilities of what can and should be integrated. One version includes integrating complementary therapies such as acupuncture, hypnosis, music/art/movement therapies, herbs, and other alternative approaches into traditional treatments for co-occurring disorders (Ziedonis 2004). Clinical programs are increasing the use of these complementary treatments, and there is a need to better understand the potential enhancement of motivational outcomes with these approaches. One of the most studied techniques is music therapy; music therapy has been demonstrated to help enhance motivation in populations of patients with mental illness and addiction, and there is even some evidence of its efficacy in inpatient dual-diagnosis settings (Ross et al. 2008). As dramatically described in the clinical case study, it was the role of the music therapist and the creative arts therapies in general that finally helped Joan turn the corner in her last inpatient stay from being stuck in a state of anger, denial, and resistance to opening up and beginning the process of transformative change toward increased motivation and recovery.

Hope

Although it may seem evident, it is worth emphasizing the importance of hope as a motivational tool. Patients with severe co-occurring disorders often activate strong emotional reactions in clinicians and treatment system staff members, leading to common responses such as anger, therapeutic nihilism, and burnout. Compound these responses with the usual inadequate addiction education in medical school and residency training, and these patients can appear to be treatment refractory and without hope of recovery. However, the great irony with addiction treatment is that it reliably works (with outcomes similar to those for other chronic conditions such as diabetes, hypertension, and asthma) when the many evidence-based psychosocial and pharmacological treatments are actually used by clinicians and treatment systems (McLellan et al. 2000). Unfortunately, the vast majority of patients with addictive disorders and co-occurring mental illness never receive optimal treatment.

Joan had become so hopeless (a function of both her mental illness and her addiction) that she was trying to kill herself. The family was so tired of the "nightmare" that they wanted to give up as well. Their response was all the more striking given how much they loved their daughter and how she had been the "special" one growing up among their children. Unfortunately, even intact families that are well-meaning and loving can be driven to the breaking point by the addiction of a loved one; desperation and frustration can lead them to act in misguided, counterproductive, hostile, and even sadistic ways. In addition, Joan's treating psychiatrist had to deal with a treatment system that viewed Joan pejoratively as a "frequent flyer," recidivist, or treatment failure.

Hope is like oxygen to our patients and their families. We need to find a way to infuse it into any clinical scenario, no matter how seemingly or actually grim the situation or prognosis may be. This applies especially to the sickest of our patients (often those with co-occurring disorders and severe and persistent mental illness) who appear to fall into a treatment-refractory category where principles of palliative care therapy seem to apply more than standard addiction treatment. The provision of external hope in the face of a seemingly hopeless situation can provide the scaffold for patients and their families to hang in there while the internal seeds of hope, motivation, and self-efficacy can be planted and have time to germinate and mature.

Suggestions for Teaching and Supervision

Several key components of supervisory guidance are mentioned here as a way to summarize and provide an algorithm for motivational treatment engagement in individuals with co-occurring disorders.

1. Start with noncoercive, intrinsically oriented approaches:
   - Respect patient autonomy.
   - Optimally foster alliance and rapport building by not engaging in early antagonism.
   - Attempt to foster maximal patient utilization of internal resources to promote greater self-efficacy and self-regulation and ultimately greater ownership of change and recovery.
   - Use Motivational Interviewing as the optimal treatment paradigm.

2. Have a low threshold to introducing more coercive interventions early in treatment:
   - This is especially important in those individuals with greater cognitive impairment and less autonomy or volitional capacity—including those with severe mental and addictive disorders.
   - Start with the least coercive approaches (e.g., SBIRT—advice to change and referral for treatment with follow-up).
   - Whenever possible, apply modified coercion, for example:
     a. Contingency management—one of the best validated psychosocial treatment modalities in addiction treatment—has coercive aspects combined with positive reinforcement and often community reinforcement approaches.
     b. The criminal justice system—drug courts (a combination of positive reinforcement + negative reinforcement + rapport with a sympathetic and fair judge and a therapeutic system of care).
   - Reserve the most coercive interventions for the most severe cases involving high-risk liability (e.g., involuntary hospitalization for acute danger to self or others, or for psychotic states).
   - Strongly consider peer-led motivational treatments with modified or attenuated forms of coercion, for example:
     a. 12-step, mutual-help recovery programs.
     b. Modified therapeutic communities.

3. Integrate treatment on multiple levels:
   - Systems of care—rather than parallel or serial paradigms.
   - Breadth of care—psychiatric, addiction, and medical.
   - Colocation of care—provide all care in one setting.
   - Combination (pharmacotherapy + psychosocial) evidentiary treatments—for mental illness, addiction, and medical illness.
   - Use of spiritually oriented treatments (i.e., 12-step programs)—not typically combined with biomedical models, especially in hospital-based treatment programs.

- Use of complementary and alternative treatments—especially creative arts therapies, with music and art therapies having some evidence base for an effect.

4. Individualization of motivational treatment approaches—use what works:
   - Combine intrinsically oriented approaches with extrinsically oriented approaches.
   - If intrinsically oriented treatments fail at first, come back to them after coercive ones have provided enough stability to allow the optimal leveraging of inner resources to increase motivation for change.
   - Be creative—use novel approaches.
5. Hang in there: provide and maintain hope for patients, families, and the treatment system.

Movie: *Rachel Getting Married*

In *Rachel Getting Married* (2008) director Jonathan Demme introduces us to a world of relentless interpersonal destruction and reconstitution in the context of a family reunion. Kym, the identified family problem, gets a pass from an inpatient addiction rehabilitation center to attend the wedding of her sister Rachel, a trained psychotherapist. The film won top honors at the 2009 Prism Awards, a collaboration with the Substance Abuse and Mental Health Services Administration, which honors entertainment that realistically portrays substance abuse and addiction, as well as mental health issues. This film accurately depicts the intersection of addiction and borderline personality disorder.

The scenes of conflict between the two sisters provide exquisite material for discussing borderline insecure attachment and chemical attachment as coexisting ways of characterizing the dually diagnosed patient. Furthermore, as Rachel and Kym keep loving and hating each other, the movie postulates that individual memories of historical events can operate as either foundations for construction or as wrecking balls for demolition of interpersonal relationships—or both.

Training supervisors also may use the film to explore the role of the psychotherapist in addressing problems in the clinician's own personal life, as reflected in Rachel's dilemmas. To what extent are we allowed to attempt to use our training during our own family disputes, such as those of Kym and Rachel? Even more fundamentally, how well does psychotherapy translate outside the office?

Rachel Getting Married is not only a brilliant study of the interface of addiction and personality disturbance, it is also a provocative treatise on the opportunities and limitations of psychotherapeutic skills when used in the therapist's own everyday life.

Key Clinical Points

- Compared with patients with only a mental illness or an SUD, those with co-occurring disorders across a broad spectrum of diagnostic types have a greater severity of illness and a worse longitudinal course of illness; thus, they pose a heightened problem with treatment engagement, motivation for change, sustained change, and overall treatment outcome.

- Regarding motivation and change in patients with co-occurring disorders, start with noncoercive, intrinsically oriented approaches but have a low threshold for introducing more coercive interventions early in treatment, especially in patients with cognitive impairment and deficiencies in volitional capacity who engage in high-risk behaviors.

- When using coercive approaches, start with the least invasive methods modified to include elements of positive reinforcement, such as contingency management, drug courts, and peer-led motivational treatments.

- If intrinsically oriented treatments fail at first, attempt to reapply these techniques after coercive interventions have provided enough stability to allow the optimal leveraging of a patient's inner resources to increase motivation for change.

- Provide and maintain hope for patients, families, and treatment system staff as a powerful motivational tool often overlooked and underutilized.

Multiple-Choice Questions

For the correct answers to these questions, including explanations of answers, please see the Answer Guide at the end of this book.

1. What percentage of patients in either mental health or addiction treatment settings has a co-occurring disorder?

   A. 10%.
   B. 25%.
   C. 50%.
   D. 90%.

2. Regarding prognosis and longitudinal outcome, in comparison with patients with only a mental illness or an SUD, those with co-occurring disorders:

   A. Have a more favorable course of illness.
   B. Have an approximately equal course of illness.
   C. Have a less favorable course of illness only in terms of poorer treatment engagement.
   D. Have a less favorable course of illness in multiple domains of psychosocial functioning.

3. Motivational Interviewing is a:

   A. Noncoercive, intrinsically oriented treatment.
   B. Coercive, intrinsically oriented treatment.
   C. Coercive, extrinsically oriented treatment.
   D. Noncoercive, extrinsically oriented treatment.

4. Motivation to change within the AA program can best be characterized by:

   A. Peer coercive approaches.
   B. Group cohesion.
   C. Spiritually oriented approaches such as connection to a "higher power."
   D. All of the above.

5. Which of the following is *not* associated with improved treatment outcomes in patients with co-occurring disorders?

   A. Employment.
   B. Greater length of time in treatment.
   C. Participation in 12-step mutual-help programs.
   D. A serial system of care model.

References

Bellack AS, DiClemente CC: Treating substance abuse among patients with schizophrenia. Psychiatr Serv 50:75–80, 1999

Brodie DA, Inoue A, Shaw DG: Motivational interviewing to change quality of life for people with chronic heart failure: a randomised controlled trial. Int J Nurs Stud 45:489–500, 2008

Brook JS, Brook DW, Gordon AS, et al: The psychosocial etiology of adolescent drug use: a family interactional approach. Genet Soc Gen Psychol Monogr 116:111–267, 1990

Brook DW, Brook JS, Rosen Z, et al: Correlates of marijuana use in Colombian adolescents: a focus on the impact of the ecological/cultural domain. J Adolesc Health 31:286–298, 2002

DiClemente CC, Nidecker M, Bellack AS: Motivation and the stages of change among individuals with severe mental illness and substance abuse disorders. J Subst Abuse Treat 34:25–35, 2008

Drake RE, Mueser KT, Brunette MF, et al: A review of treatments for people with severe mental illnesses and co-occurring substance use disorders. Psychiatr Rehabil J 27:360–374, 2004

Drake RE, O'Neal EL, Wallach MA: A systematic review of psychosocial research on psychosocial interventions for people with co-occurring severe mental and substance use disorders. J Subst Abuse Treat 34:123–138, 2008

Ferri M, Amato L, Davoli M: Alcoholics Anonymous and other 12-step programmes for alcohol dependence. Cochrane Database Syst Rev 3:CD005032, 2006

Galanter M: Network therapy for substance abuse: a clinical trial. Psychotherapy 30:251–258, 1993

Galanter M, Dermatis H, Keller D, et al: Network therapy for cocaine abuse: use of family and peer supports. Am J Addict 11:161–166, 2002

Graham AW, Fleming MF: Brief interventions, in Principles of Addiction Medicine, 3rd Edition. Edited by Graham AW, Schultz TK, Mayo-Smith MF, et al. Chevy Chase, MD, American Society of Addiction Medicine, 2003, pp 361–372

Gregoire TK, Burke AC: The relationship of legal coercion to readiness to change among adults with alcohol and other drug problems. J Subst Abuse Treat 26:337–343, 2004

Hendrickson EL: Designing, Implementing, and Managing Treatment Services for Individuals with Co-Occurring Mental Health and Substance Use Disorders: Blueprints for Action. Binghamton, NY, Haworth Press, 2006

Hser YI, Grella C, Evans E, et al: Utilization and outcomes of mental health services among patients in drug treatment. J Addict Dis 25:73–85, 2006

Johnson VE: Intervention: How to Help Someone Who Doesn't Want Help. Center City, MN, Hazelden Foundation, 1998

Kallert TW: Coercion in psychiatry. Curr Opin Psychiatry 21:485–489, 2008

Kessler RC, Nelson CB, McGonagle KA, et al: The epidemiology of co-occurring addictive and mental disorders: implications for prevention and service utilization. Am J Orthopsychiatry 66:17–31, 1996

Khantzian EJ, Dodes L, Brehm N: Psychodynamics, in Substance Abuse: A Comprehensive Textbook, 4th Edition. Edited by Lowinson JH, Ruiz P, Millman RB, et al. Philadelphia, PA, Lippincott Williams & Wilkins, 2005, pp 97–107

Martino S, Carroll K, Kostas D, et al: Dual diagnosis motivational interviewing: a modification of motivational interviewing for substance-abusing patients with psychotic disorders. J Subst Abuse Treat 23:297–308, 2002

McLellan AT, McKay JR: Components of successful addiction treatment, in Principles of Addiction Medicine, 3rd Edition. Edited by Graham AW, Schultz TK, Mayo-Smith MF, et al. Chevy Chase, MD, American Society of Addiction Medicine, 2003, pp 429–442

McLellan AT, Lewis DC, O'Brien CP, et al: Drug dependence, a chronic medical illness: implications for treatment, insurance, and outcomes evaluation. JAMA 284:1689–1695, 2000

Meyers RJ, Smith JE: Getting off the fence: procedures to engage treatment-resistant drinkers. J Subst Abuse Treat 14:467–472, 1997

Miller WR, Meyers RJ, Tonigan JS: Engaging the unmotivated in treatment for alcohol problems: a comparison of three strategies for intervention through family members. J Consult Clin Psychol 67:688–697, 1999

Mueser KT, Drake RE, Wallach MA: Dual diagnosis: a review of etiological theories. Addict Behav 23:717–734, 1998

Petry NM: A comprehensive guide to the application of contingency management procedures in clinical settings. Drug Alcohol Depend 58:9–25, 2000

Ross S: The mentally ill substance abuser, in Textbook of Substance Abuse Treatment, 4th Edition. Edited by Galanter M, Kleber M. Washington, DC, American Psychiatric Publishing, 2008, pp 537–554

Ross S, Peselow E: The neurobiology of addictive disorders. Clin Neuropharmacol 32:269–276, 2009

Ross S, Cidambi I, Dermatis H, et al: Music therapy: a novel motivational approach for dually diagnosed patients. J Addictive Dis 27:41–53, 2008

Sacks S, Banks S, McKendrick K, et al: Modified therapeutic community for co-occurring disorders: a summary of four studies. J Subst Abuse Treat 34:112–122, 2008

Substance Abuse and Mental Health Services Administration: Results From the 2003 National Survey on Drug Use and Health: National Findings (DHHS Publ No [SMA] 04–3964, NSDUH Series H-25). Rockville, MD, U.S. Department of Health and Human Services, 2004

Velicer WF, Fava JL, Prochaska JO, et al: Distribution of smokers by stage in three representative samples. Prev Med 24:401–411, 1995

Wilens TE, Faraone SV, Biederman J, et al: Does stimulant therapy of attention-deficit/hyperactivity disorder beget later substance abuse?: a meta-analytic review of the literature. Pediatrics 111:179–185, 2003

Ziedonis DM: Integrated treatment of co-occurring mental illness and addiction: clinical intervention, program, and system perspectives. CNS Spectr 9:894–904, 2004

CHAPTER 10

Integrating Addiction Pharmacotherapy and Motivational Work

Ileana Benga, M.D.

Modern psychiatry aims to conceptualize and treat patients following the biopsychosocial model, which translates into artfully combining psychopharmacology and psychotherapy. In many instances, research has shown that combining the two modalities of treatment may be more efficient than using either modality by itself, yet specific data to assess how different types of psychotherapy interact with specific medications are still lacking (Gabbard 2006). Hollon and Fawcett (2007) theorized that combining psychopharmacology with psychotherapy might be beneficial in four ways: increasing the *probability*, the *magnitude*, the *breadth of the response,* and the *acceptability* of treatment. The question remains how to combine these approaches for an optimal response.

How medication affects a specific psychotherapeutic process and how psychotherapy influences the specific relation that a patient has with the medication treatment may be looked at differently for different types of psychotherapy. For example, in *psychoanalysis,* medication may help the patient absorb the analytic work and the medication itself may become personalized, acting as a new object within the psychoanalytic framework, enriching the treatment with new transference paradigms to explore (Tutter 2006). A similar process in terms of reciprocity has been described for Cognitive-Behavioral Therapy by Wright

(2004): medication may affect the cognitive component by increasing concentration, while behavioral modification resulting from therapy may affect medication adherence. Adding medication with Dialectical Behavioral Therapy could decrease intense affect states and impulsivity (e.g., characteristic to borderline personality disorder), while the therapy may enhance compliance with medication. Even though different forms of psychotherapy with different theoretical foundations integrate medication in their own particular ways, there seems to be universal agreement that once combined, medication and psychotherapy influence one another and generate a reciprocal relationship central to the psychiatrist's work.

In Motivational Interviewing, the relationship between medication and psychotherapeutic work is especially strong. Having been widely researched, Motivational Interviewing has already been consecrated as a tool in itself for medication adherence in various conditions from diabetes to HIV infection. The core principle of Motivational Interviewing—increasing the motivation to change—facilitates the behavior change necessary for people to include the act of taking a pill, sometimes several times, in their daily routine. Moreover, DiClemente (2007) has conceptualized that different medications used to treat addictive disorders, through specific mechanisms of action, may be used as tools to move patients from a specific stage of change to the next. In this chapter, I use the context of a clinical case to open the discussion of this interdependent relationship between Motivational Interviewing and medication in the treatment of patients with substance use disorders.

Clinical Case

I first met Robert in the emergency room where I was called to evaluate him for possible admission for inpatient alcohol detoxification. I found him sitting motionless at the edge of his bed, hunched and looking down, with his hands clenched on his lap. Without seeing his eyes, I thought he was much older than the age I had learned from the referring team: "white male, in his 40s, divorced, without significant past psychiatric history other than a strong alcohol problem." Very politely, he extended his hand to greet me and he appeared embarrassed by its tremor. His breath still smelled of alcohol. Fully alert and oriented, in mild alcohol withdrawal, Robert answered my questions without any hesitation.

He was in the emergency room because his father had brought him in. He had been going through cycles—he would use alcohol, daily, for months at a time, still able to keep a job considerably below his qualifications and to care for his two minor daughters living together in a rented apartment; he then would abruptly decide that he could not deal with "[his] boring life" anymore; the "bad boy" would come out, and he would abandon all responsibilities and go away. Leaving his daughters in their grandparents' care, he would rent or buy an old car, which would become his house, and start bingeing on alcohol and sex. The cycle would end when family members or police found him and brought him to an emergency room, usually within 2 weeks. This time the cycle had been ended by his worried father—an alcoholic himself—who found him in the street "totally out of it."

Robert did not think that his alcohol use was a problem: "I can stop if I want to, but I don't want that boring life that my brothers are living." The two brothers were very accomplished professionals with apparently successful marriages. Although a talented writer, possessing an Ivy League degree in literature, Robert was no longer able to write and was struggling to function as a single father for his daughters. He acknowledged that his family was worried about his behavior. I asked what worried him regarding his current situation, trying to elicit some change talk. The only painful and worrisome thing that he could think of was the relationship with his daughters. Yet the excitement of "leaving everything behind" when running away still overshadowed the pain.

Robert was very ambivalent about another detoxification treatment. He had completed three detoxifications in the past, and after one of them, he even went for outpatient treatment to a substance abuse clinic for "a couple of weeks." There he was prescribed disulfiram, which he decided not to take, remarking, "What can a medication do, that I can't?" Using open-ended questions, I tried to learn as much as possible about his past experience with treatment. I also tried to present him with treatment options, emphasizing his ability to control the choice of treatment, whether using medication or psychotherapy. He agreed that the first step should be another detoxification, and we talked about its pros and cons. Still somewhat ambivalent, he decided to start his fourth detoxification, and I was to follow up with him the next day.

The following morning I learned that he had left the hospital; I was disappointed at the thought that the previous day's meeting had not helped. Then 2 weeks later, I received another call; this time it was not from the emergency room but from the inpatient unit, where Robert was finishing up his alcohol detoxification treatment. Surprised, I found out that he identified me as his outpatient treater, even though we had had merely one meeting, and that he was interested in outpatient follow-up care. I scheduled an appointment—he was interested to talk about treatment options and mentioned that he might even consider "some medication" to help him "at the beginning." Naturally, I was curious to find out what had happened 2 weeks prior when he decided to leave the hospital and then what made him change his mind regarding outpatient treatment, which he never valued before. His reply was that "I wasn't ready yet for the treatment, I was so angry that my father had brought me in. What pushed me to seek treatment this time, for the first time by myself, was the realization that my daughters were really harmed by my behavior. You asked me if I saw any disadvantage with what I was doing, and I told you that I was enjoying that type of life and that no one was hurt. But my daughters must have been tortured—they were leaving hundreds of messages on my cell phone every time I disappeared; I had to throw away my phone to not see that." Robert also told me that he felt comfortable with me, that I seemed to understand how difficult his position was, and that he appreciated that I did not seem to have a strong opinion about what he should do. Instead, I just presented him with alternatives that he felt he could choose from. He also had come to the realization that it was very hard for him to control his alcohol use and that he needed help. Not having a fulfilling professional and family life triggered his alcohol use, which then gave him the "courage" to run away and adopt extreme behavior. He thought that a starting point would be treatment of his alcohol problem, and he was eager to find out more about psychopharmacological options.

We spoke in detail about the pros and cons of the medications available for the treatment of alcohol dependence, and he chose disulfiram. His felt that disulfiram would help him "buy some time" when his impulses were difficult to control. He also planned to attend Alcoholics Anonymous (AA) meetings.

Taking disulfiram and coming to see me weekly, Robert did well for almost 1 month. He started to successfully reconnect with his family and with his AA sponsor, and everything seemed to be moving well; however, he then missed an appointment. Subsequently his mother (whom I had his consent to talk to) called me, crying, telling me that it had happened again—that he had disappeared after doing so well.

Another week passed, and Robert came to see me. He was angry about the disulfiram. He had stopped taking it, trying to find out whether he could trust himself enough to abstain from alcohol without it. But very soon he became overwhelmed with cravings and had "a drink or two." He isolated himself for a week, disillusioned with the treatment, with mixed feelings of shame and anger. However, he did not "take off" this time—instead he decided to come and tell me that the treatment was not working. He felt that disulfiram misled him and "took away his power."

We again went over the different options, analyzing the pros and cons of each. This time, naltrexone appeared appealing because of its known effect on cravings. He also decided between the intramuscular and tablet options and felt that the intramuscular form could give him the false impression that he would be fine for 1 month. Taking the tablet would be a "daily reminder that I'm doing something for my treatment; I need this control."

Since then, Robert's treatment has made progress. He stopped taking naltrexone several times to test how he was doing without it, and he had several slips. But he stayed engaged in treatment and managed to talk about his ambivalence. He gradually felt more in control, and after 6 months, he rented an apartment and moved in with his daughters, able to maintain a teaching job in the daytime and write poetry in the evening.

Discussion of the Clinical Case

Before discussing the specifics of Robert's case, I would like to emphasize the importance of the tone of the initial interview and the overall attitude of the interviewer. A lot of work is virtually done even before meeting the patient. It is important for the interviewer to be mindful about the importance of this first meeting—which may open the possibility of a special, durable relationship.

The double role of psychopharmacologist and psychotherapist could be difficult to manage. Prescribing medication traditionally implies assuming the role of an expert and having strong opinions about what a patient needs and why a patient needs a specific medication. This role may be in conflict with the general Motivational Interviewing philosophy, which holds that the patient is the only expert, the one who knows better than anyone else his or her specific situation and goals. If the interviewer is conflicted about his or her role, that will become obvious to the patient before any verbal communication, through the first eye contact or gesture. The education and experience that a psychiatrist has with different medications remains important and valuable if it is used as a tool and not as a goal per se; note that there are two ways to give direct advice on using medication that are consistent with Motivational Interviewing: 1) when asked for it, and 2) after asking permission to give it.

Opening the possibility of partnership, where the autonomy of the patient is maintained and where the patient has the ultimate control over treatment, keeps the psychiatrist away from an undesirable power struggle. To be *ready, willing,* and *able* should not solely be the attributes of the patient engaged in a changing process. The psychiatrist also should be *able* to provide knowledgeable advice and *willing* to learn from the patient's particular experience, while at the same time being *ready* to offer support when necessary, maintaining an overall genuine, empathic, and optimistic tone. Now that the general attitude and first expectations are established, we are ready to enter the room and meet Robert.

First Meeting: Learning and Planting the Seeds for the Future

Besides establishing a diagnosis or a differential diagnosis, an important part of the initial assessment is to be attuned to the patient's stage of change. In the process of Motivational Interviewing, the treater uses open-ended questions, reflects, affirms, summarizes, and elicits change talk whenever the possibility arises. Chances are that the patient would not move from one stage of change to another during that first meeting, but the therapist in collaboration with the patient can plant the seeds through change talk.

Another important part of the initial assessment is learning about the patient's experience: what previous treatments were or were not helpful, the reasons for medication nonadherence if any, and the patient's theory about why previous treatments worked or did not work. All this information is elicited with a nonjudgmental and empathic attitude.

In our case, Robert was stuck, repeating the same cycle of drinking, getting demoralized, isolating himself from his family, ruining his professional life, and engaging impulsively in risky behaviors. He did not see alcohol as playing an important role; rather, he blamed his "boring life" and minimized the impact of his behavior; he did not seem to have any desire to change his situation—he was there because of his father; he was in the *precontemplation* stage.

We might wonder how a therapist can help Robert when he was not even interested in starting treatment. One element was providing information about available treatment options that could help him if and when *he* decided to access them. I gave Robert an informative description of the medication options while staying sensitive to his reactions to it, explaining from my experience what medications helped patients in similar circumstances. Another element was allowing Robert to become more aware of his behavior. Finally, using change talk, Robert acknowledged the strained relationship with his children to be a major disadvantage of his behavior.

All these steps were meant to engage him in treatment and to plant the seeds for possible change later, when ready. The results of that first meeting were not obvious at all at the time, and Robert seemed to have left treatment unwilling and not yet ready for change. But the seeds for change were there.

Second and Following Meetings: Consolidating the Work

With the second visit, we were back to reassessing what stage of change Robert was in. Substantial change had taken place since the first meeting; although the patient seemed to be repeating the same cycle, he was in a different place in terms of his motivation for change.

Understanding what was accomplished in the first meeting and how Robert got "unstuck" became the foundation for further treatment. Robert had become more aware of his life predicament and had started to connect the dots between drinking and his out-of-control episodes. From our first meeting, he knew that help was available, including medication treatment.

Robert had finalized detoxification at his initiative and was trying to become engaged in outpatient treatment. This significant, initial clinical step forward is often unrecognized by treaters. Affirming and validating Robert for this accomplishment were important; they provided a way to build up his self-efficacy, a critical piece in the process of change. Robert was eager to talk about his problems and willing to evaluate the pros and cons of his behaviors. All this suggested that he had moved to the *contemplation* stage.

So how do we use medication in this stage in favor of treatment and what pitfalls should we pay attention to?

Medication becomes an instrument that can be used in different ways depending on its specific profile. In Robert's case, we first talked about the pros and cons of medications approved by the U.S. Food and Drug Administration (FDA) for the treatment of alcoholism: disulfiram, acamprosate, and intramuscular and tablet naltrexone. He decided to try disulfiram because he was concerned about not trusting his impulses. The cons he initially expressed were relying too much on the medication's effect, working less in treatment, and eventually decreasing his feelings of self-efficacy. Despite his ambivalence, he also wanted to clarify what stood in the way when he was previously offered disulfiram: he had decided not to take it earlier because he felt that it would limit his control. It is very important for both treater and patient to embark on this process of expecting ambivalence and clarifying it; undiscussed ambivalence undermines the therapeutic process.

Once a treatment plan was formulated, Robert found himself in the *preparation* stage of change, and with medication support, his move toward *action* seemed effortless. Disulfiram was now an ally and was to be evaluated in every session in terms of barriers to treatment adherence. Robert was now very concerned with side effects; moreover, at some point he perceived disulfiram as undermining his autonomy and wanted to test his capacity to stay sober without it. His cravings where building up and he relapsed. The quality of relapse was different, however; he did not wait this time to "bottom down," and he himself initiated the reconnection with treatment before becoming physiologically dependent on alcohol.

Moving from one stage to another may not always be a linear process. Before taking a step forward, we often need to deal with a step backward. Recycling—reentering the cycle of the stages of change—is to be expected and can be used as a valuable source of learning. When Robert returned after his slip, he was back to the preparation stage, ready to make a new plan. What worked one time might not work the second time around; disulfiram appeared not to be an option anymore because it had become a target of his anger, also challenging his self-efficacy.

Robert and I again discussed the psychopharmacological options of treatment, preserving his autonomy to make an informed decision. In this second preparation stage, he wanted to try a medication with a different profile, one that would diminish his cravings while allowing him the feeling of having more control over his decision to drink. The choice of naltrexone appealed to him, especially given his genetic predisposition with the positive family history of alcohol dependence.

Since then, as mentioned in the case presentation, Robert has adhered to his treatment for the most part, while making significant progress in his personal life.

Suggestions for Treatment

How medication affects the process of change—and how the process of change affects the rapport of patients with their medication—is a very subtle dance where the leader and the follower exchange places.

In conceptualizing treatment suggestions, we may look at the relationship between Motivational Interviewing and psychopharmacological treatment from several angles, each discussed in more detail below:

- Analyzing the pros and cons of using specific medications in different stages of change
- Evaluating the relationship of medication in general with the four principles of Motivational Interviewing of expressing empathy, developing discrepancy, rolling with resistance, and supporting self-efficacy
- Identifying traps to be avoided by the treater when combining the two treatments
- Summarizing the dynamic of this process in a three-dimensional model.

Analyzing Pros and Cons of Using Specific Medications in Different Stages of Change

DiClemente (2007) examined how medication can facilitate the process of change and went over some specific pros and cons of using medication to treat alcohol dependence in patients in the different stages of change, as summarized below.

In *precontemplation,* a general discussion of different treatment options can help an as-yet-uncommitted patient learn about different available forms of help, potentially moving him or her to the contemplation stage. It is also helpful for the treater, even at this stage, to begin understanding the patient's beliefs and values regarding medication use.

Contemplation is the stage of analyzing the pros and cons of behavior change, which can be integrated with the pros and cons of different medications. For example, in the treatment of alcohol dependence, *disulfiram* may buy time—a pro for some patients; however, the cons of disulfiram may include its side effects (such as increased risk of peripheral neuropathy, myocardial infarction, hepatitis, hepatic failure, and psychosis) and a general feeling of lack of control and autonomy (see the earlier section "Discussion of the Clinical Case"). *Acamprosate* is believed to prevent feelings of discomfort associated with abstinence from alcohol, which may lead to spending less time thinking about drinking. This may have pros and cons in that those feelings of discomfort may prevent change in some patients, whereas in others they may be a strong motivator for change. *Naltrexone*, with its different formulations (intramuscular injection or tablet) also may come with different pros and cons. Pros include good results for patients with a family history of alcoholism and increased control over the decision to drink by decreasing cravings, as in Robert's case. However, naltrexone is not indicated for patients with severe kidney or liver damage or for patients on opioid drugs because of its blocking effects. For the intramuscular form of naltrexone, another con (also discussed in Robert's case) could be the feeling of loss of daily control over treatment because of its monthly administration.

The same concept may be applied for any addiction for which there is available pharmacological treatment. For opiates and nicotine, there may be different nuances on how to work with an agonist, a partial agonist, or—in the case of opiates—with an antagonist. Each of these choices may have a distinct impact on the patient's feelings of self-efficacy and should be considered in light of the patient's values and goals for treatment. Offering medications with very different mechanisms of action, even opposing ones, could take the treatment in very different directions and may affect the treater's position, committing him or her to a particular course of action. This approach could jeopardize the patient's autonomy, the ability to clarify ambivalence, and the patient's values in treatment. The treater's role is to engage in a dialogue with the patient concerning the different choices available, so that ultimately the patient can make a meaningful choice.

Once the pros and cons of medication are discussed and the plan made, and while the patient moves from the *preparation* to *action* and then *maintenance* stages, it is valuable to remember that the process of change is a dynamic one—and that what is a pro today may become a con tomorrow.

When analyzing the role of medication in *relapse*, it is useful for the clinician to make the distinction between disappointment with a medication and disappointment with treatment. A treater attached to a certain medication may prevent the patient from expressing his or her disappointment. Relapse often is a great source of learning and not an impossible roadblock.

Medication and the Four General Principles of Motivational Interviewing

The four principles of Motivational Interviewing can be applied when introducing medication: expressing empathy, developing discrepancy, rolling with resistance, and supporting self-efficacy. First, in order to express empathy, the treater understands and accepts that ambivalence is natural in the process, including ambivalence about introducing a new substance into the body. Second, when the treater is engaged in developing discrepancies between current behavior and the patient's goals, it is important to make the distinction between the goal of medication adherence and the more general goal regarding addictive behavior: when Motivational Interviewing is used for medication adherence, the goal is the acceptance of medication in treatment; but when Motivational

Interviewing and medication are combined, medication is just a means to achieve the ultimate goal. Third, it is important to roll with resistance when it is encountered. Resistance to take a medication also should be differentiated from resistance to change an addictive behavior. Sometimes it is not easy to make this distinction because one type of resistance can manifest as the other; only active listening, clarification, and allowing expression of ambivalence can help distinguish between the two. Lastly, as we have seen in Robert's case, taking a medication can support self-efficacy. Whenever possible, it is valuable to affirm medication adherence in order to enhance self-efficacy.

Traps to Avoid

There are several known traps for the therapist to avoid when using Motivational Interviewing; when medication is introduced into the equation, the medication itself may play a role in this unwanted pattern:

- **The expert trap:** The treater becoming very active and enthusiastic in prescribing a specific medication places the patient in a more passive role ("Whatever you say, doc"), which is incongruent with Motivational Interviewing's philosophy.
- **The blaming trap:** Sometimes the patient may feel a general need to place blame when something does not work. This can become of concern if medication becomes the target, especially after a relapse. Reflecting and reframing the patient's concerns may help in this situation.
- **The taking sides trap:** The treater may defend the prescribed medication when the patient is ambivalent about taking it. This can make the patient defend the other side of the conflict, creating grounds for a power struggle.

Three-Dimensional Model

Flexibility in treatment is helpful for integrating three components: the particularities of the stage of change, the specific medication profile (pros and cons), and the psychological profile of the patient (i.e., the patient's readiness, willingness, and ability to change vis-à-vis his or her goals and values).

If we consider the three components to be three spatial axes (Figure 10–1), a position change in one axis requires reassessment of the position on the other two. For example, if a patient moves from precontemplation to the contemplation stage, the therapist should reassess the medication's pros and cons and the patient's psychological strengths and weaknesses in relation to the goal of the new stage.

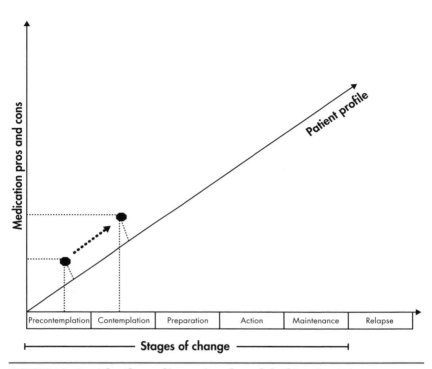

FIGURE 10–1. The three-dimensional model of treatment.

Suggestions for Teaching and Supervision

An issue common in supervision is dealing with patients' poor medication adherence. As noted earlier, ambivalence is natural in the process of change, and it may involve the patient's relationship with medication. A patient's ambivalence does not mean that treatment has been unsuccessful, but not allowing the patient to express ambivalence may make treatment unsuccessful. Therefore, nonadherence to medication treatment should prompt more exploration of ambivalence in therapy, and if necessary, the renegotiation of treatment goals—even if that means changing medication or stopping it altogether.

The supervisee (therapist) may need support when dealing with feelings of helplessness and failure once a patient has relapsed or moved to an earlier stage of change. The role of the supervisor is to emphasize that substance abuse treatment is not necessarily a linear process and that relapse is actually to be expected independently of the treater's competence. Any perceived step backward may become a precious step forward if relapse is used as a source of learning and not viewed as failure.

Another problem arises when the supervisee feels stuck between giving either insufficient input or too much direction in terms of the psychopharmacological treatment. This is a fragile balance to maintain. When there is a feeling of too much direction or overprescription, therapists should renegotiate their own agenda but at the same time clearly express clearly their concerns (Miller and Rollnick 2002).

In general, the importance of the therapist's relationship with the patient cannot be overemphasized in supervision. Medication is just an instrument and not a goal per se; more important than finding the right medication is maintaining the therapeutic relationship and preserving the flexibility of the therapeutic process.

Movie: *28 Days*

Gwen Cummings, an aspiring young writer who is drug and alcohol dependent, enters a rehabilitation facility to avoid the legal consequences of a drunk-driving car accident. The 2000 movie *28 Days* depicts her experience during the 28 days of treatment. The first meeting with her counselor finds her in the precontemplation stage, plainly uninterested in treatment: Gwen says, "I don't belong here"; "I know I drink a lot. I am a writer and that's what we do, we drink"; and "I can control myself. If I wanted to, I could."

But in an attempt to get more drugs to avoid withdrawal, she falls from her window and breaks her leg. Now physically impaired and threatened with jail for noncompliance, she realizes the severity of her condition, saying, "This is not a way to live, it's a way to die"—and she moves toward contemplation.

I chose this movie because it shows the critical transition from precontemplation to contemplation, and because Gwen has many similarities with Robert: both have a positive family history (Gwen's mother was alcoholic); both have siblings "living a boring, straight life"; and both move from precontemplation after they hit bottom with a strong injury to their self-esteem.

There is not much use of medication at the rehabilitation center in this movie, but there is a point in the patient's treatment when she asks her counselor for more help: "Give me a pill, a shot, a lobotomy, anything"—interpreted by the counselor as a need for instant gratification. We can use this movie as a teaching tool and invite speculation about what and how medication could be offered based on the patient's profile—a stubborn, egocentric, somewhat elitist female—and how to work with her from that point on.

Key Clinical Points

- Motivational Interviewing and psychopharmacology have a reciprocal relationship: psychotherapy influences medication adherence and the medication may influence progress in psychotherapy.

- Medication should be an instrument in treatment and not a goal per se.

- Psychopharmacological treatment need not jeopardize the autonomy of the patient. The patient must be able to choose and the treater should keep the patient informed about different possibilities so that an educated choice can be made.

- Different stages of change and different particularities of patient profiles require flexibility in analyzing pros and cons of medication. When combining Motivational Interviewing and psychopharmacology, the treater and patient embark on a dynamic process that requires reassessment and repositioning.

Multiple-Choice Questions

For the correct answers to these questions, including explanations of answers, please see the Answer Guide at the end of this book.

1. Which of the following statements is true, regarding when a patient engaged in Motivational Interviewing psychotherapy should be presented with the option of psychopharmacological treatment?

    A. The patient needs to be ready for change first.
    B. The patient needs to be in the preparation stage to be able to use the information about medication.
    C. The patient needs to be at least in the contemplation stage.
    D. The patient can be in any stage of change.

2. Which statement best describes the relationship between Motivational Interviewing and psychopharmacological treatment?

    A. Motivational Interviewing may be used to improve medication adherence.
    B. Medication may facilitate transition from one stage of change to the next.
    C. Both A and B are true.
    D. Neither A nor B are true.

3. Which statement is true about the relationship between medication and the Motivational Interviewing principle of supporting self-efficacy?

A. Medication may increase self-efficacy.
B. Medication may decrease self-efficacy.
C. Medication may decrease or increase self-efficacy depending on the circumstances.
D. Medication rarely affects self-efficacy.

4. Which statement is false about the following FDA-approved medications for the treatment of alcohol dependence?

A. Disulfiram can be helpful when administered to patients who want to remain in a state of enforced sobriety.
B. Naltrexone may be helpful for those with a strong family history of substance abuse.
C. Acamprosate is believed to increase feelings of discomfort associated with abstinence from alcohol.
D. Naltrexone treatment can be started when a patient is not abstinent.

5. Which of the following is false regarding patients' ambivalence?

A. Ambivalence is normal in the process of change, and it is helpful for treaters to accept it.
B. In the context of medication use, ambivalence is a sign of treatment failure.
C. A patient ready, willing, and able to change may still remain ambivalent.
D. No stage of change can be expected to be ambivalence free.

References

DiClemente CC: Alcohol dependence treatment: facilitating the process of change with medications. Addiction Professional Jan–Feb 2007

Gabbard GO: The rationale for combining medication and psychotherapy. Psychiatr Ann 35:315–319, 2006

Hollon SB, Fawcett J: Combined medication and psychotherapy, in Gabbard's Treatments of Psychiatric Disorders, 4th Edition. Edited by Gabbard GO. Washington, DC, American Psychiatric Publishing, 2007, pp 439–448

Miller WR, Rollnick S: Phase 2: strengthening commitment to change, in Motivational Interviewing: Preparing People for Change, 2nd Edition. New York, Guilford, 2002, pp 126–140

Tutter A: Medication as object. J Am Psychoanal Assoc 54:781–804, 2006

Wright JH: Integrating cognitive-behavioral therapy and pharmacotherapy, in Contemporary Cognitive Therapy: Theory, Research and Practice. Edited by Leahy RL. New York, Guilford, 2004, pp 341–366

Integrating Screening, Brief Intervention, and Referral to Treatment With Motivational Work

Christopher Cutter, Ph.D.
David A. Fiellin, M.D.

Substance use disorders are commonly encountered in nonspecialty settings and most patients with substance use problems do not present to a specialist. The role of the nonspecialist can be envisioned as a catalyst to increase the rate at which those who are at risk or have harmful substance use conditions are treated or moved from nonspecialty to specialty care. The process of identifying patients with a need for intervention or referral to treatment is often referred to as Screening, Brief Intervention, and Referral to Treatment (SBIRT). SBIRT principles are based on Motivational Interviewing and intervention practices and are designed to move an individual from the precontemplative stage to the action stage. Screening strategies for alcohol and drug use disorders often include instruments such as the CAGE questionnaire (*CAGE* being an acronym for questions about Cutting down, Annoyance by criticism, Guilty feelings, and Eye openers; Ewing 1984), the CAGE Adapted to Include Drugs questionnaire (CAGE-AID; Brown and Rounds 1995), the Alcohol Use Disorders Identification Test (AUDIT; Saunders et al. 1993), the Michigan Alcoholism Screening Test (MAST; Selzer 1971), and the Drug Abuse Screening Test (DAST; Skinner 1982; see also Staley and el-Guebaly 1990). These methods for screening for alcohol and drug problems each have differing sensitivities and specificities in primary care. For instance, the CAGE questionnaire is best used for the diagnosis of alcohol abuse and dependence in primary care, whereas the AUDIT is best used in this setting for diagnosing hazardous drinking (Brown and Rounds 1995). Hazardous drinking is defined as a quantity or pattern of alcohol consumption that puts a person at risk for health problems (Saunders et al. 1993). The National Institute on Alcohol Abuse and Alcoholism (2005) endorsed a single-item screening tool as the first step for patients seen in clinical settings: "How many times in the past year have you had X or more drinks in a day?" (X=5 for men and 4 for women.) Once a patient is noted to have a positive screening result for unhealthy alcohol use, illicit drug use, or nonmedical use of prescription medications, the goal is to help move the patient toward healthier behavior and treatment using psychoeducational strategies.

Motivational Interviewing is designed to help patients identify internal sources of motivation to support behavior change or abstinence. Brief interventions are short (5–20 minutes), focused counseling sessions that incorporate four main components: 1) motivational techniques, 2) feedback about the problems associated with alcohol and illicit drug use, 3) discussion of the adverse effects of alcohol and illicit drug use, and 4) setting recommended substance use limits. In addition, these interventions frequently include the provision of printed materials for patients, similar to those available from the National Institute on Alcohol Abuse and Alcoholism by mail or at www.niaaa.nih.gov and the National Institute on Drug Abuse at www.drugabuse.gov.

The motivational approach used in brief interventions is compatible with the five stages of change—precontemplation, contemplation, preparation, action, and maintenance—as proposed by Prochaska and DiClemente (1982). This model can help the clinician tailor the brief intervention to a patient's specific stage. A successful brief intervention will move a patient from the precontemplation stage, characterized by an unawareness of the adverse effects of alcohol or drug use, to the action stage, characterized by behavior to decrease or discontinue alcohol or drug consumption. These interventions often use the Motivational Interviewing technique of reflective listening, in which the therapist repeats or paraphrases the patient's own statements as a vehicle to work on resolving ambivalence and facilitate change. As demonstrated in the case below, the principles used in this type of counseling can be expressed in the *REDS* acronym: Roll with resistance, Express empathy, Develop discrepancies between present behavior and important goals, and Support self-efficacy (Miller and Rollnick 2002).

Clinical Case

Several weeks before presenting for treatment, Marco came in for routine physical and blood tests with his primary care physician. Marco's blood analysis revealed elevated liver function. His primary care physician ordered a hepatitis screening panel, which revealed hepatitis C infection. Subsequent tests demonstrated ongoing and chronic hepatitis C infection. Marco's primary care physician inquired about risk factors that could have led to this test result. Marco disclosed that he began abusing prescription pain medication when he received them for low back pain over 10 years ago. Shortly after his pain medication prescription ran out, Marco switched to heroin due to the high cost of illegal prescription opioids and began injecting heroin—likely the source of his hepatitis C infection.

After discussing options for treatment of hepatitis C, the physician advised Marco regarding the options for treatment of his opioid dependence and their likelihood of success: Detoxification, a systematic reduction and withdrawal of opioids, would likely take 7–10 days and result in an 85%–95% relapse rate within 6 months. Opioid agonist treatment with program-based methadone or office-based buprenorphine would likely result in 40%–70% abstinence at 3–6 months, allowing for greater engagement in psychosocial care (Fiellin et al. 2000). Marco confirmed that he was interested in a treatment program that would address both his health and opiate addiction concerns. Choosing an office-based treatment option, Marco was then referred to our office-based opioid dependency treatment program by his primary care physician.

At the time of presentation, Marco, a 45-year-old Italian American man, was engaged to be married and self-employed as a graphics designer. He was in a stable relationship of 11 years and currently lived with his fiancée. He appeared quite serious, and although cooperative, did not volunteer a great deal of information at the initial interview.

Marco reported that he had been injecting heroin for approximately 10 years with 1 year of abstinence when he was 40 years old, initiated by a hospital-based detoxification with follow-up at Narcotics Anonymous (NA) meetings. He estimated at this time that his daily heroin use cost approximately $60 per day. Most typically, Marco's use occurred in the mornings when he woke due to his intense withdrawal symptoms. He did not describe his use as a primarily hedonistic experience, but rather indicated that the emphasis was on a desire to alleviate the withdrawal symptoms and to have increased energy—that his use was a morning ritual that prepared him for his day. In fact during the initial interview, Marco reported feeling remorse about his activities for this reason, although he was deeply concerned over the effect of not being able to function without illicit opioids.

Marco reported using drugs since age 12. He reported that he initially used marijuana and alcohol to manage his distress surrounding poor academic and social performance at school. At age 15, he began using cocaine to address his increased social anxiety and difficulties making friends. When Marco was 34, he suffered a lower back injury due to a car accident. He was prescribed opioid-based pain medication for several months to reduce his back pain; however, when he was no longer able to receive this medication from his prescribers and he found they were too expensive on the street, Marco began using heroin to help him handle the intense craving and pain of opioid withdrawal that he felt whenever he tried to stop.

After his disclosure to his family 5 years ago that he was abusing heroin, Marco began detoxification at a methadone clinic and became a member of several self-help groups, including Alcoholics Anonymous (AA) and NA. Marco reported that attendance at these meetings did not diminish his drug cravings. In fact, Marco reported that the self-help meetings often triggered his drug cravings due to the "depressing stories" he heard repeatedly. Marco reported that he preferred to engage in a drug treatment that focused on the present given that he was having difficulties with substance abuse in the here and now.

A notable aspect of Marco's presentation was his candid communication style and apathetic mood. Marco even noted his absence of joy and preference for "straightforward" and often "blunt" conversation themes. It became clear that before attempting a formal psychosocial intervention, it would be necessary to understand his motivation to change in order to maximize the likelihood of success of a brief intervention. Marco had excellent insight regarding how and why he became dependent on opioids, along with the harm it was causing him physically, socially, financially, and psychologically. He saw his recent diagnosis of hepatitis C as a "wake-up call." Hence, it was not necessary to address rationalizations for drug use that could interfere with his motivation for treatment.

One of the motivational tools used with Marco was a set of four Motivational Interviewing questions:

1. What is your current level of motivation on a scale of 1–10 to remain sober?
2. Why isn't it lower than X? (X is the number that the patient identified in response to the first question; this is a technique that encourages the patient to identify motivating factors.)
3. What will it look like when you've reached your goal of sobriety?
4. What will it take to attain your sobriety goal?

Marco indicated his current motivation level was at 8 or 9. When asked why it was not lower, he reported that he had experienced severe social and financial losses in his life, along with a diminished sense of self-esteem that was harming his ability to work. He was worried that he had ruined his health by acquiring hepatitis C. Marco reported that both observing and being observed engaging in drug-using behavior provoked a particularly strong negative emotional reaction to him. Additionally, Marco reported that he was, for the first time in his life, experiencing symptoms of depression (e.g., decreased energy, decreased appetite, decreased interest, increased feelings of guilt, and recurrent feelings of sadness), which he attributed mostly to his continued heroin use. With little to no prompting, Marco was able to *develop discrepancies* between his current behaviors and his goal of becoming drug free and attaining a healthy lifestyle. Marco's response to the third question, asking him to describe sobriety, was a common response seen among opioid-dependent patients: "I just have to have enough willpower to quit, that's all." Convinced of his belief that willpower is the only method for success, it was important to *roll with resistance* and avoid arguing. This enabled Marco to reflect further that he would need a plan and medication to deal with his withdrawal symptoms. Of note, he went on to say that self-help meetings (such as NA and AA) had not been helpful to him and that he preferred to be treated without this type of intervention. Marco was slightly agitated with the fourth question inquiring about what would be needed to attain sobriety. He responded, "After all the treatment I have tried, all I know is that I have a problem. I want to quit, but my best attempts got me here in the first place. Long story short, I have no idea, with the exception of not using and having a strong desire to stop." Besides discussing various options of a concrete treatment plan, the clinician *expressed empathy* toward Marco's struggles to identify an effective treatment, which allowed the interview to *support self-efficacy,* in addition to developing Marco's trust in the therapeutic relationship.

Discussion of the Clinical Case

Marco presents with acute and chronic clinical issues of opioid dependence and depressive symptoms, respectively. Like any person's story, Marco's is unique. Aspects of Marco's story resemble innumerable case histories that take place within the United States and around the world. Office-based treatment of opioid dependence has been shown to be an effective treatment for a growing number of such patients whose ultimate goal is abstinence (Fiellin and Strain 2005).

A number of themes appear as motivational obstacles (*resistance*) and represent core struggles in Marco's life. Below are some of the statements and concepts that Marco seemed to perseverate on in early sessions:

- I'd like to quit, but nothing that I have tried ever works.
- Nobody really follows through with teaching me a hands-on application of my treatment plan.
- I'd like to get back to the way my life was before using opioids, but I don't know where to start or if it's possible.
- I'm not really sure why I need to quit altogether if I can get both things (opioid dependence and depression) under control. If I use drugs only once or twice a week, I can live a normal life.
- I've lost everything, and that thought makes me want to use even when I try to stop using.
- I don't want to involve anyone in my treatment because I don't want to bother others with my problems.

Marco's depressive symptoms are concerning for a dual diagnosis. As with many patients with substance use disorders, co-occurring psychiatric symptoms and diagnoses are common (for further discussion, see Chapter 9, "Working With Dually Diagnosed Patients"). Marco's statements also reflect a lack of motivation and faith in the treatment system. In Marco's case, he was referred for a psychiatric evaluation in order to attain diagnostic clarification regarding a comorbid psychiatric diagnosis. Major depression was then confirmed, and Marco was able to obtain the appropriate pharmacological treatment to help him move forward in treatment.

One aspect of this case that is worth noting is the potential impact of the setting on a patient's motivation to engage in treatment. Opioid-dependent patients are often referred to a methadone clinic, where a staff psychiatrist can address any co-occurring mental illness. It is incorrect to assume that the ultimate goal of methadone maintenance therapy is detoxification. Some patients are able to achieve this and some are not. The ultimate goal of methadone maintenance therapy is to avoid illicit drug use. Although treatment in a methadone program can be effective, Marco felt there might be stigma associated with receiving treatment in a substance abuse treatment clinic, and he preferred the relative anonymity of a physician's office. Additionally, Marco preferred not being in contact with several friends who are active drug users and who receive methadone treatment at local methadone clinics.

In sum, the treatment objectives of Marco's motivational drug counseling were to minimize his self-defeating attitudes and help him generate a more realistic outlook, along with enabling him to experience a sense of self-efficacy through accomplishments. At the early stages of treatment, Marco would benefit from concrete goal-oriented and problem-focused tasks that address his rehabilitation concerns. The therapy would require Marco to identify his problems and to formulate specific goals. Furthermore, his treatment would demonstrate specific skills that would enable him to routinely engage in self-mastery tasks that enhance his ability to find solutions.

Suggestions for Treatment

Patients with substance dependence may report their struggles to a primary care physician. Although referrals to a specialty treatment setting for sustained sobriety are at times indicated, there is evidence that office-based treatment interventions for substance abuse can be effective for some patients (Fiellin et al. 2006). In the case of Marco, an office-based opioid treatment approach is appropriate because he has strong negative opinions (*resistance*) regarding detoxification programs, intensive outpatient programs, and self-help group settings. In Marco's case, office-based treatment involves the treatment of opioid dependence using buprenorphine, a partial opioid agonist, for pharmacotherapy along with psychotherapy. Office-based treatment is an approach that often combines physician management with psychosocial interventions such as counseling, psychotherapy, or participation in self-help groups.

Office-based opioid treatment is not restricted to a particular medical specialty, but certain types of physicians may be more likely to practice this type of treatment. Office-based treatment is provided by treating clinicians (e.g., physicians, psychologists) who are based in routine office settings rather than a specialty clinic. Office-based treatment has increased due to availability of new medications. In addition, it provides some potential advantages:

- First, providing treatment of opioid dependence within office-based settings mainstreams the treatment of addictions. This is done so that patients with an addictive disorder will be seen as similar to those seeking treatment for other medical conditions, without having the potential stigma that might be associated if they were seen in a specialty setting.
- Second, office-based treatment allows addiction treatment services to be integrated with the care of other medical conditions, such as comorbid hepatitis C in Marco's case, thereby expanding access to patients with comorbid medical and psychiatric disorders. This approach has been shown to improve compliance with treatment recommendations (Fiellin and Strain 2005).
- Finally, because it has been difficult to expand treatment capacities through methadone clinics, it is expected that office-based strategies will be able to more rapidly expand access to needed services.

Screening and Assessment

The psychotherapist began assessing Marco through the four Motivational Interviewing questions mentioned in the "Clinical Case" section of this chapter; however, the initial sessions of therapy seek to assess a patient's level of motivation to become drug free within a specific time frame. Marco had reached the level of *contemplation* with his primary care physician visits, and moved on to the *preparation* stage by the first meeting with the psychologist. In the office-based assessment it is important to find out the following:

- What brought the patient into treatment (e.g., "I can't afford it any more"; "My parole officer told me to come in")
- What factors affect the patient's use of illicit opiates (e.g., "I'm so used to it that if I don't use, I have no energy")
- What goals the patient has for treatment (e.g., "I want to cut down on my use"; "I would like to stop using")
- What does the patient think it will take to attain sobriety in a limited time frame (e.g., "I need to stay away from my drug-using friends"; "I need something to get rid of my withdrawals")

- What the patient's current functioning is in different life domains (e.g., legal problems, medical issues)
- What the patient's preexisting coping skills are (e.g., "Talking to my partner often helps me delay use or not use"; "If I exercise, I tend to have a lot more energy throughout the day, so I don't feel like using then").

Taken together, this information is sometimes used by therapists to create a snapshot or *case formulation* of the patient's presenting problems. After allowing for some personal insight of the patient's need to seek treatment, desire for continued use, treatment goals, and coping skills, it is helpful to reintroduce the fourth question that was used at the beginning of assessment: "What will it take to attain your sobriety goal in a limited time frame?" This question is asked for the patient to develop some discrepancy between his current maladaptive drug-using behaviors and his goals to highlight behaviors that need to change if the goals are to be accomplished.

Screening for and assessing substance abuse struggles are quite common within psychotherapeutic settings. Unfortunately, research shows that substance use disorders are less likely to be recognized in non–substance abuse treatment settings, such as primary care settings (Coulehan et al. 1987; Duszynski et al. 1995). Nonetheless, strategies such as routine annual screening are supported by guidelines (U.S. Preventive Services Task Force 2004) and have been shown to be effective in large health care organizations (Aspy et al. 2008; Bradley et al. 2006).

Brief Intervention

Within the context of screening, brief therapeutic treatment, and referral to additional treatment, an integrated Motivational Interviewing counseling approach is recommended to address the complex needs of dually diagnosed patients. In particular, dually diagnosed patients' treatment needs (e.g., medical/dental, vocational, financial, housing, legal) often involve them in many dimensions of the service system. Integrating Motivational Interviewing strategies to foster patient engagement and retention in comprehensive treatment is important (Martino and Moyers 2008).

Physician Management

One strategy is an approach termed *physician management*: a brief (15–20 minutes per session), manual-guided, medically focused treatment based on group drug counseling (Umbricht-Schneiter et al. 1994). The manual for the treatment proposed for Marco focuses on reducing illicit drug use and adhering to buprenorphine use. After an initial 45-minute evaluation session, brief physician management sessions are administered on a weekly basis for 2 weeks, then biweekly for 4 weeks, then monthly. In physician management, the physician does the following:

1. Assesses the impact of alcohol and drug use on the patient's medical, psychiatric, social, vocational, and legal functioning
2. Educates the patient about alcohol and drug dependence and medication-assisted treatment
3. Encourages the patient to become or remain abstinent and adhere to medication and treatment recommendations
4. Encourages lifestyle changes, avoidance of triggers, and use of additional self-help methods
5. Identifies and addresses medical complications of alcohol and drug use
6. Refers patients to other services in the community (e.g., mental health, vocational, legal, housing, or social services).

To approximate usual drug abuse treatment, obtaining toxicology test results is helpful before or during each session.

Brief Psychotherapy

Performed by a psychotherapist, brief Motivational Interviewing–centered drug counseling (MIDC; C.J. Cutter, D.T. Barry, R.S. Schottenfeld, D.A. Fiellin, "Brief Motivational Interviewing–Centered Drug Counseling (MIDC)," unpublished manual, August 2009) is useful to patients in treatment for opioid dependence in the context of time limitations. MIDC has three theoretically consistent core components: medication adherence and management, relapse prevention, and Motivational Interviewing–enhanced drug counseling.

1. Medication compliance is the sine qua non of effective opioid dependence treatment. Simply put, in the absence of patient compliance with a prescribed medication, such as buprenorphine, the effectiveness of psychosocial interventions for opioid dependence is severely hampered. During the first weeks of treatment, the therapist assesses medication adherence at the beginning of each session and develops strategies to increase medication compliance and treatment adherence (e.g., problem solving to enhance the likelihood of attending medication appointments). Discussions of medication adherence can focus on potential side effects and patients' concerns regarding the medication. It is important to reinforce a patient's successful medication compliance through rewards, such as therapist praise.
2. Within a time-limited format, both focused and structured approaches of relapse prevention techniques have demonstrated efficacy in Motivational

Interviewing (Bothelo and Novak 1993; Mercer et al. 1992) and behavioral treatments (Rollnick et al. 1992), respectively, for substance abuse disorders. Relapse prevention involves an understanding of circumstances before and after illicit drug use. Relapse prevention interventions are designed to do the following:

a. Increase patients' understanding about the learned components of their use (e.g., triggers and rewards)
b. Help patients learn and practice using behaviors that are incompatible with drug use (e.g., avoiding places where it is easy to buy drugs)
c. Develop coping plans to avoid further relapses.

MIDC also incorporates Motivational Interviewing and Behavioral Therapy as a vehicle to effectively deliver relapse prevention techniques within a time-limited treatment setting.

3. MIDC was designed to fit a wide array of drug counseling needs. With overall goals similar to those of Motivational Interviewing, MIDC sets to create positive behavior change through understanding a patient's personal goals, and Behavioral Therapy approaches tend to be an effective component of an integrated drug counseling approach to relapse prevention. In behavioral approaches, restoring an adequate schedule of positive experiences is essential to reduce the patient's dysphoria. Altering the frequency, quality, and range of a patient's maladaptive activities (e.g., drug-using activities) and social interactions is a common method for bringing about a changed schedule of reinforcement (Piper et al. 1996). Similar to Behavioral Therapy, MIDC addresses the following:

   • Creating change in the patient's environment (e.g., having the patient drive a different route home to avoid places where it is easy to buy drugs)
   • Changing problematic environmental patterns by teaching patients skills that they can use to address these problematic patterns (e.g., drug refusal skills)
   • Enhancing positive life events and decreasing stressful environmental interactions (e.g., regularly planning positive events within the patient's daily structure).

MIDC is different from traditional behavioral therapies in that it integrates a soft Motivational Interviewing approach that focuses on building a patient's self-efficacy. Within MIDC, applying consistent Motivational Interviewing concepts such as FRAMES (Miller and Sanchez 1994) to concrete behavioral tasks, we are able to clearly identify tangible goals in a nondidactic method, while at the same time increase self-efficacy for change. The acronym

FRAMES refers to the use of **F**eedback, **R**esponsibility for change lying with the individual, **A**dvice giving, providing a **M**enu of change options, an **E**mpathic counseling style, and the enhancement of **S**elf-efficacy (Miller and Rollnick 2002). (See "Approach" section below for more on menu of change options.)

Approach

Changing the motivation of the patient and directing his or her motivation toward achievement of big treatment goals (sustained abstinence, permanent restructuring of the patient's social networks, and the development of an alternative lifestyle) is generally difficult and can rarely be achieved within a short time period (Goldsmith and Garlapati 2004). After the patient has received empathic feedback in the context of initial successes, the experience of his or her success—accompanied by a reduction in demoralization—counters pessimism and helps to change the patient's future outlook about success, and in turn, enables the patient to reformulate his or her long-term treatment goals and *menu of change options.*

Rather than focusing on general hopes about major changes in life, it is useful to focus on specific and well-defined immediate activities that produce small changes. Hence, it is highly important to generate an appropriate menu of change options. If achieved, these small changes can be rewarding and provide improved emotional functioning, reduced guilt and shame, and improved self-esteem and sense of achievement. Small changes also illustrate to the patient that his or her actions can be effective and lead to positive results. If the patient fails initially at a small attempt to change, the emotional impact of such a small failure also is not as devastating, and the problems encountered during the failed attempt are easier to analyze, understand, and overcome during the following attempt. The small changes achieved during the course of the therapy serve as the foundation for promoting larger change and are opportunities for the counselor to emphasize that more significant patient change is possible. Most important, the progress of small changes allows patients to take ownership of and *responsibility* for their change.

The key therapeutic component of short-term, office-based therapy is a series of behavioral exercises and homework assignments in the form of verbal or written agreements between the counselor and the patient. An important feature of these behavioral exercises is that they initially focus on realistic, small, and easy-to-obtain achievements (Levendusky et al. 1994). Sometimes, these initial achievements may not immediately appear to contribute substantially to the accomplishment of the greater goals of sustained abstinence and prolonged recovery. Examples of short-term behavioral goals that were used with Marco included disposing of drug paraphernalia; not using drugs for a day or two even without a commitment to extended drug abstinence; changing a daily routine related to the way drugs are obtained or used; and increasing healthy-lifestyle, self-care tasks. When patients accomplish small, well-defined goals and experience improvements in their lifestyle, mood, and sense of efficacy, they are often motivated to engage in similar efforts. In the case of Marco, he and the therapist would often discuss the increasing sense of hope surrounding his successful ability to take responsibility for change.

Behavioral, task-focused homework exercises are collaborative, simple, detailed, and written down for patients to take with them. Each contracting interaction ends with the therapist either obtaining verbal commitment from the patient to fulfill the contract or compiling a written contract that is then signed by both the patient and the therapist. The therapist suggests the most appropriate areas or activities for the contract, provides instructions and support in achieving goals, verifies the accomplishments, administers positive feedback to the patient, and discusses the patient's satisfaction with attempts to achieve contract goals.

The purpose of homework is not just for the patients to do something, but to do something that will move the therapy process along. With this in mind, when homework is assigned, specific short-term goals are set, along with collaborative predictions about how the patient will feel when that assignment is completed. The contract and homework exercise goals are behavioral in nature—for Marco, one goal would be to structure his days with positive and self-mastery activities for at least 2 days. This is very different from setting a homework goal of "experience fewer drug cravings." Structuring a patient's day may feel labor intensive and at times boring, but the goal is the behavior change.

At each session after the initial session, the therapist reviews the behavioral tasks developed in the previous session within a Motivational Interviewing framework. Specifically, the therapist reviews the patient's accomplishments (or the lack thereof), perceived obstacles and means of overcoming them (alternative plans) created by both patient and therapist, and administers empathic feedback to the patient. The empathic feedback is framed in a positive tone and includes the therapist congratulating the patient on the successful completion of a task. If the patient was not able to achieve the behavioral goals from the previous session, the therapist helps the patient understand what got in the way of successful completion. More specifically, the therapist asks the patient what his or her understanding is of what got in the way of completing the exercise, followed with asking, "What can you do, and what are your options to make sure that you complete the exercise next week?"

Ideally, Motivational Interviewing–enhanced behavioral exercise is designed to bolster the patient's *self-efficacy* and level of success by initially focusing on small, attainable goals and eventually progressing to bigger and more important goals. In the case of Marco, each goal was directly associated with sustained abstinence from drugs. The overarching goal in this brief treatment is to engage the patient in rewarding, self-mastery activities that provide viable alternatives to drug use, activities generated by the therapist and patient together with an emphasis on successful completion of small steps. Because of its emphasis on listening and behavior change, this approach encourages optimism about the possibility of change, alleviates hopelessness, increases self-efficacy, and shores up motivation to make further, broader changes toward a healthy lifestyle.

Referral to Treatment

Similar to SBIRT, MIDC has been used to help patients transition from short-term therapy to longer-term therapy in outpatient settings when they reach the action or maintenance stage of change (Madras et al. 2009). However, it is important to reassess a patient's progress on three dimensions—motivation, behavior, and stage of change—before making an appropriate referral:

1. Reassessing motivation begins with revisiting the patient's completion of therapy goals. Once that is established, using Motivational Interviewing–consistent questions such as the four mentioned earlier in the "Clinical Case" section often helps determine the level of motivation for and desire for continued self-improvement.
2. Identifying major and minor behavior changes that impact the patient's life medically, vocationally, financially, interpersonally, and legally is recommended.
3. It is useful to collaboratively assess the patient's stage of change within each session.

Once all three dimensions are identified, the treatment team can discuss all helpful referral options with the patient, emphasizing that the decision is up to the patient. This approach is seen as a final exercise in supporting a patient's self-efficacy, so that belief in his or her personal ability to change (as in changing the type of treatment, in this case) becomes a self-fulfilling prophecy (Saunders et al. 1993).

Suggestions for Teaching and Supervision

Teaching brief interventions:

- Provide an overview of the stages of change.
- Provide information regarding the appropriate goal for each stage.

- Provide information regarding the appropriate tools to use at each stage.
- Contrast confrontational approaches and Motivational Interviewing.
- Discuss strategies used to elicit motivational statements.
- Describe reflective listening.
- Introduce the mnemonics REDS and FRAMES.
- Discuss the evidence in support of brief interventions.
- List the components that are used in successful brief interventions.
- Conduct role-play exercises.

Supervising brief interventions:

- Provide teaching cases.
- Provide structured clinical encounter notes.
- Make audio and/or video recordings of interventions.
- Listen to audiotapes and/or watch videos with the trainee, stopping periodically to provide corrective feedback.
- Praise correct implementation of REDS, FRAMES, Motivational Interviewing, and reflective listening techniques.

Movie: *Trainspotting*

In the movie *Trainspotting* (1996), the actor Ewan McGregor portrays a young man, Mark Renton, and his struggles with heroin in Edinburgh, Scotland. Renton has periodic moments in his life when he develops an intense level of motivation to become sober. However, his attempts are thwarted by the lack of a treatment plan and consistently being tempted to use heroin through the influence of drug-using friends. Renton's brief episode of abstinence is quickly erased by his drug use in response to psychosocial and legal stressors. After 2 weeks of abstinence, Renton resumes using heroin. He describes heroin as the best experience that this world has to offer, and says that when you are not on it, you often worry about the day-to-day stresses of life. He continues to say, "Why choose life when you have heroin?" and describes several examples showing that when a person is on heroin, he stops caring about the outside world. After another detoxification, Renton is finally motivated to maintain abstinence, primarily by his desire to leave his drug-using life behind him.

Within this film, we see Renton struggling with motivational vicissitudes and lack of a comprehensive psychosocial treatment plan to address his opioid dependence. Renton would have benefited from attention to his motivational states and treatments tailored to move him through those stages. For instance, the ambivalence he demonstrates could be portrayed to him in sessions highlighting the *discrepancy* between his desires and actions. A clinician would need to *avoid argumentation* and *roll with the resistance* manifested by his statements about needing a rationale to choose life when there is heroin. Likewise, support would need to be provided for the *self-efficacy* he demonstrates in his attempts to identify strategies to maintain his abstinence. Opioid agonist treatment with methadone or buprenorphine would certainly be among the *menu of treatment options* offered to him at the time of his relapse following detoxification.

Key Clinical Points

- Screening asymptomatic patients to identify addictive disorders is appropriate because of the prevalence of these disorders, the benefits of early treatment, the presence of screening tools with good operating characteristics, and the presence of effective treatments.

- Brief interventions, based on the Stages of Change model, can be effective in changing behavior and working on patients' motivation to seek treatment.

- Office-based treatments for addictive disorders can incorporate combined psychosocial and pharmacological treatments provided by one or more clinicians. These interventions begin with screening, incorporate components of Motivational Interviewing, may be preferred by some patients due to reduced stigma and increased availability, and are effective for some patients.

Multiple-Choice Questions

For the correct answers to these questions, including explanations of answers, please see the Answer Guide at the end of this book.

1. The best screening tool for harmful and hazardous drinking to use in primary care practices is the:

   A. DAST.
   B. AUDIT.
   C. CAGE questionnaire.
   D. MAST.

2. According to the National Institute on Alcohol Abuse and Alcoholism recommendations, effective screening for alcohol problems can be accomplished with as little as:

   A. One question.
   B. Two questions.
   C. Three questions.
   D. Four questions.

3. In attempting to assess a patient's motivation and elicit motivational statements, it is important to ask, "What is your current level of motivation on a scale of 1–10 to remain sober?" If the patient provides an answer indicating partial motivation, such as "6," the clinician should follow up with:

   A. "Why is it so high?"
   B. "Why is it 6 and not 2?"
   C. "Why is it 6 and not 10?"
   D. "It sounds like you are not really that motivated."

4. The REDS acronym stands for:

   A. Reject resistance, Express empathy, Develop discrepancy, accept ambivalence, and Support sobriety.
   B. Rock and roll, Experience, Drugs, alcohol, System.
   C. Recognize responsibility, Express empathy, Develop discrepancy, advice giving, and Support self-efficacy.
   D. Roll with resistance, Express empathy, Develop discrepancy, and Support self-efficacy.

5. Methadone and buprenorphine:

   A. Can both be provided for treatment of opioid dependence from physicians' offices.
   B. Are only used for detoxification.
   C. Are effective against both opioids and cocaine.
   D. Both result in 40%–70% abstinence from opioids at 3–6 months.

References

Aspy CB, Mold JW, Thompson DM, et al: Integrating screening and interventions for unhealthy behaviors into primary care practices. Am J Prev Med 35:S373–S380, 2008

Bothelo RJ, Novak S: Dealing with substance misuse, abuse, and dependency. Prim Care 20:51–70, 1993

Bradley KA, Williams EC, Achtmeyer CE, et al: Implementation of evidence-based alcohol screening in the Veterans Health Administration. Am J Manag Care 12:597–606, 2006

Brown RL, Rounds LA: Conjoint screening questionnaires for alcohol and other drug abuse: criterion validity in a primary care practice. Wis Med J 94:135–140, 1995

Coulehan JL, Zettler-Segal M, Block M, et al: Recognition of alcoholism and substance abuse in primary care patients. Arch Intern Med 147:349–352, 1987

Duszynski KR, Nieto FJ, Valente CM: Reported practices, attitudes, and confidence levels of primary care physicians regarding patients who abuse alcohol and other drugs. Md Med J 44:439–446, 1995

Ewing JA: Detecting alcoholism: the CAGE questionnaire. JAMA 252:1905–1907, 1984

Fiellin DA, Strain EC: Office-based treatment with buprenorphine and other medications, in The Treatment of Opioid Dependence. Edited by Strain EC, Stitzer MI. Baltimore, MD, Johns Hopkins University Press, 2005, pp 251–276

Fiellin DA, Reid MC, O'Connor PG: Screening for alcohol problems in primary care: a systematic review. Arch Intern Med 160:1977–1989, 2000

Fiellin DA, Pantalon MV, Chawarski MC, et al: Counseling plus buprenorphine-naloxone maintenance therapy for opioid dependence. N Engl J Med 355:365–374, 2006

Goldsmith RJ, Garlapati V: Behavioral interventions for dual-diagnosis patients. Psychiatr Clin North Am 27:709–725, 2004

Levendusky PG, Willis BS, Ghinassi FA: The therapeutic contracting program: a comprehensive continuum of care model. Psychiatr Q 65:189–207, 1994

Madras BK, Compton WM, Avula D, et al: Screening, brief interventions, referral to treatment (SBIRT) for illicit drug and alcohol use at multiple healthcare sites: comparison at intake and 6 months later. Drug Alcohol Depend 99:280–295, 2009

Martino S, Moyers TB: Motivational interviewing with dually diagnosed patients, in Motivational Interviewing in the Treatment of Psychological Problems. Edited by Arkowitz H, Westra HA, Miller WR, et al. New York, Guilford, 2008, pp 277–303

Mercer D, Carpenter G, Daley D, et al: Group Drug Counseling Manual. Philadelphia, PA, University of Pennsylvania, 1992

Miller WR, Rollnick S: Motivational Interviewing: Preparing People for Change, 2nd Edition. New York, Guilford, 2002

Miller WR, Sanchez VC: Motivating young adults for treatment and lifestyle change, in Alcohol Use and Misuse by Young Adults. Edited by Howard GS, Nathan PE. Notre Dame, IN, University of Notre Dame Press, 1994, pp 51–81

National Institute on Alcohol Abuse and Alcoholism: Helping Patients Who Drink Too Much: A Clinician's Guide (NIH Publ No 05–3769). Rockville, MD, U.S. Department of Health and Human Services, 2005

Piper WE, Rosie JS, Joyce AS, et al: Time-Limited Day Treatment for Personality Disorders: Integration of Research and Practice in a Group Program. Washington, DC, American Psychological Association, 1996

Prochaska JO, DiClemente CC: Transtheoretical therapy: towards a more integrative model of change. Psychotherapy: Theory, Research, and Practice 19:276–288, 1982

Rollnick S, Heather N, Bell A: Negotiating behaviour change in medical settings: the development of brief motivational interviewing. J Ment Health 1:25–37, 1992

Saunders JB, Aasland OG, Babor TF, et al: Development of the Alcohol Use Disorders Identification Test (AUDIT): WHO Collaborative Project on Early Detection of Persons With Harmful Alcohol Consumption—II. Addiction 88:791–804, 1993

Selzer ML: The Michigan Alcoholism Screening Test (MAST): the quest for a new diagnostic instrument. Am J Psychiatry 127:1653–1658, 1971

Skinner HA. The drug abuse screening test. Addict Behav 7:363–371, 1982

Staley D, el-Guebaly N: Psychometric properties of the Drug Abuse Screening Test in a psychiatric patient population. Addict Behav 15:257–264, 1990

Umbricht-Schneiter A, Ginn DH, Pabst KM, et al: Providing medical care to methadone clinic patients: referral vs on-site care. Am J Public Health 84:207–210, 1994

U.S. Preventive Services Task Force: Screening and behavioral counseling interventions in primary care to reduce alcohol misuse: recommendation statement. Ann Intern Med 140:554–556, 2004

Engaging in Self-Help Groups

Marianne T. Guschwan, M.D.

This chapter focuses on the application of motivational principles to the engagement of patients in mutual/self-help groups. To start, I define mutual/self-help, clarify the difference between formal treatment and self-help, and then explain several types of self-help groups. Clinical cases and tips for teaching and supervising on this subject are presented, including an excerpt from a television series. As in the other chapters, review questions end the chapter.

Mutual-help groups, also known as self-help groups (or mutual/self-help groups), are support groups that are led and organized by members. There is an important distinction to make between professional treatment and self-help. The former involves trained and licensed clinicians providing treatment with a formalized structure. It involves well-defined provision of treatment as well as well-defined expectations of the patient (American Psychiatric Association 1995). The responsibility of the patient is to show up at a certain time and place and to pay (or have an insurance company pay) for treatment. Group and individual therapy are provided. Certainly, the patient needs to do more than show up in order to benefit from the treatment; however, patients do not have to find their own groups for therapy nor try to figure out on their own what is expected of them. In contrast, self-help is available free of charge (for the most part), is guided by peers who have endured the same problem, and is offered in a less structured way. There are no defined starting and ending dates. The patient is provided guidelines but is not required to do any one thing in particular.

Why is it important to make this distinction between professional treatment and self-help? From a policy point of view, insurance companies would like to view self-help as the sole form of addiction treatment that they cover because it costs them nothing. In addition, some data suggest that introducing self-help as part of professional treatment yields better outcomes than either approach on its own (Montgomery et al. 1995). Finally, it is important to explain to patients what treatment options exist for them.

Self-help in the addiction field has most popularly meant Alcoholics Anonymous (AA), but the concept has broadened to include several anonymous groups encompassed under the moniker "12-step groups," such as Narcotics Anonymous (NA), Marijuana Anonymous (MA), Cocaine Anonymous (CA), and so on. Other, less well-known self-help groups that have evolved from 12-step groups include Self Management and Recovery Training (known as SMART Recovery), Rational Recovery (available for a fee), Women for Sobriety, Secular Organizations for Sobriety (also known as Save Our Selves), and Moderation Management. Each group has its own set of principles guiding an individual in how to live his or her life without substances.

Clearly the most widely known self-help group is AA, with over 2 million members and over 100,000 meetings held weekly throughout the world (General Service Office of Alcoholics Anonymous 2007). Meetings are free. Those that are "open" are available to anyone who wants to attend even if just as an observer wanting more information (e.g., a family member or perhaps a student). AA was developed in 1935 and evolved from the principles of a Christian fellowship called the Oxford Group. This is important for clinicians to recognize because there are references to God and to practices similar to those professed in Christian religions. Those practices were formalized in the 12 steps, which form the basis of AA and other Anonymous groups (e.g., NA, CA, MA). Patients often raise this as a resistance to going to meetings (more about how to address this later; see "Case 1" discussion). The basic philosophy of AA is that the person is powerless over drinking, and to deal with this problem, the individual must acknowledge this powerlessness and turn his or her will over to "a Higher Power" (General Service Office of Alcoholics Anonymous 2007). AA's Twelve Steps are included in Table 12–1.

SMART Recovery, established in the early 1990s, is focused on helping individuals achieve behavior change. Rather than viewing addiction as a disease, the program views addiction as a maladaptive behavior. Rather than professing powerlessness, the program empowers the individual and teaches self-reliance. It emphasizes four areas (called the "Four Points") in the process of recovery: 1) building motivation, 2) coping with urges, 3) problem solving, and 4) lifestyle balance. It is based on the Cognitive-Behavioral Therapy principles of Albert Ellis, an approach also known as Rational Emotive Behavioral Therapy. SMART Recovery emphasizes an individual's control over himself or herself and his or her

---

TABLE 12–1.   The Twelve Steps of Alcoholics Anonymous

Step 1:   We admitted we were powerless over our alcohol—that our lives had become unmanageable.

Step 2:   Came to believe that a Power greater than ourselves could restore us to sanity.

Step 3:   Made a decision to turn our will and our lives over to the care of God *as we understood Him.*

Step 4:   Made a searching and fearless moral inventory of ourselves.

Step 5:   Admitted to God, to ourselves and to another human being the exact nature of our wrongs.

Step 6:   Were entirely ready to have God remove all these defects of character.

Step 7:   Humbly asked Him to remove our shortcomings.

Step 8:   Made a list of all persons we had harmed, and became willing to make amends to them all.

Step 9:   Made direct amends to such people wherever possible, except when to do so would injure them or others.

Step 10: Continued to take personal inventory and when we were wrong promptly admitted it.

Step 11: Sought through prayer and meditation to improve our conscious contact with God *as we understood Him,* praying only for knowledge of His will for us and the power to carry that out.

Step 12: Having had a spiritual awakening as the result of these steps, we tried to carry this message to alcoholics, and to practice these principles in all our affairs.

Note.   The Twelve Steps and a brief excerpt from the book *Alcoholics Anonymous* are reprinted with permission of Alcoholics Anonymous World Services, Inc. ("AAWS"). Permission to reprint a brief excerpt from the book, *Alcoholics Anonymous,* and the Twelve Steps does not mean that AAWS has reviewed or approved the contents of this publication, or that AAWS necessarily agrees with the views expressed herein. AA is a program of recovery from alcoholism only—use of the Twelve Steps in connection with programs and activities which are patterned after AA, but which address other problems, or in any other non-AA context, does not imply otherwise.

Source.   Reprinted with permission from Alcoholics Anonymous: Alcoholics Anonymous, 4th Edition. New York, Alcoholics Anonymous World Services, 2002, pp. 59–60.

problems as opposed to the individual being powerless (the premise of AA). More than 300 weekly face-to-face meetings are held worldwide in addition to online meetings. Meetings are free and open to all who wish to participate. Literature is available for a fee. Although it is often considered an alternative to AA, many people use it as an adjunct to AA (SMART Recovery 2009).

Women for Sobriety, founded in 1976 by psychologist Jeanne Kirkpatrick, promotes a "New Life" program. It is based on 13 statements focused on positive thinking and life change (Table 12–2). The underlying focus is to help recovering women take better care of themselves physically and mentally in addition to spiritually. The founder's experience with AA was that repetition of a person's story in 12-step meetings had detrimental effects. Shame and guilt were revisited, which were demoralizing to the participant. The author developed her program based on the emotional needs of women in recovery (Women for Sobriety 2009).

The guiding principle of AA is one of mutual attraction, not coercion, so the notion of requiring attendance is contrary to this basic idea. Motivational Interviewing has a similar guiding principle in that it involves working with patients' intrinsic motivation—not coercion—to help. It assumes that ambivalence is the norm (Miller and Rollnick 1991). The goal of the therapist in Motivational Interviewing is to help patients develop their own reasons for change.

Clinical Cases and Discussion of Cases

The following case examples illustrate the common resistances the clinician might encounter in clinical practice, and the subsequent discussions suggest ways to utilize Motivational Interviewing to facilitate change.

Case 1

A 40-year-old single white male with cocaine dependence is referred for psychiatric follow-up after completing an intensive outpatient rehabilitation program. He had entered treatment after getting into some trouble at work— showing up late for meetings and not completing work on time. Although he attended 12-step group meetings during the rehabilitation program, he states he prefers to have aftercare with an individual therapist because he found CA to be too religious.

This is a common reason that patients give for not wanting to attend 12-step groups. It is important for the clinician to acknowledge the Christian roots of AA. However, although it has religious roots, the program does not espouse a particular organized religion. And although the 12 steps often reference God,

TABLE 12–2.   Women for Sobriety "New Life" Program

1. I have a life-threatening problem that once had me.

    I now take charge of my life and my disease. I accept the responsibility.

2. Negative thoughts destroy only myself.

    My first conscious sober act must be to remove negativity from my life.

3. Happiness is a habit I will develop.

    Happiness is created, not waited for.

4. Problems bother me only to the degree I permit them to.

    I now better understand my problems and do not permit problems to overwhelm me.

5. I am what I think.

    I am a capable, competent, caring, compassionate woman.

6. Life can be ordinary or it can be great.

    Greatness is mine by a conscious effort.

7. Love can change the course of my world.

    Caring becomes all important.

8. The fundamental object of life is emotional and spiritual growth.

    Daily I put my life into a proper order, knowing which are the priorities.

9. The past is gone forever.

    No longer will I be victimized by the past. I am a new person.

10. All love given returns.

    I will learn to know that others love me.

11. Enthusiasm is my daily exercise.

    I treasure all moments of my new life.

12. I am a competent woman and have much to give life.

    This is what I am and I shall know it always.

13. I am responsible for myself and for my actions.

    I am in charge of my mind, my thoughts, and my life.

To make the program effective for you, arise each morning fifteen minutes earlier than usual and go over the Thirteen Acceptance Statements. Then begin to think about each one by itself. Take one Statement and use it consciously all day. At the end of the day, review the use of it and what effects it had that day for you and your actions. Keeping a daily journal is helpful during this time.

Source.   Reprinted with permission from Women for Sobriety, Inc. Copyright © 1976, 1987, 1993. www.womenforsobriety.org.

it is "as we understand God." Some patients take that to mean the power of nature, such as exemplified in the ocean, the mountains, the sunrise, or the sunset.
It is interesting to note that although many patients may report the emphasis
on religion as their reason for resistance to engaging in AA and similar 12-step
programs, in polls taken in the United States more than 90% of respondents
report that they believe in God (Bezilla 1993).

Rolling with resistance is an important technique in this scenario. The clinician can explore with the patient what the patient's past experience with religion has been. While acknowledging that spirituality is an important part of
AA, the clinician may challenge the religiosity defense of the patient. Another
important aspect to explore is the patient's past experience in AA, if any. If it
has been limited, the clinician might encourage another trial (for more suggestions, see Case 2 and discussion).

Supporting self-efficacy is important—allowing the patients to take charge
of what they want to do, such as trying other meetings or perhaps trying an alternative to 12-step groups. As outlined earlier, several alternative self-help
groups exist depending on the situation with the patient. For example, Women
for Sobriety is an alternative for women. There is literature available from the
group Men for Sobriety, but that organization is not as well established. Many
fewer groups exist for the Women for Sobriety program compared with the 12-
step programs. However, there is the opportunity to connect with a buddy who
can facilitate using the 13 guiding principles of Women for Sobriety.

Case 2

A 45-year-old female advertising executive is referred for an evaluation of anxiety. In the history, she reveals heavy alcohol use and reports trying AA in the
past. She acknowledges that alcohol is a problem for her; however, she resists going to meetings because she feels she could not relate to the people in the group.

The Motivational Interviewing principle of expressing empathy is important in this scenario. If patients state that they did not find people they could
relate to, the clinician may suggest trying AA meetings in different locations
and at different times to see whether patients are able to find a meeting with
people they identify with. With further exploration, the clinician may find the
patient identifying feelings of shame about their addiction and related experiences. Patients who experience substance use disorders are often the victims of
trauma—sexual or physical abuse (Jacobsen et al. 2001). Often patients engage
in sexually promiscuous behavior while using substances. In other circumstances, the patient may be the perpetrator of abuse (either sexual or physical).
Patients may manifest this shame as a resistance to talking with others in a
group about the problems they have encountered regarding substance misuse,

such as trading sex for drugs, engaging in prostitution to support themselves, or perhaps being the victim of physical abuse. Using Motivational Interviewing to engage patients in self-help groups, the clinician must be able to meet patients where they are in their resistance or ambivalence and allow them to be heard. This may take time and gentle probing when surrounding issues of shame. Although advice giving is not within the framework of Motivational Interviewing, it is helpful for the clinician to be aware of what might be solutions to some of the obstacles that patients present. Attending same-sex meetings may help the patient with shame feel more comfortable sharing.

Other patients have difficulty speaking in a group and may meet criteria for social phobia or other anxiety disorders. In these instances, the clinician may need to take a more proactive role and possibly suggest medication when indicated. Another helpful approach to suggest is that the patient attend meetings with a friend (even someone who may not have a problem with alcohol). If the patient does attend AA with a supportive nonalcoholic friend, be sure to advise the patient to attend an *open* meeting where those who do not identify themselves as alcoholic are allowed to attend. Closed meetings are for alcoholic individuals only.

Case 3

A 35-year-old recently married man presented to treatment after an altercation with his wife. He has a history of marijuana, alcohol, and cocaine dependence. The patient had made attempts to be in therapy but would leave when he became angry with the therapist. His past history is notable for treatment in a therapeutic community. His family history is notable for his father, who was dependent on heroin and cocaine, and his mother, who is a recovering alcoholic actively involved in AA.

Developing discrepancy is a useful Motivational Interviewing principle in this scenario. Given that substance use disorders are genetically influenced, it is not uncommon for patients to have a parent who also has had an addiction. This often drives some people to abstain from substances; however, those who become like their parents (i.e., develop an addiction) may have difficulty in getting well even though their parents may have, such as by attending AA. The patient may also strongly identify with a nonsober parent and have difficulty getting well because of what it would mean for the relationship with that parent. Often a patient will choose a substance-using partner who may or may not be in recovery. In utilizing the technique of developing discrepancy, remember to include exploration of what effect using and not using will have on the patient's relationships. It is helpful for the patient to look at his or her reasons for not attending AA; for example, in the case above the patient may remark, "My mother attends AA, but look at her craziness."

Suggestions for Treatment

Often, resistance to AA (or other self-help group) is ultimately an expression of ambivalence about giving up drugs or alcohol. Using Motivational Interviewing helps to clarify the resistance and hopefully move the patient into action. As the clinician engages patients toward action, it is helpful to know about the different self-help groups. However, in Motivational Interviewing, the *patient* should be suggesting the treatment plan. The clinician should encourage patients to do research and present the reasons that a specific alternative is better for them. Those who are truly in the action phase will do the work—get information and attend a group's meetings. If the patient continues to give reasons for not going, the clinician must evaluate where the patient is in the stages of change and utilize Motivational Interviewing to move the patient along toward action.

Every addicted patient's fantasy is to be able to use the substance socially, every once in a while, like a nonaddicted individual. It is difficult for addicted patients to accept the loss of the substance—relinquishing use is a mourning process. Using a substance is also a coping mechanism, something to get patients through the tough times, as well as to celebrate the happy times. As patients become more aware that the mechanism is not working for them, their motivation to change increases. It is the clinician's role then to promote self-efficacy—the patient's belief that he or she *can* change—and to guide the patient into doing what will help him or her change.

Suggestions for Teaching and Supervision

To facilitate students' empathy for addicted patients, an instructor may require students to attend a self-help group meeting. The most widely available are 12-step groups. The visits may be accomplished in different ways: The students could attend a specific, prechosen, outsider-friendly meeting in small groups or pairs. Or students could search on their own for an open 12-step meeting to attend (please be sure to educate them about attending only *open* meetings, not *closed* ones, because the latter are for members only). After attending the group meeting, students can write up and/or discuss their experiences with each other. Table 12–3 provides a listing of groups that students may consider visiting. An alternative approach is for the instructor to give students the list of groups in Table 12–3 and ask them to write about their experiences. Some of the less common self-help groups may not be readily available

TABLE 12–3.   Self-help group contact information

Group	Phone	Web site
Alcoholics Anonymous	212-870-3400	www.aa.org www.aaonline.net
Marijuana Anonymous	Toll free: 800-766-6779	www.marijuana-anonymous.org www.ma-online.org
Men for Sobriety	215-536-8026	www.womenforsobriety.org (same contact information as for Women for Sobriety)
Moderation Management	212-871-0974	www.moderation.org
Secular Organizations for Sobriety (or Save Our Selves)	323-666-4295	www.sossobriety.org
SMART Recovery	Toll free: 866-951-5357 440-951-5357	www.smartrecovery.org
Women for Sobriety	215-536-8026	www.womenforsobriety.org

in all areas or may not welcome outsiders. In discussing their findings, students may gain insight into what patients may experience when told to go to AA without other instruction.

Another important issue in teaching about 12-step groups is the question of the clinician's role in addressing spiritual issues with patients. It is important to note that there are data to support the notion that clinicians often do not have the same spiritual beliefs as their patients. As noted in the discussion of Case 1 earlier, Gallup poll data have indicated that over 90% of Americans do express a belief in God (Bezilla 1993). This finding has been consistent for the past 60 years (Winseman 2005). Physicians may be less likely to endorse this belief (Daaleman and Frey 1999). Even if a clinician's spiritual or religious beliefs do not present an obstacle, there may be other resistances to exploring spiritual issues with patients, such as discomfort with this mode of inquiry, feeling inadequately trained to address spiritual matters, not having enough time, and concern about the patient's reaction to such an inquiry (Chibnall and Brooks 2001). Showing supervisees how their beliefs and attitudes may impact their approach to spiritual issues may help overcome some of the difficulties in addressing this important area with patients.

Television Series: *South Park*'s "Bloody Mary" Episode

The "Bloody Mary" episode of the *South Park* television series presents a unique opportunity to teach about addiction by countering some of the stereotypical perceptions of alcoholism and AA. In the episode, Stan's father is pulled over while the kids are in the car. He is noted to be drunk. He goes to court and is told to go to AA by the judge.

Teaching Point 1: The Disease Model of Addiction

During the AA meeting, alcoholism is discussed as a disease. The character then gives up any attempt at controlling his drinking, explaining that he has a disease and implying that he cannot help it. He takes on the sick role and starts drinking excessively. He is told that he can't cure the disease himself and that it's deadly.

This brings up the important concept of why addiction is viewed as a disease. Data show that alcoholism is a genetically influenced condition (such as diabetes and hypertension), suggesting that alcoholism is not just a moral failing or a personal weakness as some people may perceive it to be. Often a medical student's first introduction to addiction is through an encounter with a patient who repeatedly presents to the emergency room intoxicated and never seems to get better, fostering a sense of hopelessness about the patient's prognosis. Often judgments are made about this type of patient that can interfere with the clinician's care of the patient. It is important to take every opportunity to teach students that addiction is a treatable illness and that relapses happen just as they do with other chronic relapsing illnesses, such as diabetes, hypertension, and asthma.

Teaching Point 2: Powerlessness

The other notion of AA that is mocked in the television show is the idea that the individual is powerless (therefore Stan's father continues to drink). This is an important teaching point, because many patients bristle at the idea that they are powerless. Others may question the idea that an individual can be truly powerless and yet somehow stop drinking. Although powerlessness is a factor in alcoholism, it is helpful to clarify the concept as powerlessness that intensifies after the first drink. Criteria for alcohol dependence in the *Diagnostic and Statistical Manual of Mental Disorders* (DSM-IV-TR; American Psychiatric Association 2000) emphasize the inability to control drinking. Certainly because of cravings, an alcoholic individual may have more difficulty resisting having a drink than a nonalcoholic person. AA helps the individual to not take that first drink.

Teaching Point 3: AA as a Cult

In the television episode, a member in the AA meeting says, "The most fun thing I do is go to meetings." Stan's father refers to AA as a cult. This episode ridicules the way that meetings are emphasized and the fact that AA professes a spiritually based way of thinking or approaching life. Patients may resist going to AA meetings because AA seems like a cult to them. However, one of the key elements of AA is that it is a program of attraction, not recruitment—whereas in a cult, members are actively recruited. Another key difference between AA and cults is that there are no absolute rules in AA except that the individual have a desire to quit drinking. Meetings are an important part of the program; however, as people progress in the program, service to others takes on a greater role.

Teaching Point 4: Moderation Management

The episode ends with Stan's father cutting down on his drinking. Although alcoholic individuals fantasize about being able to drink socially, the very notion that the individual could do that is contrary to the definition of alcoholism. A significant number of people, perhaps 40% of those who choose to drink, at some point have a problem related to alcohol. However, not all of those people develop alcoholism; some of them are able to either stop drinking on their own or cut down on the amount they drink. There is evidence that physicians doing brief interventions with heavy drinkers can decrease drinking in those individuals. Remember that one of the DSM-IV-TR criteria is having a persistent desire and/or repeated unsuccessful attempts to stop drinking. So perhaps Stan's father falls into a different category: of being a problem drinker—but not being alcohol dependent.

Teaching Point 5: Alcohol Abuse Versus Alcohol Dependence

Stan's father was pulled over for driving under the influence. Does he meet criteria for alcohol dependence? Well, we don't know enough about his history for that. Does he meet criteria for alcohol abuse? We don't know enough information about this either. DSM-IV-TR criteria for abuse state that there must be repeated problems as a result of the use—not just one isolated incident. It is likely that someone who is caught driving while intoxicated has done so repeatedly, therefore meeting that criterion. However, it is not just the getting caught that is the problem; it's the behavior. It is also possible that this was the first time Stan's father did this and that he may use it as an opportunity to curb his drinking, and certainly change his behavior so that he does not drink and drive again. It is helpful to remind students that although understanding the criteria for abuse and dependence are useful guidelines in suggesting proper treatment, intervention is needed if the patient is consuming large quantities of alcohol and/or doing dangerous things while intoxicated—regardless of whether the patient meets diagnostic criteria for a substance use disorder. Counseling patients about safe levels of drinking (on average one drink per day for women and two drinks per day for men; U.S. Department of Agriculture and U.S. Department of Health and Human Services 2005) and the consequences of drinking are important parts of brief interventions that have been shown to help reduce drinking in at-risk patients (Babor et al. 2007).

Key Clinical Points

- There are differences between self-help groups and professional treatment.

- Involvement in self-help groups helps patients remain sober.

- Clinicians' knowledge of different types of self-help groups is useful in utilizing the principles of Motivational Interviewing to overcome resistances within addicted patients.

- Clinicians' awareness of their own biases regarding spirituality is important in helping motivate patients to engage in self-help groups.

Multiple-Choice Questions

For the correct answers to these questions, including explanations of answers, please see the Answer Guide at the end of this book.

1. The following is NOT an example of a mutual/self-help group for patients with substance use disorders:
   A. AA.
   B. SMART Recovery.
   C. Women for Sobriety.
   D. Recovery International.

2. The following BEST describes mutual/self-help:
   A. Substance use disorder treatment.
   B. AA.
   C. Peer support that functions as an adjunct to formal substance use disorder treatment.
   D. A social club.

3. The best way to handle a patient who declares "AA is too religious for me" is to:

   A. Roll with resistance and explore further why the patient feels this way.
   B. Reply, "AA is not religion."
   C. Insist that the patient attend 90 meetings in 90 days, as prescribed by AA.
   D. Insist the patient attend SMART Recovery meetings instead.

4. The following is a statement that is an example of expressing empathy in response to a patient telling you that he or she is not interested in AA because he or she is not religious:

   A. "I know how you feel. I don't believe in God, either."
   B. "I can understand that because you felt mistreated by nuns in grade school you are skeptical of anything that has to do with God."
   C. "You shouldn't let the past influence your choices now."
   D. "Try SMART Recovery instead."

5. The following statement is true:

   A. Ninety-five percent of people worldwide believe in God.
   B. Over 90% of physicians endorse the statement, "I believe in God."
   C. Over 90% of Americans endorse the statement, "I believe in God."
   D. One hundred percent of SMART Recovery participants believe in God.

References

American Psychiatric Association: Substance-Related Disorders Position Statement (APA Document Reference No 950011). Washington, DC, American Psychiatric Association, 1995. Available at: http://www.psych.org/Departments/EDU/Library/APAOfficialDocumentsandRelated/PositionStatements/199511.aspx. Accessed February 19, 2010.

American Psychiatric Association: Diagnostic and Statistical Manual of Mental Disorders, 4th Edition, Text Revision. Washington, DC, American Psychiatric Association, 2000

Babor TF, McRee BG, Kassebaum PA, et al: Screening, Brief Intervention and Referral to Treatment (SBIRT): toward a public health approach to the management of substance abuse. Subst Abus 28:7–30, 2007

Bezilla R (ed): Religion in America: 1992–1993. Princeton, NJ, Princeton Religion Research Center (The Gallup Organization), 1993

Chibnall JT, Brooks CA: Religion in the clinic: the role of physician beliefs. South Med J 94:374–379, 2001

Daaleman TP, Frey B: Spiritual and religious beliefs and practices of family physicians: a national survey. J Fam Pract 48:98–104, 1999

General Service Office of Alcoholics Anonymous: A.A. Fact File. New York, AA World Services, 2007

Jacobsen LK, Southwick SM, Kosten TR: Substance use disorders in patients with posttraumatic stress disorder: a review of the literature. Am J Psychiatry 158:1184–1190, 2001

Miller WR, Rollnick S: Ambivalence: the dilemma of change, in Motivational Interviewing: Preparing People to Change Addictive Behavior. New York, Guilford, 1991, pp 36–50

Montgomery HA, Miller WR, Tonigan JS: Does Alcoholics Anonymous involvement predict treatment outcome? J Subst Abuse Treat 12:241–246, 1995

SMART Recovery: Introduction page. Available at: www.smartrecovery.org. Accessed September 30, 2009

U.S. Department of Agriculture and U.S. Department of Health and Human Services: Alcoholic beverages, in Dietary Guidelines for Americans. Washington, DC, US Government Printing Office; 2005, pp 43–46

Winseman AL: Americans Have Little Doubt God Exists. December 13, 2005. Available at: http://www.gallup.com/poll/20437/americans-little-doubt-god-exists.aspx. Accessed February 19, 2010.

Women for Sobriety: Introduction page. Available at: www.womenforsobriety.org. Accessed September 30, 2009

CHAPTER 13

Adolescents

Ramon Solhkhah, M.D.
Georgia Gaveras, D.O.

Working in pediatric settings, for both physical and mental health, can present unique challenges to the clinician. Children and adolescents often require complex interventions to provide the necessary comprehensive and developmentally sensitive treatment. Brief interventions are particularly useful in working with youths with behavioral, developmental, or social problems. Among the brief interventions, Motivational Interviewing is often used (Dunn et al. 2001; Erickson et al. 2005). Motivational Interviewing was developed by Miller and Rollnick (1991, 2002) and its utility has been well described in the treatment of a wide group of disorders in adults, primarily substance abuse and dependence (Miller and Rollnick 2002).

Given the dearth of evidence-based practices in the treatment of many of these disorders, Motivational Interviewing and its structured derivative, Motivation Enhancement Therapy (MET), are often employed. (MET is further discussed in Chapter 16, "The Science of Motivational Interviewing"). To date, Motivational Interviewing and MET have been used in the treatment of adolescents with a wide variety of disorders and behaviors, including alcohol use disorders in the emergency room setting (Bailey et al. 2004; Monti et al. 2007), alcohol use disorders in the college setting (Marlatt et al. 1993), adolescent smoking (Brown et al. 2003; Colby et al. 1998, 2005), avoidance of dental care (Skaret et al. 2003), diabetes care (Channon et al. 2007), poor dietary adherence (Berg-Smith et al. 1999), pediatric obesity (Acosta et al. 2008; Barlow et al. 2007; Schwartz et al. 2007), antisocial and criminal behavior (Knopes 2004; Knott

2004), lack of contraception use (Cowley et al. 2002), lack of HIV transmission prevention (Brown and Lourie 2001), behaviors risking HIV transmission in HIV-positive youths (Naar-King et al. 2006, 2008), and adolescent marijuana abuse and dependence (Dennis et al. 2002, 2004; Diamond et al. 2002; Martin and Copeland 2008; Martin et al. 2005; Sampl and Kadden 2001).

In working with adolescents, the clinician needs to consider several aspects inherent in the use of Motivational Interviewing and MET. First of all, therapy should be developmentally sensitive (Carroll et al. 2001; Sindelar et al. 2004). Next, it must be personalized to the teenager that the clinician is working with (D'Amico et al. 2008; Deas 2008). Lastly, it is often helpful to use these approaches in conjunction with the Stages of Change model as originally described by Prochaska and DiClemente (1984) (Dennis et al. 2002; Dilallo and Weiss 2009).

The stages of change identify five areas an individual may inhabit in relation to a behavioral, psychosocial, or even medical disorder: precontemplation, contemplation, preparation, action, and maintenance (Prochaska and DiClemente 1984). In this chapter, the following case illustrates the various stages in a substance-abusing adolescent patient seen in an outpatient setting.

Clinical Case

Carrie was a 15-year-old girl who was brought to the emergency room of a large urban hospital by her mother for escalating substance abuse. She had been abusing marijuana and alcohol for 3 years and crystal methamphetamine for 6 months. Her longest period of sobriety was approximately 6 months, during which she regularly attended Alcoholics Anonymous (AA) and Narcotics Anonymous (NA) meetings. That ended recently when her family moved and she transferred to a new school. In the emergency room, she was diagnosed with polysubstance dependence and oppositional defiant disorder. She was not admitted to the hospital but was referred for follow-up in the child and adolescent psychiatry outpatient department.

The use of MET began in the emergency room in the initial interview. By using open-ended questions regarding her substance use, Carrie was able to discuss her use as a bond in her friendships. She felt that she had nothing in common with her parents, and she had no siblings; her social circle consisted entirely of people who used drugs. The interviewing clinician sympathized with her concerns about finding new friends at her new school and agreed with Carrie's assertion that she wanted to find people with common interests. Carrie admitted that drugs could be dangerous but would shut down when the risks of drug use were discussed. She refused to acknowledge the physical repercussions possible with drug use, and the therapist chose not to make this a focus because it risked alienating her. Fortunately, the therapeutic alliance could continue because the same clinician met with the patient in the outpatient setting.

In precontemplation, the patient is not yet even considering the possibility of change (Miller and Rollnick 1991). In this case, Carrie saw drug use as a social bond, the benefits of which outweighed any risks. In her eyes, there was no real incentive to change her behavior even though she had been brought to the emergency room by her parents. As adolescents struggle with what Erik Erikson (1980) calls *identity versus role confusion,* the individual no longer solely considers the values of his or her parents or other authority figures in the determination of self. The input from peers at this point outweighs consequences levied by the parents.

At this point, Carrie came to her appointments with her mother because there was no other transportation available to her, but she asked that her mother not be present for sessions. She would later say that she wanted only individual sessions because her mother might taint the therapist's perceptions. Carrie would talk about parties and using drugs with her friends. Although she did not view substance use as anything more than a common interest, like writing or watching movies, she did recognize that she did not use when alone. Carrie would assert her independence in many aspects—she was bright, creative, and talented—but deferred to her friends when it came to making plans or obtaining drugs. This became a focus of several sessions in which the therapist used open-ended questions to express empathy and develop Carrie's perception of discrepancies in her concepts of friendship and how drugs are involved. Although initially scheduled for weekly sessions, she asked to come in two times per week, to which both her family and therapist agreed. After several more sessions, Carrie admitted that she wanted to come in more often because it gave her an excuse not to see her friends. She would complain to them that her parents were forcing her to go to therapy more often, whereas in reality, she requested the increased frequency. This was her shift from precontemplation to the contemplation stage (Walker et al. 2006).

In using open-ended questions and reflective listening, the therapist allowed Carrie to identify what she considered to be negative consequences of her behavior rather than attempt to educate or admonish her on the decisions she had made thus far. After the ambivalence about her substance use was established, Carrie began to acknowledge the trouble that she was having with her parents as well as with herself. Again, in trying to establish her own identity, she began to question how much of that would be dictated by her peers and others.

Carrie recognized that when she did not do drugs she received positive feedback and even motivated herself to go to classes more often and complete homework. At the same time, she missed her social circle and felt that it was not worth the isolation she experienced to stop taking drugs in favor of praise from her teachers and parents. At this time, an admittedly fortuitous opportunity arose for Carrie. She had entered a local writing competition and her short story was selected as a finalist along with a dozen others in the state. She admitted that she was proud of her accomplishment and realized that she was most productive and creative when she hadn't been using. This insight was the beginning of her realization of reasons for change. The result from the writing competition was a concrete and immediate reward for Carrie that the therapist was able to use as a basis for more changes. Carrie's friends were passively congratulatory, but Carrie later admitted they never asked again of the results of the competition. Although she did not win, she was encouraged by her teachers to enroll in an advanced writing course that could possibly qualify as college credit in the future. Carrie had never thought of college as an option and in the past had remarked that she did not think that it was a necessity for her. She was now excited about the possibility of going to college "out of state and leaving [her] family."

Carrie was an intelligent young woman for whom college was a realistic goal. Affirming her accomplishments, the therapist further solidified the alliance with the patient, who was beginning to show pride in her accomplishments. Although she said that the intention of going to college out of state was motivated by a desire to leave her family, Carrie later admitted that she felt the most pride about the writing competition when talking with her parents. She said that she felt as she had when she was "a little girl." Asked to explain why this was a positive feeling in light of her desire for independence, Carrie stated that she felt acceptance and love from her parents for who she was, for what felt like the first time since she was a child.

Carrie moved into the next stage of change, preparation, when she decided that she would like to try abstaining from drugs and alcohol as a "test." She knew that this would be difficult to do if she continued to spend time with the same group of friends, so she decided to enroll in a local after-school writing workshop at a community college near her home. Her parents were very resistant at first for fear that being around college students would open up a new venue for Carrie to use drugs. This became an opportunity for Carrie to involve her family in her treatment, and at their first family session Carrie presented her idea and plan for remaining abstinent. She, with help from her therapist, had conceived a timetable for Carrie's week to which her parents agreed.

After several more weeks, Carrie said that she would be attending a party being thrown by some of her high school friends. She said she was nervous because she had not used drugs for 20 days and felt that she had been doing well. She discussed with her therapist the reasons why she wanted to go to the party and eventually admitted to feeling lonely. This was the first time that Carrie had discussed any mood problems since she began treatment. In the end, she opted out of the party, and in the subsequent weeks, talked more about the mood component of her substance use. She discussed her resentment toward her father, who although still married to her mother, was never home. She also talked about her negative self-image and that her last group of friends had been the ones who accepted her regardless of her appearance.

This marked the beginning of her taking action to change her behaviors—when she decided to stay away from the party and continue working on abstinence from substances. In skipping the party and avoiding her old friends' invitations to spend time together after school, they had drifted away and she no longer felt as though she belonged in that social circle, but she had not become part of a different one. She eventually came to realize that she would need to work on the underlying issues that had been discovered. In part, those issues were the reasons she had been using and needed to be addressed if she were going to continue to be abstinent. Eventually, her parents engaged in family therapy and they began to attend Al-Anon meetings while Carrie went to AA and NA meetings again. Carrie continued to do well in school and eventually found a niche in the dramatic arts department at her school, where she helped write and design sets for school plays. She later remarked to her therapist that she never thought she'd be a "drama club geek." This marked the maintenance phase of her sobriety. She continued to address issues in family and individual therapy and terminated treatment shortly before going to college. She did, in fact, go to college out of state, where she continued treatment with a counselor at college.

Discussion of the Clinical Case

This case exemplifies several of the principles of Motivational Interviewing/ MET. Most notably and specific to adolescents is the therapist's restraint in preaching the ill effects of drugs and alcohol (Gance-Cleveland 2007). The social implications of stopping Carrie's drug and alcohol use were more important than any physical or emotional effects of the substances. While Carrie sought to determine her own identity, she was rejecting input from authority figures such as her parents and physicians. With Motivational Interviewing/MET, she was able to realize that she was basing her identity on her peers and their influences and ideals. The fear of social rejection kept her from using her own interests and talents as a basis for her developing identity. This realization led her to question her actions and behaviors as being ineffective and actually keeping her from reaching goals that she then had set for herself. When she was able to come to this conclusion on her own, she was empowered to ask more questions about drugs as well as to take steps toward furthering her writing. She also began to work on repairing relationships that she had let suffer, including that with her parents. Importantly, Carrie was able to take these steps at a crucial time that allowed her to complete high school and move on to college. It is easy to imagine that without treatment, her drug use could have led to unrealized goals and underachievement.

Suggestions for Treatment

Research on the techniques of MET has ranged from research on its use as a single, brief intervention in the emergency room setting (Tait and Hulse 2003; Tait et al. 2005) to its use as multisession, manualized therapy (Barrowclough et al. 2001; Diamond et al. 2002). The four principles of Motivational Interviewing as described by Miller and Rollnick (2002) are expressing empathy, developing discrepancies, rolling with resistance, and supporting self-efficacy. These principles all build on the primary adolescent developmental task of individuation—the process "in which adolescents develop separate identities from their parents or caregivers" (Sampl and Kadden 2001, p. 26).

The first principle of *expressing empathy* requires the use of active listening by clinicians with accurate reflection of the thoughts expressed by the teenager (Grenard et al. 2006). The clinician should avoid confrontation and instead strive to understand the adolescent and to let the patient feel accepted.

Next, the clinician works to *develop discrepancies* in the statements made by the teens. Most often this occurs by pointing out ways that the behavior in question is interfering with the adolescent's stated life goals. Again, the manner should be nonjudgmental and nonconfrontational, with the clinician using words and ideas that the adolescent himself or herself has expressed (Smith and Hall 2007). The goal is to create cognitive dissonance in the teenager's mind. This may be accomplished by reflecting back on negative effects such as poor school performance, academic failure, legal consequences, and so forth (Diamond et al. 2002).

Another principle is framed as *rolling with resistance*. This notion is not dissimilar to principles of martial arts whereby an individual uses opponents' strength and momentum against them. The clinician uses the resistance of the teenager to highlight contradictions; demonstrate understanding and acceptance of the individual with nonconfrontational, nonjudgmental statements and inquiries; and focus on empathic responses (Solhkhah 2003). Intermixed with the principle of rolling with resistance is the notion of avoiding argumentation. Clinicians can often find themselves dragged into an argument with teenagers, as opposed to a Motivational Interviewing/MET–based intervention (Tait et al. 2004). This trap needs to be avoided with most patients, but particularly with teenagers, in whom identity issues and struggles with authorities are part of the normal developmental milieu (Helstrom et al. 2007).

Lastly, the therapist works to bolster the teenager's *self-efficacy*. This can be accomplished by reminding the youth of previous successes in dealing with the problem behavior (e.g., times in the past when the person stopped using drugs or alcohol, times when he or she lost weight) or identifying times or strategies used when he or she mastered other life struggles. Self-efficacy also can be fostered by reinforcing little successes in the current treatment toward effecting change (Diamond et al. 2002).

Clinicians can fall into many traps when working with teenagers, so it's best to be aware of potential pitfalls. Most important, the clinician needs to avoid the "I'm the expert" way of thinking. Teens rebel against authority and particularly against parental figures. A corollary to this approach is to avoid being too chummy with kids. The clinician needs to be respectful, nonjudgmental, and empathic—and sure to maintain boundaries. Another common mistake is to focus on too many details and to respond with questions asking for elaboration rather than making reflective statements.

When clinicians work with teenagers in a Motivational Interviewing/MET framework, the initial goals focus on the teen being able to verbalize self-efficacy in four areas:

1. Recognize the presence of a problem
2. Express some concern over the presence of that problem or the impact of the problem on some aspect of his or her life

3. Verbalize some intention to change that behavior
4. Express optimism and hope that he or she will be able to overcome this problem area in his or her life.

Most commonly, clinicians new to the Motivational Interviewing/MET approach facilitate resistance rather than rolling with it. Warning signs of resistance include the patient arguing or disagreeing with the clinician. Teenage patients may also ignore or interrupt the clinician. Another sign of resistance is minimizing the scope of the problem or denying its existence. When these signs occur, and they often do, clinicians can refocus by using simple reflective statements, shifting focus, or highlighting personal control. As described by Hopfer (1999), more advanced techniques include using a *reframe*—presenting risk in behavior in a much more prominent role, reframing a weakness as a strength, or using an "agreement with a twist" (i.e., using a reflective statement followed by a reframe). Signs that a teen is truly ready to change are often demonstrated by the teen appearing more quiet and pensive, the teen being less argumentative and asking more questions of the clinician, and lastly by increased talk of a future without the behavior in question (Hopfer 1999).

Suggestions for Teaching and Supervision

When teaching and supervising aspects of Motivational Interviewing/MET, it is important to remember a couple of key points. First, remind the student or supervisee not to forget their role in enhancing the patient's motivation for change. Often, the clinician's primary role is to be cheerleader and offer a sympathetic ear. Also, instruct the student to avoid simple solutions to complex problems. If simple solutions had worked, the teenage patient likely would not have had to see a clinician in the first place.

Movie: *Antwone Fisher*

Antwone Fisher (2002) is an excellent movie to highlight principles of Motivational Interviewing/MET in working with adolescents and young adults. The film, directed by and starring Denzel Washington (as psychiatrist Jerome Davenport), is based on the true story of a young Navy sailor, Antwone Fisher, who is forced to see a psychiatrist after a violent outburst. During the treatment with the psychiatrist, the young man (played by Derek Luke) reveals a history of a horrific childhood including foster care, trauma, abuse, neglect, and exposure to violence. Just about any one of the scenes between Antwone and Dr. Davenport highlights the Motivational Interviewing/MET principles, including empathic responses, rolling with resistance, development of discrepancies, and support of self-efficacy.

Key Clinical Points

- Motivational Interviewing/MET is an evidenced-based intervention suitable for working with teenagers with a wide variety of disorders.

- When working with adolescents, the clinician must always be developmentally sensitive.

- Clinicians need to constantly work to promote self-efficacy in teenagers to maintain trust and enhance the therapeutic relationship.

Multiple-Choice Questions

For the correct answers to these questions, including explanations of answers, please see the Answer Guide at the end of this book.

1. Which of the following is NOT a sign of resistance?

    A. Arguing.
    B. Questioning.
    C. Ignoring.
    D. Minimizing.

2. According to Erik Erikson, the developmental stage that hallmarks adolescence is:

    A. Trust versus mistrust.
    B. Initiative versus guilt.
    C. Identity versus role confusion.
    D. Integrity versus despair.

3. Teenagers verbalize self-efficacy in each of the following ways, EXCEPT:

    A. Expressing concern for a problem or effects of the problem.
    B. Expressing optimism for overcoming the problem.

C. Recognizing the presence of a problem.

D. Being told the expert opinion on a topic by a clinician.

4. Motivational Interviewing/MET has been studied in work with adolescents with all of the following disorders, EXCEPT:

A. Adolescent substance abuse.

B. Pediatric obsessive-compulsive disorder (OCD).

C. Adolescent HIV transmission prevention.

D. Avoidance of dental care.

5. All of these are signs that a teenager is ready to change, EXCEPT:

A. Asking more questions.

B. Labeling substance use as problematic.

C. Being argumentative.

D. Increasing talk about the future.

References

Acosta M, Manubay J, Levin F: Pediatric obesity: parallels with addiction and treatment recommendations. Harv Rev Psychiatry16:80–96, 2008

Bailey K, Baker A, Webster R, et al: Pilot randomized controlled trial of a brief alcohol intervention group for adolescents. Drug Alcohol Rev 23:157–166, 2004

Barlow SE; Expert Committee: Expert committee recommendations regarding the prevention, assessment, and treatment of child and adolescent overweight and obesity: summary report. Pediatrics 120 (suppl 4):S164–S192, 2007

Barrowclough C, Haddock G, Tarrier N, et al: Randomized controlled trial of motivational interviewing, cognitive behavior therapy, and family intervention for patients with comorbid schizophrenia and substance use disorders. Am J Psychiatry 158:1706–1713, 2001

Berg-Smith SM, Stevens VJ, Brown KM, et al: A brief motivational intervention to improve dietary adherence in adolescents: The Dietary Intervention Study in Children (DISC) Research Group. Health Educ Res 14:399–410, 1999

Brown L, Lourie K: Motivational interviewing and the prevention of HIV among adolescents, in Adolescents, Alcohol and Substance Abuse: Reaching Teens Through Brief Intervention. Edited by Monti P. New York, Guilford Press, 2001, pp 244–274

Brown RA, Ramsey SE, Strong DR, et al: Effects of motivational interviewing on smoking cessation in adolescents with psychiatric disorders. Tob Control 12 (suppl 4):IV3–IV10, 2003

Carroll K, Libby B, Sheehan J, et al: Motivational interviewing to enhance treatment initiation in substance abusers: an effectiveness study. Am J Addict 10:335–339, 2001

Channon SJ, Huws-Thomas MV, Rollnick S, et al: A multicenter randomized controlled trial of motivational interviewing in teenagers with diabetes. Diabetes Care 30:1390–1395, 2007

Colby SM, Monti PM, Barnett NP, et al: Brief motivational interviewing in a hospital setting for adolescent smoking: a preliminary study. J Consult Clin Psychol 66:574–578, 1998

Colby S, Monti P, Tevyaw T, et al: Brief motivational intervention for adolescent smokers in medical settings. Addict Behav 30:865–874, 2005

Cowley CB, Farley T, Beamis K: "Well, maybe I'll try the pill for just a few months…": brief motivational and narrative-based interventions to encourage contraceptive use among adolescents at high risk for early childbearing. Fam Syst Health 20:183–204, 2002

D'Amico E, Miles J, Stern S, et al: Brief motivational interviewing for teens at risk of substance use consequences: a randomized pilot study in a primary care clinic. J Subst Abuse Treat 35:53–61, 2008

Deas D: Evidence-based treatments for alcohol use disorders in adolescents. Pediatrics 121 (suppl 4):S348–S354, 2008

Dennis M, Titus J, Diamond G, et al: The Cannabis Youth Treatment (CYT) experiment: rationale, study design and analysis plans. Addiction 97 (suppl 1):16–34, 2002

Dennis M, Godley S, Diamond G, et al: The Cannabis Youth Treatment (CYT) Study: main findings from two randomized trials. J Subst Abuse Treat 27:195–196, 2004

Diamond G, Godley SH, Liddle HA, et al: Five outpatient treatment models for adolescent marijuana abuse: a description of the Cannabis Youth Treatment interventions. Addiction 97 (suppl 1):70–83, 2002

Dilallo J, Weiss G: Motivational interviewing and adolescent psychopharmacology. J Am Acad Child Adolesc Psychiatry 48:108–113, 2009

Dunn C, Deroo L, Rivara FP: The use of brief interventions adapted from motivational interviewing across behavioral domains: a systematic review. Addiction 96:1725–1742, 2001

Erickson SJ, Gerstle M, Feldstein SW: Brief interventions and motivational interviewing with children, adolescents, and their parents in pediatric health care settings: a review. Arch Pediatr Adolesc Med 159:1173–1180, 2005

Erikson E: Identity and the Life Cycle. New York, WW Norton, 1980

Gance-Cleveland B: Motivational interviewing: improving patient education. J Pediatr Health Care 21:81–88, 2007

Grenard J, Ames S, Pentz M, et al: Motivational interviewing with adolescents and young adults for drug-related problems. Int J Adolesc Med Health 18:53–67, 2006

Helstrom A, Hutchinson K, Bryan A: Motivational enhancement therapy for high-risk adolescent smokers. Addict Behav 32:2404–2410, 2007

Hopfer CJ: Motivational interviewing: workshop on building skills in the treatment of substance-dependent adolescents. Presented at the 46th Annual Meeting of the American Academy of Child & Adolescent Psychiatry, Chicago, IL, October 19–24, 1999

Knopes DR: Motivating change in high-risk adolescents: an intervention focus on the deviant friendship process. Dissertation Abstracts International: Section B: The Sciences and Engineering 65 (2-B)B, 2004

Knott JM: Self-efficacy and motivation to change among chronic youth offenders: an exploratory examination of the efficacy of an experiential learning motivation enhancement intervention (doctoral dissertation, University of Oregon, 2004). Dissertation Abstracts International 65(02):411A, 2004

Marlatt GA, Somers JM, Tapert SF: Harm reduction: application to alcohol abuse problems. NIDA Res Monogr 137:147–166, 1993

Martin G, Copeland J: The adolescent cannabis check-up: randomized trial of a brief intervention for young cannabis users. J Subst Abuse Treat 34:407–414, 2008

Martin G, Copeland J, Swift W: The Adolescent Cannabis Check-Up: feasibility of a brief intervention for young cannabis users. J Subst Abuse Treat 29:207–213, 2005

Miller WR, Rollnick S: Motivational Interviewing: Preparing People to Change Addictive Behavior. New York, Guilford, 1991

Miller WR, Rollnick S: Motivational Interviewing: Preparing People for Change, 2nd Edition. New York, Guilford, 2002

Monti PM, Barnett NP, Colby SM, et al: Motivational interviewing versus feedback only in emergency care for young adult problem drinking. Addiction 102:1234–1243, 2007

Naar-King S, Wright K, Parsons J, et al: Transtheoretical model and condom use in HIV-positive youths. Health Psychol 25:648–652, 2006

Naar-King S, Lam P, Wang B, et al: Brief report: maintenance of effects of motivational enhancement therapy to improve risk behaviors and HIV-related health in a randomized controlled trial of youth living with HIV. J Pediatr Psychol 33:441–445, 2008

Prochaska JO, DiClemente CC: The Transtheoretical Approach: Crossing Traditional Boundaries of Therapy. Homewood, IL, Dow Jones-Irwin, 1984

Sampl S, Kadden R: Motivational Enhancement Therapy and Cognitive Behavioral Therapy for Adolescent Cannabis Users: 5 Sessions (Cannabis Youth Treatment [CYT] Series, Vol 1; DHHS Publ No 01–3846). Rockville, MD, Center for Substance Abuse Treatment, Substance Abuse and Mental Health Services Administration, 2001

Schwartz RP, Hamre R, Dietz WH, et al: Office-based motivational interviewing to prevent childhood obesity: a feasibility study. Arch Pediatr Adolesc Med 161:495–501, 2007

Sindelar H, Abrantes A, Hart C, et al: Motivational interviewing in pediatric practice. Curr Probl Pediatr Adolesc Health Care 34:322–339, 2004

Skaret E, Weinstein P, Kvale G, et al: An intervention program to reduce dental avoidance behaviour among adolescents: a pilot study. Eur J Paediatr Dent 4:191–196, 2003

Smith D, Hall J: Strengths-oriented referrals for teens (SORT): giving balanced feedback to teens and families. Health Soc Work 32:69–72, 2007

Solhkhah R: The intoxicated child. Child Adolesc Psychiatr Clin N Am 12:693–722, 2003

Tait R, Hulse G: A systematic review of the effectiveness of brief interventions with substance using adolescents by type of drug. Drug Alcohol Rev 22:337–346, 2003

Tait R, Hulse G, Robertson S: Effectiveness of a brief-intervention and continuity of care in enhancing attendance for treatment by adolescent substance users. Drug Alcohol Depend 74:289–296, 2004

Tait R, Hulse G, Robertson S, et al: Emergency department-based intervention with adolescent substance users: 12-month outcomes. Drug Alcohol Depend 79:359–363, 2005

Walker D, Roffman R, Stephens R: Motivational enhancement therapy for adolescent marijuana users: a preliminary randomized controlled trial. J Consult Clin Psychol 74:628–632, 2006

CHAPTER 14

Older Adults

Susan D. Whitley, M.D.

Substance misuse in older adults is a growing problem with enormous costs to individuals and society. The majority of older adults with problems related to substance use present in settings other than addiction treatment centers; in those settings it seems likely that many will be in the precontemplation or contemplation stage regarding the need to change behaviors. Health care and social service professionals must be alert to potential problems and be equipped to intervene when problems are identified.

Studies estimate that as many as 15% of men and 12% of women age 60 and older who are treated in the primary care setting regularly drink in excess of limits recommended by the National Institute on Alcohol Abuse and Alcoholism (NIAAA) (Center for Substance Abuse Treatment 1998). Surveys estimate that 6%–11% of hospitalized elderly patients exhibit symptoms of alcohol misuse, as do 20% of elderly patients admitted to psychiatric wards and 14% of elderly patients seen in emergency rooms (National Institute on Alcohol Abuse and Alcoholism 1998). Substance use and misuse contribute to accidents as well as to worsening of chronic medical illness and mental illness. As the population in the United States ages, the scope of this problem can be expected to grow, increasing the imperative that clinicians be prepared.

Illicit drug use also occurs, but this is less common in older adults. A study of geriatric psychiatry inpatients found just 4% with substance use disorders (other than alcohol abuse), with 3% misusing prescription drugs and only 1% using illicit drugs (Edgell et al. 2000). The misuse of prescription drugs is relatively more common, although the scope of the problem is difficult to estimate. People age 65 and older are the largest consumers of prescription medications, accounting for consumption of one-quarter of the prescription drugs sold in the United States (Culberson and Ziska 2008). Adverse consequences from prescription drug use can occur even when the individual does not intend to misuse them. Older adults using benzodiazepines are particularly vulnerable to risks such as daytime sedation, cognitive impairment, and falls (Fick et al. 2003). Nonprescription use of opiate pain relievers is uncommon, with estimates from the National Survey on Drug Use and Health of approximately 1% among people ages 50 and older (Blazer and Wu 2009). Unintentional misuse, however, is harder to quantify. Other medications, including sleep aids and antihistamines, carry a risk for adverse effects in older adults. Problems may be compounded by interactions with other medications or concomitant use of alcohol, even at low levels.

Routine screening for alcohol and prescription drug abuse is recommended; however, multiple barriers exist. Provider biases and a low index of suspicion contribute to underidentification of these problems. In addition, diagnostic criteria may be misleading and contribute to underdiagnosis. Medical and psychiatric comorbidities may distract family members and health care providers from the true nature of a substance use problem. Sleep problems, depressed mood, and memory deficits may all be worsened by substance use but also may be falsely attributed to the normal aging process. Finally, once a problem has been identified, many providers may feel unprepared to address it.

Despite strong recommendations in favor of screening, there has been limited study of treatment options in the older adult population. Employing the tools of Motivational Interviewing to address problematic alcohol use has been well studied and validated in the general population. Translation of these techniques to the population of older adults makes empirical sense. While further research is ongoing, expert guidelines as well as a small selection of published studies, discussed later in the section "Suggestions for Treatment," strongly support the use of Motivational Interviewing in the population of older adults.

In this chapter, I focus on the more common misuse of alcohol and prescription drugs, although providers also must remain alert to the possibility of illicit drug use. The same techniques of screening and intervention can be applied to older individuals regardless of the substance being used.

Clinical Case

Kate is a 66-year-old female presenting for follow-up regarding hypertension. While reviewing her chart, you recall that her blood pressure at the previous visit was somewhat elevated (152/92) after years of excellent control with hydrochlorothiazide. During the previous visit, she mentioned that she was hav-

---

TABLE 14–1. The CAGE questionnaire

C   Have you ever felt you should *cut down* on your drinking?

A   Have people *annoyed* you by criticizing your drinking?

G   Have you ever felt bad or *guilty* about your drinking?

E   Have you ever had a drink first thing in the morning to steady your nerves or get rid of a hangover (*eye opener*)?

Source.   Ewing 1984.

ing difficulty sleeping and felt this was the likely explanation for her increase in blood pressure. She also admitted to forgetting to take her medication some mornings because she was more tired than usual. You counseled her about medication compliance and scheduled a follow-up visit in 2 months. She has no other medical problems.

At today's visit, her blood pressure is again elevated. You notice bruises on both knees. When questioned, she explains that she fell at home while walking to her bedroom from the living room in the evening 1 week ago. She had no dizziness or loss of consciousness and explains, "I must just be getting clumsy." Her sleep remains poor, and she continues to forget to take her blood pressure medication some mornings.

A quick review of her social history reminds you that she is a retired schoolteacher, widowed, and living alone. You inquire about her adult daughter who lives close by and she reports that they have been seeing less of each other because her daughter is busy with a new job and a new boyfriend. She admits to feeling lonely. She used to spend time as a volunteer with children at a local after-school program; however, today she indicates that she is not doing this as much because she does not have the energy. Flipping through the chart, you notice in her admission paperwork that she is an ex-smoker, has reported no history of depression, and has answered *no* to all CAGE questions (Table 14–1).

Concerned about her apparent forgetfulness and the recent fall, you decide to investigate further. You ask if she has tried anything to help with her sleep problem. She reveals that several months ago, she started having a drink at night to help her relax. She is now having 1 or 2 drinks nightly, as this is the only thing that helps her fall asleep. On some nights she also takes one of the "little white pills" that her neighbor shared with her. You decide to readminister the CAGE questionnaire. You do so in a conversational and open-ended manner to invite dialogue. She indicates that she has not felt the need to cut down on her drinking. Her daughter has expressed some concern, and the patient does find it annoying when her daughter asks about her drinking. As a result, she has made an effort to conceal her drinking but denies feeling guilty. She is adamant that she only drinks in the evening to help herself relax and fall asleep. She does not express any concern about taking sleeping pills as "my neighbor's doctor prescribed them." She does sometimes fall asleep in front of the television, and this is likely what happened on the night she fell.

TABLE 14–2. Triggers for screening
Sleep complaints
Cognitive impairment
Seizures
Malnutrition, muscle wasting
Liver function abnormalities
Altered mood: depression, anxiety, irritability
Poor hygiene, self-neglect
Unexplained gastrointestinal complaints (nausea, vomiting)
Slurred speech
Altered gait or poor coordination
Falls or unexplained bruising

Source.   Adapted from Center for Substance Abuse Treatment 1998.

Discussion of the Clinical Case

Screening for alcohol and prescription drug misuse is recommended as part of routine physical exams in all older adults and should be repeated when certain physical symptoms are present (Table 14–2) and during major life changes or transitions (Center for Substance Abuse Treatment 1998). In this case, the sudden poor control of a previously stable medical issue (hypertension), sleep disturbance, and the patient's falling are red flags for a possible substance use problem.

Use of a standardized screening instrument is preferable and multiple screening tools have been validated in the older adult population. The CAGE questionnaire (Ewing 1984; see Table 14–1) is easy to administer and can be adapted to screen for problematic use of other drugs; see also the CAGE Adapted to Include Drugs questionnaire (CAGE-AID; Brown and Rounds 1995). In older adults, an answer of *yes* to any of the CAGE questions should trigger further assessment. Another option, the Alcohol Use Disorders Identification Test (AUDIT), is a 10-item, self-administered, written screening tool that has been validated in multiple primary care settings (Reinert and Allen 2007). The Michigan Alcoholism Screening Test—Geriatric Version (MAST-G; Blow et al. 1992) and its short version (S-MAST-G; Blow et al. 1998; Figure 14–1) were developed specifically for use in older adults. It is advisable to become familiar with a few tools and decide on the one most suitable to your practice. Cognitive impairment may interfere with the screening process. Obtaining collateral information from family or friends is helpful.

Short Michigan Alcoholism Screening Test—
Geriatric Version (S-MAST-G)

	YES (1)	NO (0)
1. When talking with others, do you ever underestimate how much you actually drink?	_____	_____
2. After a few drinks, have you sometimes not eaten or been able to skip a meal because you didn't feel hungry?	_____	_____
3. Does having a few drinks help decrease your shakiness or tremors?	_____	_____
4. Does alcohol sometimes make it hard for you to remember parts of the day or night?	_____	_____
5. Do you usually take a drink to relax or calm your nerves?	_____	_____
6. Do you drink to take your mind off your problems?	_____	_____
7. Have you ever increased your drinking after experiencing a loss in your life?	_____	_____
8. Has a doctor or nurse ever said they were worried or concerned about your drinking?	_____	_____
9. Have you ever made rules to manage your drinking?	_____	_____
10. When you feel lonely, does having a drink help?	_____	_____

TOTAL S-MAST-G SCORE (0–10) _____

FIGURE 14–1.   Short Michigan Alcoholism Screening Test—Geriatric Version (S-MAST-G). Copyright © 1991 The Regents of the University of Michigan.

Scoring: 2 or more "yes" responses indicative of alcohol problem.

For further information, contact Frederic Blow, Ph.D., at University of Michigan Mental Health Services Outcomes & Translation Section, 4250 Plymouth Road, SPC 5765, Ann Arbor, MI 48109-5765.

Source.   Blow et al. 1998.

Defining the problem of alcohol or prescription drug misuse may be difficult, especially in older adults. Safe drinking levels are not as clear for older adults, but are clearly lower than for the general population. NIAAA guidelines indicate that healthy women of any age as well as healthy men over age 65 who drink more than 3 drinks per day (or more than 7 per week) are at increased risk for alcohol-related problems (National Institute on Alcohol Abuse and Alcoholism 2005). Lower tolerance, slower metabolism, and increased risk for interaction with prescription medications add up to a lower level of drinking that can be considered safe in older adults. Lower limits or abstinence are advisable for patients who take medications that interact with alcohol or who have a health condition exacerbated by alcohol.

Many clinicians, especially psychiatrists, rely on the latest criteria from the *Diagnostic and Statistical Manual of Mental Disorders* (DSM) for the diagnosis of substance use disorders (American Psychiatric Association 2000). Use of DSM criteria for the diagnosis of substance abuse and dependence, however, will result in failure to identify many patients who are at risk for adverse consequences from drinking or drug use. Using the categories of at-risk and problem drinking will decrease false-negatives and increase the flexibility in describing drinking problems in older adults (Table 14–3). People who do not meet DSM criteria for alcohol abuse or dependence might still have a problem that requires intervention.

When problem alcohol or drug use is present, a high index of suspicion for psychiatric comorbidity is warranted. Studies indicate that as many as 30% of older adults abusing alcohol have a primary mood disorder (Koenig and Blazer 1996). Follow-up questions about mood, sleep, appetite, feelings of guilt, low energy, impaired concentration, hopelessness, and suicidality should be included. A standard screening instrument, such as the nine-item depression scale of the Patient Health Questionnaire (PHQ-9), is an alternative (Kroenke et al. 2001). When primary depression is suspected it should generally be treated concurrently with the substance use problem. Substance-induced symptoms may not require treatment if the patient successfully stops using.

The information collected indicates that your patient is having 7–14 drinks weekly, more than NIAAA-recommended levels for an older female. She is experiencing negative consequences including worsening of a chronic medical condition, falls, insomnia, and possibly major depression. This adds up to a diagnosis of problem drinking. Her initial statements indicate that she is precontemplative regarding the need to change, but she appears open to further discussion.

Suggestions for Treatment

The following suggestions for treatment are based on recommendations summarized in the Substance Abuse and Mental Health Services Administration's Treatment Improvement Protocol 26 (Center for Substance Abuse Treatment 1998) and reflect a combination of expert guidelines plus the author's own opinion and clinical experience. Many of these recommendations are based on work done at the University of Michigan and are elaborated in the textbook *Alcohol Problems in Older Adults: Prevention and Management* (Barry et al. 2001). The book also includes a "Health Promotion Workbook for Older Adults" with many useful clinical tools in both English and Spanish.

Once a problem has been identified, Motivational Interviewing offers a tool for both further assessment and intervention. If more intensive interven-

TABLE 14–3.　Patterns of alcohol consumption in older adults

Abstainers and light drinkers

Drink no alcohol or less than 3 drinks per month

Alcohol use does not affect health or result in negative consequences

Moderate drinkers

Drink 1 to 2 standard drinks per occasion

Drink three or fewer times per week

Alcohol use does not affect health or result in negative consequences

When appropriate, consume NO alcohol (such as before driving, while operating machinery, and so forth)

At-risk drinkers

Drink more than 3 drinks per occasion

Drink more than 7 standard drinks per week

No current problems, but at risk for negative health or social consequences

Lower threshold for those with medical or psychiatric comorbidities

Problem drinkers

More hazardous levels of consumption

Clear negative health or social consequences

Dependent drinkers

Physical dependence on alcohol may be present

More serious health and social consequences

Source.　Adapted from Center for Substance Abuse Treatment 1998.

tion becomes necessary, you will have established a treatment alliance and set the stage to move patients toward the needed level of care. By tailoring interventions to the patient's readiness for change, you can reduce the risk of prematurely labeling a problem or rupturing the treatment alliance. Depending on the treatment setting and the patient's readiness for change, your intervention may take place in a single session or become an ongoing discussion over several months.

Motivational Interviewing for changing substance use behaviors has been well studied and validated in the general population (Dunn et al. 2001; Vasilaki et al. 2006). Although fewer studies have been carried out in older adults, existing evidence is favorable. The first major study of the efficacy of Brief Motivational Interviewing in problem drinkers age 65 and older is Project GOAL

(Guiding Older Adult Lifestyles) (Fleming et al. 1999). This study demonstrated that two 10- to 15-minute interventions delivered by physicians in primary care settings reduced the total number of drinks per week, the frequency of binge drinking, and the frequency of excessive drinking compared with levels in a control group receiving only general health information. These differences persisted up to 1 year. Interviews with older adult substance users indicate a higher level of satisfaction with client-centered approaches than with confrontational approaches (West and Graham 1999). Case studies of older adults successfully treated with Motivational Interviewing–based interventions are also present in the literature (Royer et al. 2000).

Another small study of Brief Motivational Interviewing interventions in primary care patients age 65 and older demonstrated reduction in drinking levels but no difference in outcomes such as emergency room visits, hospitalizations, office visits, injuries, or mortality (Mundt et al. 2005). Further studies are needed to demonstrate the benefit of these interventions as well as their impact on health care utilization and longer-term outcomes. It is likely that similar interventions can be used successfully in other treatment settings, such as general psychiatry, but again further study is needed.

These brief interventions are targeted for at-risk or problem drinkers and do not apply to alcohol-dependent individuals. If a patient is in danger of immediate health consequences or has symptoms of alcohol withdrawal, your level of concern must be higher. Involve family members immediately and refer the patient to an addiction specialist if possible.

Use a nonjudgmental tone to create an atmosphere of collaboration. The level of shame may be higher among older adults, making risky behaviors harder to uncover and discuss. Older adults may be reluctant to openly question your authority as a health care professional. Be alert to nonverbal indicators of discomfort. Avoiding labels, avoiding confrontation, and accepting ambivalence all will assist you in engaging this patient. It is not about making the perfect statement; rather, focus on maintaining a respectful dialogue and be attentive to the flow of the conversation.

Use the early part of the interview to establish rapport and gather more information. Ask questions to identify the patient's goals, priorities, and current level of concern about the situation. Follow up with reflections and summary statements. Once the patient's concerns and goals are identified, they can be used later to develop discrepancy with current behaviors and to develop a plan of action. Appropriate questions or statements could include the following (these and other sample questions and statements throughout this section are based on the clinical case discussed earlier in this chapter):

- "What concerns you about your blood pressure becoming difficult to control?"
- "How worried are you about your sleep problem?"

- "What made you curtail your volunteer work?"
- "It sounds like you are feeling lonely and your mood has been down."

Specific advice is best given after asking permission to give it or when the patients asks for it. When possible, make a clear matter-of-fact statement about the patient's current level of drinking. Discuss where the patient's drinking behavior fits into population norms for his or her age group. Be sure to include the definition of a standard drink as part of this description. You might say something like:

- "The amount you are drinking is higher than what is considered safe for a woman your age and may put you at risk for problems."
- "As we age, our bodies don't handle alcohol as well. Even 1 or 2 drinks might affect you more than it did when you were younger."

An intervention based on the principles of Motivational Interviewing requires discussion of both the positive and negative aspects of drinking. Change occurs when perceived risks outweigh benefits. This discussion will serve to further develop discrepancy and provide material for a decisional balance (discussed in further detail in Chapter 4, "Contemplation"). Engage in an empathic discussion of the patient's reasons for drinking and seek to understand the role of alcohol as a coping strategy. Social isolation, boredom, and negative family interactions are common triggers. You might ask questions like:

- "So, drinking helps you to relax and sleep better?"
- "Does drinking help you cope when you feel lonely or bored?"

Discuss the consequences of drinking. Focus on patient-driven concerns elicited earlier in the interview. Whenever possible, link concerns to the chief complaint and any other pertinent medical problems. Gently interject your own concerns about current or potential adverse consequences of drinking, while continuing to highlight concerns generated by the patient. Again, advice and expert opinion are best offered after asking permission or when the patient requests it. Examples of statements to make are:

- "We are having trouble controlling your blood pressure and that puts you at risk for serious health problems."
- "You have mentioned that you don't see as much of your daughter as you used to."
- "You are spending less time in activities you used to enjoy, such as volunteer work."
- "Drinking alcohol or taking sleeping pills can often make sleep problems worse even when it feels like it is helping."

- "I am concerned that the amount you are drinking could be making some of these problems worse."

Tie this information together into reasons to cut down or quit. It is best to have the patient choose his or her reasons to cut down or quit. You may be worried about the patient's health, but the patient may be more motivated by the cost of drinking, so you can use that as an effective motivator. Whenever possible, elicit and reinforce statements of self-motivation and self-efficacy, and reflect these statements back to the patient. Maintaining independence, physical health, financial security, and mental capacity can be key motivators in this age group (Center for Substance Abuse Treatment 1998). Say something like:

- "It seems that you are concerned about your high blood pressure and your sleep problem. Cutting down on drinking may be one way to help improve these problems."
- "You have quit smoking in the past, so I know you can make changes that are important for your health."
- "The amount that you are drinking may be contributing to your low mood and lack of energy. I wonder what would happen if you cut down?"

Even when delivered in a nonjudgmental manner, these statements may evoke a defensive reaction. If the patient is resistant do not push; instead, roll with the resistance. Maintain an atmosphere of respect where future discussion can take place. Scheduling a return visit may be the most important goal of your session. You might say:

- "I understand you don't see your current level of drinking as a problem. Let's continue to work on your blood pressure and sleep problems and see what happens."

In light of the risks associated with prescription drug use, consensus guidelines recommend against long-term use of benzodiazepines or sleep aids in older adults (Center for Substance Abuse Treatment 1998; National Institutes of Health 1990). When these agents are used, cautious selection of agents with the safest side-effect profile is advised.

If the patient is open, make a recommendation that he or she cut down on drinking. Older adults with serious health problems and those taking multiple prescription medications should be advised to abstain. Others may be advised to reduce their drinking to recommended limits. Provide guidance while allowing the patient to chose a target goal. Once a goal is agreed on, consider providing a written prescription of this agreement. This could be accomplished by asking:

- "What do you think is a reasonable goal?"
- "I am concerned that your blood pressure is out of control, and I recommend that you cut down on your drinking to see whether that helps."
- "Given all that we have talked about, I suggest that you limit your drinking to 1 drink per night. How does that sound to you?"

If time allows, further discussion of potential triggers can be helpful. Anticipate difficult situations and discuss strategies for dealing with them. Discuss seeking social opportunities that do not involve alcohol. Ask something like:

- "What activities would help you feel less alone?"
- "What would it be like to have a conversation with your daughter about finding ways to spend more time together?"

If the patient's history is not clear or cognitive impairment is suspected, consider getting collateral information from the family. Involving family members in treatment is encouraged whenever possible. This must be done with care to balance the goals of increasing the patient's self-esteem and placing the choice for change with the patient. Ask the patient questions such as:

- "Who else is worried about you?"
- "What does your daughter say about your current problems?"

End by summarizing the session. Review the agreed-on drinking limit, highlight reasons for change, elicit statements of self-efficacy, and schedule a follow-up visit. In more ambivalent patients, the medical complaint can be the agreed-on reason for follow-up, but it also will serve as an opportunity to continue your intervention.

Suggestions for Teaching and Supervision

When teaching and supervising trainees in a Motivational Interviewing approach for elderly patients who may be using substances, it is important to emphasize the following:

- Advise routine screening for drug and alcohol misuse in all older adults and rescreen when red flags are present.
- Become familiar with one or two screening tools.
- Be alert for comorbid mental illness, especially depression.

- Review all medications used, including nonprescription medications.
- Avoid long-term use of sedatives in the elderly.
- Establish trust and acceptance as key goals of any patient interaction.

Movie: *Requiem for a Dream*

One of the most widely recognized portrayals of an older adult misusing substances is the Academy Award–nominated performance of Ellen Burstyn in *Requiem for a Dream* (2000). The character of Sara Goldfarb is a widow dealing with life's disappointments, including her son's addiction to heroin. She becomes obsessed with the idea of appearing on television in her favorite red dress, which is now a bit snug on her. What could be safer than the collection of pills ("purple in the morning, blue in the afternoon, and orange in the evening") prescribed by a helpful physician?

Her drug-induced decline into a world populated by hallucinations of an angry refrigerator may offer an extreme example, but the number of older adults experiencing ill effects from the use of prescribed medications cannot be ignored. Intentionally or not, many older adults take more pills than prescribed, miss doses, or mix drugs prescribed by various physicians. The addition of alcohol or illicit drugs can increase the damage. The personal costs include adverse physical and mental health consequences and accelerated decline in function. The cost to society, including added health care costs, is difficult to quantify. It becomes imperative for health care professionals in all settings to think about the potential for harm with every prescription written and remain alert for evidence of the adverse effects of substance use in our older patients.

Key Clinical Points

- Routine screening for alcohol and prescription drug misuse is recommended in older adults.

- Safe drinking limits are lower in older adults compared with limits in the general population, and even lower when medical or psychiatric comorbidity is present.

- Sleep problems, depressed mood, and memory problems should not be routinely attributed to normal aging.

- The efficacy of Motivational Interviewing has been demonstrated in older adults.

Multiple-Choice Questions

For the correct answers to these questions, including explanations of answers, please see the Answer Guide at the end of this book.

1. NIAAA guidelines recommend that a healthy male older than age 65 drink:
   A. No more than 4 drinks in a day.
   B. No more than 14 drinks in a week.
   C. No more than 3 drinks in a day, and no more than 7 drinks in a week.
   D. No alcohol whatsoever under any circumstances.

2. A 66-year-old male reports drinking 1 mixed drink after dinner most nights, sometimes 2 or 3 on weekend evenings or special occasions, never totaling more than 7 per week. He has adequately controlled diabetes. On multiple occasions he has driven his car home after parties where he has consumed 3 drinks, but denies any traffic accidents. Based on this information, the patient has a diagnosis of:
   A. Moderate drinking.
   B. At-risk drinking.
   C. Problem drinking.
   D. Alcohol dependence.

3. Which of the following older adult patients is most likely to require acute medical care?
   A. A 78-year-old female drinking 2 drinks daily. She has no medical or psychiatric problems.
   B. A 72-year-old female drinking 1 drink every second day to help her fall asleep. She lives with her supportive husband and reports a history of anxiety and diabetes, for which she is in treatment.
   C. A 67-year-old male drinking 4–5 drinks daily. He reports a past history of heavy daily drinking and withdrawal seizures as well as delirium tremens.
   D. A 68-year-old female being treated with medications for hypertension, mild depression, and insomnia. She reports drinking 1 drink nightly. She denies negative consequences from alcohol use.

4. Which of the following screening tools for substance abuse was specifically developed for use in older adults?

   A. CAGE.
   B. AUDIT.
   C. MAST-G.
   D. All of the above.

5. Which of the following should trigger further evaluation of drinking and drug use behavior in an older adult?

   A. A complaint of insomnia.
   B. Unexplained bruising.
   C. Poor hygiene.
   D. All of the above.

References

American Psychiatric Association: Diagnostic and Statistical Manual of Mental Disorders, 4th Edition, Text Revision. Washington, DC, American Psychiatric Association, 2000

Barry KL, Oslin DW, Blow FC: Alcohol Problems in Older Adults: Prevention and Management. New York, Springer, 2001

Blazer DG, Wu LT: Nonprescription use of pain relievers by middle-aged and elderly community-living adults: National Survey on Drug Use and Health. J Am Geriatr Soc 57:1252–1257, 2009

Blow FC, Brower KJ, Schulenberg JE, et al: The Michigan Alcoholism Screening Test—Geriatric Version (MAST-G): a new elderly specific screening instrument (abstract). Alcohol Clin Exp Res 16:372, 1992

Blow F, Gillespie B, Barry K, et al: Brief screening for alcohol problems in elderly population using the Short Michigan Alcoholism Screening Test-Geriatric Version (SMAST-G). Alcohol Clin Exp Res 22:20-25, 1998

Brown RL, Rounds LA: Conjoint screening questionnaires for alcohol and other drug abuse: criterion validity in a primary care practice. Wis Med J 94:135–140, 1995

Center for Substance Abuse Treatment: Substance Abuse Among Older Adults (Treatment Improvement Protocol Series, No 26; DHHS Publ No 98-3179). Rockville, MD, Substance Abuse and Mental Health Service Administration, 1998. Available at: http://www.ncbi.nlm.nih.gov/bookshelf/br.fcgi?book=hssamhsatip&part=A48302. Accessed February 25, 2010.

Culberson JW, Ziska M: Prescription drug misuse/abuse in the elderly. Geriatrics 63:22–31, 2008

Dunn C, Deroo L, Rivara FP: The use of brief interventions adapted from motivational interviewing across behavioral domains: a systematic review. Addiction 96:1725–1742, 2001

Edgell RC, Kunik ME, Molinari VA, et al: Nonalcohol-related use disorders in geropsychiatric patients. J Geriatr Psychiatry Neurol 13:33–37, 2000

Ewing JA: Detecting alcoholism: the CAGE questionnaire. JAMA 252:1905–1907, 1984

Fick DM, Cooper JW, Wade WE, et al: Updating the Beers criteria for potentially inappropriate medication use in older adults: results of a US consensus panel of experts. Arch Intern Med 163:2716–2724, 2003

Fleming MF, Manwell LB, Barry KL, et al: Brief physician advice for alcohol problems in older adults: a randomized community-based trial. J Fam Pract 48:378–384, 1999

Koenig HG, Blazer DG II: Depression, in Encyclopedia of Gerontology: Age, Aging, and the Aged. Edited by Birren JE. San Diego, CA, Academic Press, 1996, pp 415–428

Kroenke K, Spitzer RL, Williams JB: The PHQ-9: validity of a brief depression severity measure. J Gen Intern Med 16:606–613, 2001

Mundt MP, French MT, Roebuck MC, et al: Brief physician advice for problem drinking among older adults: an economic analysis of costs and benefits. J Stud Alcohol 66:389–394, 2005

National Institute on Alcohol Abuse and Alcoholism: Alcohol and Aging (Alcohol Alert No 40). 1998. Available at: http://pubs.niaaa.nih.gov/publications/aa40.htm. Accessed August 24, 2009

National Institute on Alcohol Abuse and Alcoholism: Helping Patients Who Drink Too Much: A Clinician's Guide (NIH Publ No 05–3769). Rockville, MD, National Institute on Alcohol Abuse and Alcoholism, 2005. Available at: http://pubs.niaaa.nih.gov/publications/Practitioner/CliniciansGuide2005/clinicians_guide.htm. Accessed August 24, 2009

National Institutes of Health Consensus Development Conference Statement: The treatment of sleep disorders in older people. Consens Statement 8:1–22, 1990

Reinert DF, Allen JP: The Alcohol Use Disorders Identification Test: an update of research findings. Alcohol Clin Exp Res 31:185–199, 2007

Royer CM, Dickson-Fuhrmann E, McDermott CH, et al: Portraits of change: case studies from an elder-specific addiction program. J Geriatr Psychiatry Neurol 13:130–133, 2000

Vasilaki EI, Hosier SG, Cox WM: The efficacy of motivational interviewing as a brief intervention for excessive drinking: a meta-analytic review. Alcohol Alcohol 41:328–335, 2006

West PM, Graham K: Clients speak: participatory evaluation of a nonconfrontational addictions treatment program for older adults. J Aging Health 11:540–564, 1999

CHAPTER 15

Changing the Culture

Petros Levounis, M.D., M.A.

Clinicians these days do much more than treat patients. Motivating people and helping them change is a ubiquitous request. From managing interdisciplinary teams to directing units, divisions, departments, and hospitals, we are often called on to fill leadership positions. We are routinely recruited for such roles primarily because of our training in human behavior and our profound interest in what other people have to say. Although we sometimes frown on administrative and managerial tasks—"I did not go to medical school to learn how to hold meetings!"—a number of us are finding that the principles discussed in this book apply to a wide range of activities beyond the psychotherapeutic dyad. Furthermore, managing people from a humanistic perspective can be as rewarding and gratifying as treating patients.

Whether motivating a team to experiment with a new work schedule or planting the seed of ambivalence in an addict's mind, the path to the contemplation stage of change is similar. Negotiating a new contract (either of an employee or of your own) may not be all that different from convincing a patient to come to the emergency room. Ultimately, basic motivational skills such as expressing empathy and rolling with resistance can go a long way toward helping people change their behavior in many clinical and nonclinical situations.

In this chapter, I first introduce a case study of an attempt to change the culture of a health care organization. The case is discussed by examining how disciplines other than psychiatry and psychology address motivation and change. I then apply concepts and suggestions on motivating individuals from the world of clinical service (the subject of the previous chapters of this book) to the task of changing the larger culture of a system of individual human beings.

Case Study

A few years ago, I was asked to lead a consultation team for Recovery Central, a community mental health organization that wanted to increase its number of admissions, and consequently, improve its flailing finances. We quickly realized that the problem was not external (there were plenty of patients presenting for treatment) but internal. Several patients were deemed by staff as untreatable or undesirable and thus were turned away. The majority of them were patients who had been treated at the facility in the past but relapsed. A staff member proudly told me: "We do not readmit here. What's the point? We have no interest in providing a revolving door for people who cannot take advantage of what we have to offer." And this attitude was shared widely by the rest of the staff. Our task was clear: we needed to help the organization change its culture from "just say no" to "just say yes."

We identified a number of staff misconceptions about the clinical course of substance use disorders and other mental illnesses. The idea of addiction as a chronic relapsing illness was far from familiar to everyone. We also made a list of other logistical barriers that had to be deconstructed and obstacles that had to be overcome so that patients would be easily admitted to the facility and receive proper care. We invited mental health experts to give in-service seminars and grand rounds lectures, mandated attendance to the training events, and made sure that everyone understood why their attitudes were outdated, uninformed, misguided, or just plain wrong. They needed to change. We wrote tests to check the staff's knowledge, had the staff take the tests (once again, this was mandated), and put their scores in their permanent personnel files. We asked supervisors to review all cases that were deemed inappropriate for admission and incentivized the desired change by giving staff a bonus based on the number of patients admitted.

A year later, staff could recite diagnostic criteria for major depressive disorder, list the stages of change, and even talk about Motivational Interviewing. However, the number of admissions showed only modest improvement, and ultimately returned to baseline. Supervisors' reviews of denied cases seemed to reflect that they essentially agreed with the staff's original choices of rejecting returning patients. The entire exercise of our consultation received high praise from everyone—they liked us! Evaluations revealed that the staff members were very impressed with our qualifications and expertise. They found us "dynamic," "visionary," and "inspirational." But change was not achieved. What went wrong?

Discussion of the Case

Everything went wrong. Wait a minute—that's not entirely correct. We taught the staff a lot of good theories (not unlike the ones in the book you are holding in your hands), and we provided them with practical, hands-on exercises. We checked the impact of our efforts with reviews and feedback mechanisms. But it seems that we missed the mark.

Motivating people to change is not a task unique to the world of psychotherapy. Coaching in sports, inspiring troops in military campaigns, teaching, and parenting share similar ambitions and, quite often, similar techniques. In the corporate world, successfully motivating employees has become the very core mission of business administration, management, and leadership. A basketball coach may be able to dismiss a player more easily than a professional corporate coach can fire a client, but their basic goal and process of motivating people to achieve excellence remain essentially the same. Let's review some traditional explanations of what might have happened at Recovery Central.

Military: The Art of War (Circa 500 B.C.)

In *The Art of War*, one of the oldest and most popular treatises on military strategy, Sun Tzu suggests that motivating troops requires that the commander and the army be one with the *Tao* (Tzu 500 B.C./2003). He goes on to explain that being one with the Tao in this case means that people and their superiors work toward common goals. Although this idea seems self-evident, it is in stark contrast to the alternative strategies of the carrot and the stick, which are the bread and butter of today's approach to motivating people. James Flaherty (2005) gave another name for the carrot-and-stick tactics of motivation; he called them the *amoeba theory of management*. Do you remember the amoeba experiments from high school biology labs? You could make an amoeba move in a particular direction by either poking it with a needle from the back or placing a piece of sugar in front of the protozoon (Figure 15–1). The problem here is that these techniques ignore the internal desires, fears, hopes, and goals of the amoeba itself. And people are not amoebas. Trying to motivate people by fear and punishment (needle) ultimately leads to resentment and revolution; hoping to lead by charisma and infatuation (sugar) leads to disillusionment and secrecy, as we explain below in the "Business: Charisma Versus the Brutal Facts (2000s)" section.

Had we appreciated Sun Tzu's perspective, we might have invested more in listening than talking at Recovery Central. We clearly employed a top-down instead of bottom-up approach. Effective motivation and lasting change depend on gaining an understanding of the staff's needs and building a relationship based on common goals.

Sociology: The Hawthorne Effect (1920s)

In a series of studies with factory workers conducted at the Hawthorne Works manufacturing facility in Illinois between 1924 and 1932, productivity improved dramatically during the experiment but returned to baseline after the researchers

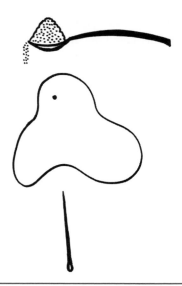

FIGURE 15–1.   The amoeba theory of management.
The amoeba moves in the desired direction by being either poked with a needle or rewarded with sugar.
Source.   Adapted from Flaherty 2005. Graphic by Lukas Hassel.

left the plant (Mayo 1949). The classic interpretation of this finding is that the workers were motivated and worked harder just because they were being studied. Perhaps they feared that they were under greater scrutiny, or they responded to the experimental conditions by working as a team toward a higher goal, or they felt that they were being heard by the higher-ups. The *Hawthorne effect* is essentially the social equivalent to the well-described pharmacological placebo effect.

At Recovery Central, the staff may have responded to our consultation with a combination of fear and good intentions, which resulted in the modest improvement in attitude and number of admissions. However, the positive outcomes were short-lived.

Education:
What You Expect Is What You Get (1960s)

In the 1960s, Rosenthal and Jacobson (2003) expanded the ideas of the Hawthorne studies to the worlds of education and parenting. They conducted an experiment with a group of elementary school teachers as their unsuspecting subjects. At the beginning of the school year, the researchers told the teachers that some students were particularly bright; they were the "academic spurters" as compared to the rest of the class. In fact, the so-called gifted students were selected randomly and any difference between the two groups existed solely in the teachers' minds. At the end of the school year, the designated academic spurters scored considerably higher on standard IQ tests than the children who were deemed less gifted. Rosenthal and Jacobson named this self-fulfilling prophecy the *Pygmalion effect* after the mythological sculptor who fell in love with his own ivory creation.

Perhaps our expectations of the staff at Recovery Central were not high enough to effect change. More correctly, we may have hoped that they would change in the direction we wished, but we failed to allow ourselves to believe that they were truly willing (or even capable) of changing.

Sports:
The Self-Determination Theory (1980s)

From a sports psychology perspective, motivation for achieving athletic goals traditionally has been seen as driven by two forces: 1) external rewards and 2) internal resolve. The external force is based on the ideas of operant conditioning, not unlike Flaherty's amoeba theory (Flaherty 2005)—people learn from the consequences of their actions and respond to environmental cues by seeking reward and avoiding punishment. The internal force was not fully appreciated until the 1984 Olympics in Los Angeles, when the field of sport and exercise psychology became a scientific discipline in earnest. The *self-determination theory*, formally introduced by Edward L. Deci and Richard M. Ryan in the 1980s, postulates that an athlete's behavior is primarily self-endorsed and self-determined, thus shifting the focus of motivational efforts from external to internal considerations (Deci and Ryan 1985). If the Hawthorne and Pygmalion effects point to the power of social placebos, self-determination theory reminds us that humans still maintain a degree of autonomy and free will.

At Recovery Central, the consulting team appreciated neither the cultural context of the organization nor the staff's own needs for competence and self-actualization. We steadfastly insisted on a highly directive approach that suffocated both nurturing and nature.

Business:
Charisma Versus the Brutal Facts (2000s)

Since the 1990s, the work of Jim Collins has informed and transformed the way we think about motivation and change in the business arena (Collins 2001,

2005, 2009; Collins and Porras 1995). He boldly states that "expending energy trying to motivate people is largely a waste of time" (Collins 2001). Helping people face brutal facts is far more helpful than giving inspirational pep talks. Based on extensive research in what makes today's companies succeed or fail, he challenges the traditional idea that a strong, charismatic, highly motivating, and visionary leader is an essential factor for positive change. In fact, charismatic leaders tend to shield—and more importantly, be shielded from—the frequently unpleasant truth, thus becoming less effective in the long run than their less charismatic counterparts.

It is unlikely that the staff members at Recovery Central were fully forthcoming about the messy realities of their everyday work when talking with the consultation team, whose members included Ivy League professors with considerable ego strengths (if not egos) and personality pizzazz. Remember how we were evaluated as impressive and inspirational? Charisma might have been more of a liability than an asset for effecting change.

Suggestions for Change

From a Transtheoretical Model of Change (Prochaska and DiClemente 1984) and Motivational Interviewing (Miller and Rollnick 2002) perspective, our consultation at Recovery Central essentially failed primarily because we misdiagnosed the stage of change. More correctly, we did not even attempt to identify the stage of change at the organization. We behaved as though Recovery Central were fully ready for a new approach to treatment, when the reality was quite different. The system was more in the precontemplation than the preparation stage of change.

Is it possible to apply our clinical expertise in motivation and change gained from working with individual patients to changing the culture of a system? I believe so. Then how do we do it? First, we embrace the basic premise of Motivational Interviewing that change is natural and intrinsic to humans—and by extension, human systems. By adopting a spirit of collaboration and expressing genuine empathy for the struggles of the people in a system that needs change, we can adapt the techniques and strategies of Motivational Interviewing to the larger task of changing an entire cultural structure. Without repeating the treatment suggestions detailed in the previous chapters of this book, I now discuss a few motivational methods that may be particularly helpful in working with systems, based on the stages of change.

Precontemplation

The essence of working with an organization at the precontemplation stage is planting the seed of ambivalence. Specifically, we try to identify any discrepancy between where the system is and where we would like it to be. For example, at Recovery Central the staff may have had no interest in admitting "repeat offenders" or "frequent flyers," but they still may have wanted to offer a solution to these patients' problems. Few people like to be mean, and given the opportunity, the staff would have liked to have been able to offer a mutually acceptable alternative to admission. Another way to approach assessing a system at this stage is to ask for a description of a typical day. In going through the details of daily life, people invariably report both what they experience and what they wish they could experience. Capitalizing on the smallest discrepancy between reality and perfection, and eventually driving a wedge through it, is an effective way to move the system from precontemplation to contemplation.

Contemplation

At the contemplation stage of change, systems are asked to perform a cost-benefit analysis—based on the brutal facts of the organization's realities. A two-by-two table is constructed: the columns identify positive and negative outcomes, whereas the rows depict what things would look like with and without the proposed changes (this is an example of a decisional balance sheet, discussed further in Chapter 4, "Contemplation"). For example, a church that is considering accepting same-sex marriages may benefit from such a decisional analysis. Traditionally, when we try to change a system we tend to focus on the quadrant of negative outcomes that may occur if things don't change—and sometimes the wonderful things that will happen if things do change. However, investigating all four quadrants moves the process of change more effectively. Exploring a congregation's fears of negative publicity or divine retribution if lesbians and gays start getting married may reveal little basis for these concerns. Ironically, the church may get a step closer to preparation for same-sex marriages by allowing the dissenting opinions to be fully heard.

Preparation

Before appreciating the need for motivational approaches to change—and developing effective methods for evoking intrinsic motivation—helpers of all sorts tend to say: "Come see me when you are ready." Such rebuttal often stems less from a disinterest in helping with the task than from a lack of technology to work with people and systems in earlier stages of change. Traditional coaching and consulting feel much more competent, and thus comfortable, with the task of motivating people who are already prepared to change. From H.A. Dorfman's (2003) *Coaching the Mental Game: Leadership Philosophies and Strategies for Peak Performance in Sports—and Everyday Life* to Max Messmer's (2001)

Motivating Employees for Dummies, the world is full of inspirational advice—provided the person is prepared to receive it. Nonetheless, our expertise in clinical settings can still provide unique insights and recommendations in changing a culture. In the preparation stage, motivational work focuses on developing a realistic action plan that anticipates problems and identifies solutions. However, during this time there is danger of a system reverting to the contemplation stage of change when hit by unforeseen complications and frustrating obstacles. For example, overwhelmed by the magnitude of the task, a country that seemed to be fully prepared to change its health care system may start rethinking the wisdom of its resolve. Ambivalence has crept back in. In this case, recruiting contemplation stage strategies may be the most effective approach.

Action

Living in a new home is stressful—even if the new home is better than the old one. Adjusting to the new realities of the action phase can be logistically complex and emotionally taxing. For example, a newspaper that recently moved its entire production online may face severe demoralization of its workforce despite the accompanying financial stabilization. Cognitive-behavioral methods of identifying, avoiding, and/or coping with triggers of relapse can be very helpful both for patients and for organizations in transition. In addition, this stage may be the right time for consolidation of intrinsic motivation with extrinsic coercion. For journalists whose organizations are now in the black after years of being in the red, appreciating that financial well-being does not necessarily occur at the expense of quality can open the door to new ideas. Ultimately, these journalists may embrace the unique opportunities of the electronic medium instead of always longing for the good old days of smelling ink on paper.

Maintenance

Maintaining and consolidating the gains of the changed behaviors often require a combination of motivational, cognitive, behavioral, regulatory, disciplinary, and social approaches. After the excitement of a triumphant transformation subsides, systems have to brace for the long run. For example, a law enforcement system that has successfully managed to change its culture and eliminate racial profiling from its practices may find it difficult to sustain the motivation of its members to continue fighting crime without profiling. Especially under stressful conditions, the old ways of thinking, feeling, and behaving feed on disappointments and frustrations, gain strength, and threaten the system with relapse. A multifaceted program based on the following lays the foundation for effective maintenance:

- An unrelenting vigilance for early signs of recurrence
- Anticipation and planning in case of relapse
- Continuous care to support self-efficacy and self-correction.

Furthermore, long-term success also calls for the system to be courageous enough to open up, go outside its strict boundaries, break walls of silence, and engage its members with the larger community. For the police force in our example to sustain its cultural shift, a number of community stakeholders (sometimes disenfranchised and angry) have to be involved, heard, and genuinely understood.

Relapse

As difficult as it is not to be disappointed, it is best to accept relapse as part of the process of change. We often say that *addiction is a chronic, relapsing illness*—and the same principle of acceptance applies to larger systems that struggle to sustain their new identity and culture. In the previous section, I alluded to the importance of vigilance, anticipation, and preparation for relapse. When it does occur, it is essential to return and reengage in the process of change as quickly as possible. Furthermore, identifying the elements that might have triggered the relapse and seizing the opportunities to do things differently next time may result in additional improvements and stronger stabilization of the changed culture. For example, consider a city that has managed to nearly eliminate graffiti from its subway system by empowering its subversive citizens to engage in sports and the arts. Funding for the innovative programs disappears and graffiti returns. The sooner the city council returns to the drawing board and develops alternative lower-cost programs (perhaps based on patronage from charity and community organizations), the higher the likelihood will be of successful reentry to the action stage of changing the face of the city's transportation system.

*　　*　　*

One of the greatest challenges for both clinical and nonclinical motivational work is limiting the ambition of the helper. People who hold advice-dispensing positions tend to be quite efficient and effective in achieving change in their own lives and thus expect immediate change in others. More often than not, simply identifying the stage of change; helping an individual or culture move a little forward; supporting her, him, or it at the new stage; and following up is enough. Faster, more ambitious timetables run the risk of overreaching. Ultimately, a humanistic approach that focuses on communication, collaboration, and the intrinsic motivation of people to change is often the key to success at any stage of change.

TABLE 15–1.   Douglas McGregor's Theory X and Theory Y

Managerial attitudes can be classified according to the assumption that people:

Theory X	Theory Y
Are lazy	Are motivated and creative
Inherently dislike work	Find work as natural as play
Require coercion to put forth adequate effort	Are committed and self-directed
Avoid responsibility	Seek responsibility
Resist change	Welcome change

Source.   McGregor 2005.

The spirit of Motivational Interviewing is based on this humanistic orientation in contrast to the more traditional attitudes toward motivation and change. Douglas McGregor (2005) crystallized the two approaches and described two very different attitudes toward workforce motivation; he called them Theory X and Theory Y (Table 15–1). Theory X assumes that people only work for money and security, whereas Theory Y embraces individuals' own search for fulfillment as the foundation of motivation. Successfully changing the culture of a system relies heavily on a Theory Y attitude.

Suggestions for Teaching and Supervision

Teaching and supervising a trainee in psychotherapy is surprisingly similar to advising a consultant who is working to change the culture of a system. The basic principles—and challenges—outlined in this book are relevant to both settings. However, consultants who seek advice for a project have subtly different expectations of their teachers than psychotherapy students have of their supervisors. Both groups appreciate practical information, but in general, psychotherapy students are more history oriented and like to analyze "what went wrong," whereas consultants are somewhat more results oriented and like to work on "what to do about it." Both perspectives are essential and both groups can benefit from each other's orientation and focus.

Let's look at two examples of teaching and supervision. A third-year psychiatry resident who struggled with the treatment of a masseur with borderline personality disorder came to me for advice. The resident wanted me to help her explore the innumerable half-truths that the patient kept bringing to the sessions—and the significant countertransference she experienced. When the focus of supervision shifted from relentlessly investigating massage table sagas and psychotherapy couch squabbles to helping the masseur build concrete life skills, both the resident and her patient experienced a sense of improvement, advancement, and relief. In another situation, a junior consultant asked me to supervise him on how to improve communication among staff at a drug rehabilitation center. He clearly expected me to help him create a new organizational structure and teach him how to develop innovative, morale-boosting incentives. I suggested that before drawing up specific strategies and plans, we should look at the personalities of the leadership team and the group dynamics of the line staff. In both cases, the intention was to nudge the students out of their comfort zones—for the resident, this meant speeding things up; for the consultant, slowing things down.

Movies: *The Devil Wears Prada* and *The September Issue*

In *The Devil Wears Prada* (2006), fashion maven Miranda Priestly, played brilliantly by Meryl Streep, is the head of *Runway,* the most influential magazine in the fashion industry. From the first few scenes of the movie, viewers see that her attitude is squarely Theory X. Her managerial style is clearly domineering—even tyrannical at times—with complete focus on the job and no concern, or appreciation, for the people who work for her. In *Runway*'s world of produce or perish, all motivation is extrinsically driven; cruelty and fear abound.

Another way to view Miranda Priestly's managerial style is through Blake and Mouton's (1964) managerial grid model of leadership. Their model classifies managerial style based on the leader's concern for production versus concern for people (Table 15–2). Clearly, Miranda Priestly lives comfortably in the autocratic quadrant. However, in a unique sequel to this fictional portrayal, we are given the opportunity to look at some of the reality behind the imaginary tale.

The September Issue (2009) is a documentary film about Anna Wintour, the legendary editor-in-chief of the fashion magazine *Vogue,* the magazine on which *The Devil Wears Prada* is based. Anna does resemble Miranda (or vice versa if you like) both physically and emotionally, but Anna pays far more attention to collaborating with her colleagues and fostering the autonomy of her devoted staff. Despite the cinematographer's focus on capturing the most frictional aspects of life with Anna, it is obvious that she strives for balance between concern for production and attention to people—in other words, task orientation and human needs. In essence, the famed Anna Wintour is not the autocratic leader portrayed in *The Devil Wears Prada,* but rather a successful team leader, as identified in Table 15–2.

TABLE 15–2.　Blake and Mouton's managerial grid model of leadership

Commitment to people and task varies from low to high, resulting in five types of leaders:

Leader type	People	Task
Country-club leaders	High	Low
Laissez-faire leaders	Low	Low
Middle-of-the-roaders	Middle	Middle
Autocratic leaders	Low	High
Team leaders	High	High

Source.　Blake and Mouton 1964.

Key Clinical Points

- The Transtheoretical Model of Change and Motivational Interviewing concepts, developed to facilitate change in individuals, can be applied to changing the culture of systems of individuals.

- In the precontemplation stage, plant the seed of ambivalence.

- In the contemplation stage, explore both the positive and the negative prospects of life with and without the proposed change in culture.

- In the preparation stage, develop a realistic action plan that anticipates problems and identifies solutions.

- During the action stage, consolidate intrinsic motivation with extrinsic coercion.

- In the maintenance stage, use a multitude of motivational and psychosocial approaches to sustain the desired change.

- If relapse occurs, accept it as an opportunity to reengage, rethink, and reemerge stronger than before.

- Throughout the process of change, focus on communication, collaboration, and the intrinsic motivation of individuals.

Multiple-Choice Questions

For the correct answers to these questions, including explanations of answers, please see the Answer Guide at the end of this book.

1. A Greek family rethinks its cooking strategies. On one hand, the health benefits of a lower-fat diet are well understood and appreciated. On the other, *fasolakia ladera* are not really *ladera* unless they happily swim in a sea of olive oil. Ambivalence and tension reign in the family. What's the stage of change?

   A. Precontemplation.
   B. Contemplation.
   C. Preparation.
   D. Action.

2. Confucius said: "Our greatest glory is not in never falling but in rising every time we fall." This quote is most helpful in:

   A. Preparation.
   B. Action.
   C. Maintenance.
   D. Relapse.

3. Three friends are stranded in an elevator without their cell phones. One of them keeps buzzing the alarm bell and screams for help while another looks for a way out. The third friend waits for the other two to figure it out. This is an example of the:

   A. Hawthorne effect.
   B. Pygmalion effect.
   C. Self-determination effect.
   D. All of the above.

4. According to Jim Collins's analysis of successful companies, a leader's charisma is:

   A. More likely to be a liability than an asset.
   B. More likely to be an asset than a liability.
   C. Irrelevant to success or failure.
   D. More important than the facts in motivating people.

5. Margaret Mead said: "Never doubt that a small group of thoughtful, committed citizens can change the world. Indeed, it is the only thing that ever has." This attitude is most consistent with:
   A. Theory W.
   B. Theory X.
   C. Theory Y.
   D. Theory Z.

References

Blake R, Mouton J: The Managerial Grid: The Key to Leadership Excellence. Houston, TX, Gulf Publishing, 1964

Collins J: Good to Great: Why Some Companies Make the Leap…and Others Don't. New York, HarperCollins, 2001

Collins J: Good to Great and the Social Sectors: A Monograph to Accompany Good to Great. Boulder, CO, Jim Collins, 2005

Collins J: How the Mighty Fall: And Why Some Companies Never Give In. Boulder, CO, Jim Collins, 2009

Collins J, Porras JI: Built to Last: Successful Habits of Visionary Companies. New York, HarperCollins, 1995

Deci EL, Ryan RM: Intrinsic Motivation and Self-Determination in Human Behavior. New York, Plenum, 1985

Dorfman HA: Coaching the Mental Game: Leadership Philosophies and Strategies for Peak Performance in Sports—and Everyday Life. Lanham, MD, Taylor Trade Publishing, 2003

Flaherty J: Coaching: Evoking Excellence in Others. Oxford, UK, Elsevier, 2005

Mayo E: Hawthorne and the Western Electric Company, The Social Problems of an Industrial Civilisation. London, Routledge, 1949

McGregor D: The Human Side of Enterprise, Annotated Edition. New York, McGraw-Hill, 2005

Messmer M: Motivating Employees for Dummies. New York, Wiley, 2001

Miller WR, Rollnick S: Motivational Interviewing: Preparing People for Change, 2nd Edition. New York, Guilford, 2002

Prochaska JO, DiClemente CC: The Transtheoretical Approach: Crossing Traditional Boundaries of Therapy. Homewood, IL, Dow Jones-Irwin, 1984

Rosenthal R, Jacobson L: Pygmalion in the Classroom: Teacher Expectation and Pupils' Intellectual Development. Norwalk, CT, Crown House, 2003

Tzu S: The Art of War (circa 500 B.C.). Translated by Lionel Giles and edited by Dallas Galvin. New York, Barnes and Noble Classics, 2003

CHAPTER 16

The Science of Motivational Interviewing

Michelle Acosta, Ph.D.
Deborah L. Haller, Ph.D., A.B.P.P.
Karen Ingersoll, Ph.D.

In recent years, there has been an increasing trend for clinicians to become fluent in the delivery of evidence-based treatments. But what are evidence-based treatments and how do they differ from standard care?

Evidence-based treatments are those that have been studied scientifically and have been found to be effective in controlled studies. Controlled studies are ones in which near-optimal results might be expected because all clinicians are well trained, follow a treatment protocol, and are closely supervised. The effectiveness of the evidence-based treatment compared with that of a standard treatment (or with that of another evidence-based treatment) is determined by assessing the extent to which predetermined outcomes are met for patients treated using each approach. When patient outcomes are better for those receiving the experimental treatment, we say that this treatment has promise or efficacy. When the outcomes for the experimental treatment are comparable to those attained by other approaches, we have showed that the experimental treatment is as good as approaches already in use (standard care).

Although this research approach, often termed a *clinical trial*, has been used to study pharmacotherapies for many years, its application to psychotherapies is more recent. Even so, there are rigorous methods available to evaluate psychotherapies. Motivational Interviewing is one type of psychotherapy that has been studied in a number of clinical trials. Motivational Interviewing includes some well-articulated strategies, processes, and objectives that lend themselves to measurement. The tone, or *spirit*, of Motivational Interviewing is somewhat harder to measure, as it is more abstract and subjective; trained evaluators and supervisors are needed to identify this in treatment sessions.

Clinicians may ask whether or not such rigorous inquiry of treatment approaches is necessary. We would argue that indeed it is. As consumers of mental health services, patients have the right to receive the interventions that have the greatest chance of succeeding. We expect this in other areas of medicine, and psychiatry is no exception. Moreover, third-party payers are increasingly requiring that clinicians employ evidence-based treatments (i.e., those that have been shown to bring about measurable changes) and employ objective assessments of change. In addition, many clinicians want feedback about their own performance in order to hone their skills and maximize their ability to help their patients. Finally, clinical program managers want to know which treatment approaches are most likely to achieve the best outcomes in the shortest period of time and at the lowest cost. Information provided from clinical trials can help to answer these questions and improve patient outcomes, therapist skills, and program development.

Numerous clinical trials have shown that Motivational Interviewing works for various clinical populations and a wide range of problems. Its popularity in clinical programs has increased significantly in recent years, with many substance abuse programs adopting it as a treatment option. However, there are multiple barriers to the successful implementation of Motivational Interviewing in clinical settings. If the implementation is part of a clinical trial, treatment programs may be suspicious of research, viewing it as more for the benefit of the researchers than of patients or staff. If implementation is through a clinical trial or an expert trainer, the pressure for clinicians to develop new and/or complex skill sets and to be closely monitored in their delivery of a new treatment may feel threatening. In substance abuse treatment, Motivational Interviewing may represent a radical departure from traditional drug counseling approaches that employ strategies such as confrontation. For the clinician to modify his or her own belief system in order to effectively adopt this approach may be unappealing for some substance abuse clinicians. For Motivational Interviewing to be successfully adopted by clinicians and integrated into treatment programs, these barriers must be overcome.

For programs that are considering participating in Motivational Interviewing–based research or bringing in an expert trainer, it is important to develop a good working relationship with researchers or trainers. It is helpful if clinicians are interested in learning new skills for themselves that will be sustainable once the project ends. It can be helpful if both program staff and clinicians believe that Motivational Interviewing is effective, and therefore, worth using. With these considerations in mind, the objectives of this chapter include:

1. Clarifying how Motivational Interviewing differs from other approaches
2. Demonstrating that Motivational Interviewing is worthy of further consideration
3. Identifying the steps toward becoming a competent Motivational Interviewing clinician and/or researcher
4. Understanding what outcomes are measured to assess change (and how they are measured) when using Motivational Interviewing.

Finally, we hope that this introduction to Motivational Interviewing research is sufficient to encourage further pursuit of this area by clinicians and researchers alike.

How Do I Know What Motivational Interviewing Is (and Isn't)?

In order for clinicians to better understand how Motivational Interviewing works, the Motivational Interviewing approach and spirit must be differentiated from those of other therapies, as summarized below:

- Motivational Interviewing is a person-centered approach. Although the relationship is important, it is not the focal point of discussion. Rather, respect for the patient and his or her decision-making abilities is shown through listening, reflecting, and being nonjudgmental.
- Like dynamic approaches, Motivational Interviewing recognizes the importance of resistance and ambivalence, although these are dealt with differently. Confrontation, interpretation, and a focus on the past and emotion are consistent with dynamic therapies, but inconsistent with Motivational Interviewing.
- Motivational Interviewing also has supportive aspects yet differs from supportive therapy in that it is strategic and goal oriented. Both approaches are encouraging and hopeful, however.
- Compared with Cognitive-Behavioral Therapy (CBT), Motivational Interviewing is more about the spirit, or tone, of the sessions and less about specific exercises and strategies. For example, Motivational Interviewing strives to elicit solutions from the patients, as opposed to instructing the patient in ways to solve his or her problems.

- Both traditional drug counseling and Motivational Interviewing employ feedback on a routine basis; however, the tone tends to differ. Whereas patients in drug counseling may be confronted about positive drug test results, those in Motivational Interviewing would be encouraged to view such results as a sign of ambivalence about changing their drug use behavior. In addition, drug counseling tends to be pathology based, labeling patients as addicts, mentally ill, or personality disordered. In contrast, Motivational Interviewing tries to stay away from labeling.
- Drug counseling and Motivational Interviewing do have several elements in common, including being goal-directive and attempting to identify barriers to change and ways to overcome them.

Table 16–1 compares and contrasts the techniques and strategies that characterize Motivational Interviewing with those of other common treatment approaches. Although some Motivational Interviewing–defining constructs may occur during other types of treatment as well, if they are not characteristic of those treatments they remain unchecked in the table. Conversely, many of the constructs that typify other interventions often are combined with pure Motivational Interviewing, yielding a blended intervention. However, in order to make the distinctions between intervention approaches as clear as possible, we have elected to focus on pure Motivational Interviewing in this instance. Nevertheless, it should be recognized that nearly all published, evidence-based studies involve adaptations of Motivational Interviewing (AMIs), as opposed to pure Motivational Interviewing, and this table is merely for illustrative purposes.

Does Motivational Interviewing Work?

Motivational Interviewing has been studied extensively and has been shown to be efficacious for a variety of problems. Most studies have focused on reducing substance use (including tobacco, alcohol, and drugs), reducing HIV transmission risk, improving treatment compliance, reducing gambling, reducing disordered eating, and improving healthy diet and exercise behaviors. Recent studies have also examined Motivational Interviewing as a treatment for psychiatric disorders.

Motivational Interviewing sometimes has been studied as a brief, free-standing (one or two sessions), motivational prelude to other treatment. More frequently, AMIs have been studied. Adaptations are when Motivational Interviewing is combined with other intervention components such as feedback, CBT, education, relapse prevention, or skills building.

The research literature on Motivational Interviewing has increased exponentially in the past decade. Due to the strength of evidence supporting its

TABLE 16–1. Comparing elements of Motivational Interviewing (MI) with those of other treatment approaches

Therapeutic construct	MI	Dynamic	Supportive	CBT	DC
Person centered	✓	✓			
Reflection	✓	✓			
Nonjudgmental	✓		✓		
Focuses on resistance/ ambivalence	✓	✓			
Options oriented	✓				
Goal directed	✓			✓	✓
Uses confrontation		✓		✓	✓
Focuses on interpretation		✓			
Instructive/directive				✓	✓
Focuses on skills building				✓	

Note. CBT = Cognitive-Behavioral Therapy; DC = traditional drug counseling.

efficacy, Motivational Interviewing and its most common adaptation, Motivation Enhancement Therapy (MET), have been listed as evidence-based practices in two prominent compendia of evidence-based treatments for substance use disorders: 1) the National Registry of Evidence-Based Programs and Practices (www.nrepp.samhsa.gov; sponsored by the U.S. Department of Health and Human Services, Substance Abuse and Mental Health Services Administration) and 2) the National Quality Forum (www.qualityforum.org; sponsored by the U.S. Department of Health and Human Services' Centers for Medicare and Medicaid Services, and the Assistant Secretary for Planning and Evaluation). In addition, three recent meta-analyses combined findings from a wide range of studies using Motivational Interviewing and found that the effect size of Motivational Interviewing, or the strength of Motivational Interviewing, depends on the target behavior (Burke et al. 2003; Hettema et al. 2005; Rubak et al. 2005). These meta-analyses are described below.

- Burke et al. (2003) reviewed 30 clinical trials of AMIs across several risk behaviors and found that Motivational Interviewing was generally efficacious, with small to medium effect sizes. Overall, AMIs improved patient success rates from 33% to 50% (from one-third of patients making the desired change to one-half of patients doing so). In addition, AMIs doubled drug and alcohol abstinence rates, from 20% to 40% (from one in five patients to two in five patients achieving abstinence), and reduced drinking in patients by 56%. These treatment effects were durable, decreasing only slightly from 20 to 67 weeks of follow-up. Finally, AMIs were efficient, meaning that the change produced by AMIs in two sessions was equivalent to the change achieved by other psychotherapy methods in eight sessions across a variety of target behaviors.

- A second meta-analysis (Hettema et al. 2005) examined studies with at least a pre-post design as well as randomized controlled trials. Across all studies, the total number of participants was 14,267; the number of participants in individual studies ranged from 21 to 952, with an average of 198 patients per study. About half (55%) of the patients were men and they were approximately 34 years old; 43% were members of ethnic minorities. In this review of 72 studies, the average effects of Motivational Interviewing and AMI interventions were large at the end of treatment (effect size $d=0.77$), but generally decreased to having a medium effect size at follow-up ($d=0.31$ at 4–6 months and $d=0.30$ at 6–12 months). In addition to changes in outcomes, Motivational Interviewing and AMI interventions increased treatment retention, treatment adherence, and patient motivation, as perceived by treatment staff. The researchers concluded that Motivational Interviewing is effective for a number of risk behaviors. However, process variables, including therapist behaviors, may affect outcomes.

- A third meta-analysis, of 72 trials, compared the impact of Motivational Interviewing on health behaviors with the impact of brief advice (Rubak et al. 2005). Motivational Interviewing had a significant effect on several disease markers, including body mass index value, total blood cholesterol level, systolic blood pressure level, blood alcohol concentration, and standard blood ethanol content, but not on the number of cigarettes smoked per day or hemoglobin A_{1c} level (a marker for diabetes). Motivational Interviewing demonstrated an effect in 74% of the clinical trials assessed, regardless of the interventionist's profession (psychologist, physician, nurse, etc.). In addition, the likelihood of Motivational Interviewing being efficacious increased as the number of minutes per session and the number of encounters per patient increased. The authors concluded that Motivational Interviewing is more beneficial than brief advice for a broad range of target behaviors.

How Does Motivational Interviewing Work?

Although the connection between process and outcome has not yet been firmly established, significant progress has been made in identifying the mechanisms of action in Motivational Interviewing. Most studies focused on describing the "active ingredients" in Motivational Interviewing have examined therapist and patient processes that are presumed to relate to change in Motivational Interviewing, based on Miller and Rollnick's descriptions in the two editions of their definitive book (Miller and Rollnick 1991, 2002). Although still limited, the literature in this area is growing and providing some consistent answers about how Motivational Interviewing works. When therapists display a high degree of acceptance, egalitarianism, empathy, warmth, and Motivational Interviewing spirit, they may facilitate the formation of a helpful therapeutic alliance and the engagement of patients in the process.

In one study examining these mechanisms, therapists' interpersonal skills—including the aforementioned acceptance, egalitarianism, empathy, warmth, and Motivational Interviewing spirit—were positively related to patient involvement. Similarly, the relationship between therapists' interpersonal skills and Motivational Interviewing–inconsistent behaviors was negative (Moyers et al. 2005b). These findings indicate that therapists' interpersonal skills directly facilitated patient collaboration, and that therapists with these skills did not undermine patient engagement even when they displayed some behaviors inconsistent with Motivational Interviewing. Another study (Thrasher et al. 2006) found that both a higher ratio of reflections to questions and the number of affirmations were associated with higher antiretroviral therapy adherence among HIV patients at the end of treatment, whereas closed-ended questions were negatively associated with adherence.

Similarly, Catley et al. (2006) assessed the Motivational Interviewing quality of a smoking counseling intervention using the Motivational Interviewing Skills Code (Moyers et al. 2003). An averaged Motivational Interviewing global score composed of ratings for therapists' acceptance, egalitarianism, warmth, genuineness, empathy, and Motivational Interviewing spirit, along with counts of behavior with higher Motivational Interviewing consistency (including providing advice with permission, affirming, emphasizing choice and control, reframing, supporting, and using open-ended questions and reflections), were related to greater frequency of patient *change talk* (statements about recognizing problems; expressing concern, desire, intention, or optimism for change). Higher Motivational Interviewing consistency also was related to a higher average global score of patients' expressions of affect, cooperation, self-disclosure, and engagement. Motivational Interviewing–inconsistent behaviors were unrelated to patient change talk or global scores. However, specific behaviors were related to some outcomes, in the predicted direction. Behavior counts of affirmations, open-ended questions, reflections, and support were positively related to a therapist-patient collaboration and treatment benefit. Behavior counts of giving advice without permission showed a negative correlation with change talk.

In a study of Motivational Interviewing skills in a college peer intervention, investigators used the Motivational Interviewing Treatment Integrity scale (Moyers et al. 2005a) to assess the relationship between facilitator skills and drinking-related outcomes (Tollison et al. 2008). Closed-ended questions were associated with decreased contemplation, and open-ended questions were associated with increased contemplation. More simple reflections were associated with increased drinking, but this relationship was attenuated by a greater proportion of complex reflections.

Taken together, these studies suggest that therapist characteristics such as empathy, warmth, egalitarianism, and spirit foster greater patient involvement, and that specific therapist behaviors such as using more complex reflections and more affirmations are related both to better therapist-patient relationships and to better patient outcomes.

Several studies have assessed patient resistance and its relationships to therapist behaviors and to outcomes. Although not directly examining Motivational Interviewing, an early study exploring the relationship of therapist behavior to patient resistance found that resistance varied depending on therapist behaviors, with educational or confrontational behaviors eliciting more resistance, and patient-centered behaviors eliciting less resistance (Patterson and Forgatch 1985). In an extension of this research, Miller et al. (1993) investigated the relationship of resistance to outcome and found that the more time the patient showed resistance in the session, the poorer the outcome for reducing drinking. The reverse was also true; patients who showed little resistance manifested improved drinking outcomes up to 12 months later.

Several studies also have found that change talk is related to outcomes. Patients who decreased their drug use and maintained this change showed increasing commitment language across a Motivational Interviewing session (Amrhein et al. 2003). Further, Strang and McCambridge (2004) rated patient speech for change talk and found that action-oriented change talk, presumably representing commitment, was related to subsequent decreases in marijuana use at 3-month follow-up. Moyers et al. (2007) found that patient change talk and counterchange talk were related to substance abuse outcomes in the expected directions. Moyers and Martin (2003) found that the more the therapist affirmed, emphasized control, asked permission before raising concerns, and made reflections, the more patients engaged in total change talk during the session.

Moyers and Martin (2006) studied the conditional probabilities of different classes of patient speech occurring following various forms of therapist speech in MET sessions. They found that when therapists performed in a Motivational Interviewing–consistent manner, there was an immediate increase in the probability that patients would produce change talk in the next utterance. In contrast, therapists warning or advising without permission increased the immediate probability of patients producing counterchange-talk resistance. Additionally, change talk sometimes followed other therapist behaviors that are part of the basic Motivational Interviewing style such as posing open-ended questions and making reflections, as well as strategies such as giving information, providing feedback, providing opinions, and uttering simple conversational fillers. The researchers then investigated whether patient change talk during three types of substance abuse treatment sessions predicted drinking outcomes (Moyers et al. 2007). They rated sessions of 12-step facilitation, CBT, and MET from a large multisite clinical trial (Project MATCH Research Group 1993) using the Motivational Interviewing Skills Code. Using the outcome definitions from Project MATCH (Matching Alcoholism Treatment to Client Heterogeneity), they considered the impact of patient change talk and counterchange talk on the percentage of days patients were abstinent and the number of drinks they had per drinking day, taking into account baseline values on both of these drinking variables. When examining predictors of change, the study found that change talk and counterchange talk improved the statistical model's ability to predict the percentage of days abstinent, with counterchange talk being a significant predictor. In addition, adding change talk and counterchange talk also improved the statistical model's ability to predict the number of drinks per drinking day, with both change talk and counterchange talk acting as significant predictors in the expected directions. The authors concluded that the causal chain tested in their series of studies demonstrates that therapist behaviors evoke change talk, that counterchange talk and change talk are different constructs, and that they are simultaneous predictors of outcome.

In sum, although the literature on how Motivational Interviewing works is still emerging, some findings are consistent to date. Empathy and Motivational Interviewing spirit (collaboration, evocation, and autonomy) both relate to engaging patients and building therapeutic alliances. Several studies have found that open-ended questions, reflections, and affirmations encourage change talk, whereas closed-ended questions do not. In addition, those behaviors considered to be consistent with Motivational Interviewing—such as asking permission to give advice, affirming, emphasizing patient choice and control, and making supportive statements—have been related to more change talk as well as to more positive substance abuse outcomes in several studies. Some aspects of a model of how Motivational Interviewing works are emerging already, although many questions remain about the directionality and causality of current hypotheses.

How Do I Learn Motivational Interviewing?

People from various professional backgrounds—clinicians and nonclinicians—have learned to deliver Motivational Interviewing effectively. Most studies have trained mental health or medical clinicians, but others have trained people as diverse as graduate students, dieticians, probation officers, and medical patients. Miller and Moyers (2006) identified eight stages in learning Motivational Interviewing:

1. Learning about the philosophy of Motivational Interviewing, particularly the notions of collaboration, evocation, and autonomy
2. Learning basic patient-centered counseling skills including reflections, affirmations, summaries, and open-ended questions
3. Adding a more Motivational Interviewing–specific approach to this person-centered style, including recognizing and reinforcing change talk
4. Being mindful of change talk and encouraging change talk when appropriate (an expansion of stage 3)
5. Learning how to roll with resistance and conceptualize resistant behavior as a normative part of the change process
6. Learning to help patients develop a change plan
7. Learning to help patients become committed to their change plan
8. Learning to integrate the Motivational Interviewing approach effectively with other intervention approaches based on a patient's needs.

Given the extensive work needed to achieve mastery in Motivational Interviewing, it seems logical that becoming proficient may take time. Most training begins with a workshop, often lasting 2 days, conducted by an expert in Motivational Interviewing. There is a network of clinicians who are certified to train others in Motivational Interviewing, who are called MINT trainers (Motivational Interviewing Network of Trainers). Training typically includes didactics, experiential exercises, and role-play. Unfortunately, a study indicated that a 2-day training period is not enough for clinicians to become proficient in Motivational Interviewing (Miller and Mount 2001). A later study showed that although the initial training is important, only those clinicians who received continued supervision via telephone and/or feedback on audiotaped practice sessions were able to achieve mastery (Miller et al. 2004). This finding suggests that although attending a workshop might be a good starting place, to truly learn Motivational Interviewing, clinicians may require ongoing supervision from someone with Motivational Interviewing mastery.

How Do I Know I'm Doing It Right?

One of the ways in which clinical research differs from standard care is the extent to which the clinician is evaluated. In standard care, clinicians either monitor themselves or are evaluated by supervisors, usually by providing supervisors a brief account of the intervention and patient progress. In contrast, most research studies use other people, including supervisors and outside raters, to evaluate clinician performance. Supervision in research studies is often audio-taped or videotaped and feedback is provided to the clinician. Outside raters listen to or watch session tapes and complete rating measures, though typically do not provide feedback directly to study clinicians. The reason that clinicians are evaluated so much more thoroughly in research studies is to ensure *treatment fidelity*. Treatment fidelity concerns how well clinicians can learn the intervention and how accurately they can deliver the intervention according to the treatment manual, study protocol, or theoretical approach. Treatment fidelity is important in clinical research for a variety of reasons. First, if clinicians are unable to learn the intervention, it suggests that the intervention is not feasible. Second, if clinicians do not deliver the intervention appropriately, it will be impossible to know whether patient outcomes are a function of the intervention or are due to other factors. In addition, if clinicians are unable to perform the intervention in a standardized way (i.e., if all clinicians do not carry out the intervention in the same way), then other researchers and clinicians will not be able to replicate the results of the study.

The first step to ensure treatment fidelity is training the clinicians. As stated above, initial training typically consists of a workshop. After training, clinician skills are evaluated and often clinicians are given *pilot* or test patients and monitored closely to make sure that they are performing the intervention as directed. Once clinicians achieve mastery, they are allowed to begin delivering the intervention with ongoing supervision. Clinicians are supervised and rated via audiotape or videotape or via in-person observation. Raters use a standardized measure to evaluate clinician tapes or observed sessions. There are many tools available for raters to use (Table 16–2), and they vary in length and content. Raters are typically well trained in Motivational Interviewing and have a good working knowledge of the intervention. Most measures of fidelity require the rater to review the tape and then evaluate the clinician on a number of items. In addition, some measures require that the clinician keep a tally of specific clinician behaviors in session.

The rating scales presented in Table 16–2 are general Motivational Interviewing–style tools. However, rating scales may be adapted to incorporate different items from the intervention, using the intervention manual as a guide. Clinicians also may use the manual or other standardized intervention materials to assist in intervention delivery. Although most studies provide manuals to assist in training and ensure fidelity, a recent meta-analysis of Motivational Interviewing studies indicated that studies that did not use a manual for Motivational Interviewing yielded better patient outcomes (Hettema et al. 2005). Unfortunately, many clinicians have difficulties learning an intervention without a manual or guide, especially if the intervention incorporates other strategies (e.g., CBT) in addition to Motivational Interviewing. Manuals and

TABLE 16–2. Tools to assess adherence to and competence of using Motivational Interviewing interventions

Scale	What it consists of	What it measures
Yale Adherence and Competence Scale (YACS; Carroll et al. 2000)	50-item scale to assess elements common to all psychotherapies, with 9 additional MI-specific items	3 general ratings—assessment, general support, and goals for treatment; 3 specific ratings—clinical management, 12-step facilitation, and cognitive-behavioral management; assesses both adherence (how often a technique was used) and competence (how well the technique was executed)
Independent Tape Rater Scale[a]	Adapted from YACS; 39-item scale using 7-point Likert responses	3 ratings—MI-consistent interventions, MI-inconsistent interventions, and general substance abuse counseling interventions
Motivational Interviewing Skills Code (MISC; Moyers et al. 2003)	3 views of the audio/videotape for 3 different scales using a 7-point Likert scale after each review	3 ratings—Global Therapist Rating (acceptance, egalitarianism, empathy, genuineness, warmth, and spirit of MI), Global Patient Rating (affect, cooperation, disclosure, and engagement), and Global Interaction Rating (level of collaboration and benefit of the interaction)
Motivational Interviewing Treatment Integrity (MITI; Moyers et al. 2005a) scale[b]	Consists of 2 global ratings on a 7-point Likert scale and behavior counts	Global ratings on MI spirit and empathy and tallies for behaviors: giving information, MI adherent, MI nonadherent, questions (closed and open), reflection (simple and complex)
Motivational Interviewing Supervision and Training Scale (MISTS; Madson et al. 2005)	Behavior count of therapist responses and 16-item global ratings of quality, MI fidelity, and effectiveness of therapist interventions on a 7-point Likert scale	Behavior counts of therapist responses include open questions, reflection, affirmations, etc., and 16 global ratings on aspects of MI including simple and complex reflection, rolling with resistance, and MI spirit
Behavior Change Counseling Index (BECCI; Lane et al. 2005)	11-item checklist with items rated on a 5-point Likert scale	Ratings in 4 domains of MI: agenda setting and permission seeking, the why and how of change in behavior, the whole consultation, and talk about target

Note.　MI = Motivational Interviewing.

[a]Ball SA, Martino S, Corvino J, et al: "Independent Tape Rater Guide." Unpublished psychotherapy tape rating manual. New Haven, CT, Department of Psychiatry, Division of Substance Abuse, Yale University School of Medicine, 2002.
[b]Moyers TB, Martin T, Manuel JK, et al: "The Motivational Interviewing Treatment Integrity (MITI) Code, Version 3.0." Unpublished coding manual. University of New Mexico, Center on Alcoholism, Substance Abuse, and Addictions, 2007.

periodic retraining also are useful in preventing *drift*, which occurs when clinicians drift back to their own style and away from the intervention approach. In addition to ensuring that clinicians remain well trained and adherent to the intervention, researchers also are concerned with something called *contamination*. Contamination occurs when a clinician is exposed to, and incorporates, elements of the other intervention condition in his or her delivery of the intended intervention. Researchers try to prevent this from occurring in multiple ways, including having clinicians deliver different interventions at separate sites. In addition to close monitoring of the clinicians, patients or participants are often asked about or given measures to assess their perceptions of the intervention and/or the clinician.

How Do I Know When Motivational Interviewing Is Working for My Patients (Are My Patients Changing)?

As with most interventions, there are several ways to assess whether Motivational Interviewing is working, both for individual patients and for groups of patients. One of the most common ways researchers and clinicians determine whether or not an intervention is working is to track patients' specific goal-oriented outcomes. In standard care, individual goal-oriented outcomes are those outcomes that patients hope to change or improve. For example, a patient may want to reduce his or her drinking or may want to reduce symptoms of depression. In standard care, individual goal-oriented outcomes are often tracked regularly on treatment plans or through the regular use of objective assessments, including clinical instruments like the Beck Depression Inventory (BDI; Beck et al. 1996) or urine toxicology screens. If patients show change in their goal-oriented outcomes (e.g., lower scores on the BDI), then the clinician might infer that the intervention is working. However, it is difficult to determine the extent to which an intervention is working for the individual, or the extent to which external factors may be influencing outcomes. One way to feel more confident that the intervention is the active agent of change is to examine change in a group of patients or to compare two groups of patients receiving different interventions. Group outcomes may be tracked by collapsing individual goal-oriented outcomes. For example, in an alcohol treatment program, the investigator might track the number of days abstinent from alcohol across all patients. However, this approach is sometimes difficult in

TABLE 16–3. Tools to assess change process

Scale	Description	What it measures
URICA (McConnaughy et al. 1983)	32 items rated on a 5-point Likert scale	Scores on each of 4 stages of change: precontemplation, contemplation, action, and maintenance; also scores on readiness to change
Stages of change algorithm (Velicer et al. 1995)	3–5 stepped questions	Places person within a single stage of change: precontemplation, contemplation, preparation, action, or maintenance
SOCRATES (Miller and Tonigan 1996)	19 items rated on a 5-point Likert scale	Scores for recognition, ambivalence, and taking steps
Decisional Balance Scale (Velicer et al. 1985)	10–20 items depending on change behavior, rated on a 5-point Likert scale	Scores for pros of change and cons of change
Treatment Motivation Scale (Knight et al. 1994)	29 items rated on a 5- or 7-point Likert scale	Scores for overall treatment readiness

Note. SOCRATES = Stages of Change Readiness and Treatment Eagerness Scale; URICA = University of Rhode Island Change Assessment. These scales are in the public domain and provided in Appendixes A and B in Chapter 4, "Contemplation."

more general standard care settings, because individual patients often have different goal-oriented outcomes.

In addition to goal-oriented outcomes, patients may exhibit change in process outcomes. Process outcomes include patient attendance or retention in treatment, the therapeutic alliance, or satisfaction with services. In addition to these general process outcomes, there are process outcomes specific to Motivational Interviewing. These include stage of change or readiness to change. As reviewed in Chapters 3 through 7, the stages of change are precontemplation, contemplation, preparation, action, and maintenance (Prochaska and DiClemente 1983). Precontemplation is when patients either do not believe they have a problem—or recognize the problem but do not want to change. Contemplation is when patients begin to think about changing their problematic behaviors, and preparation is when patients begin to plan or take their first steps toward change. Action is when patients begin to fully engage in behavior change, whereas maintenance occurs when the behavior change has been sustained for some period of time. Patients may enter treatment in one of the early stages of change (e.g., precontemplation or contemplation), and one way to evaluate an intervention is to determine whether or not patients are advancing through the stages of change. For individual patients, the clinician may compare the patient's stage of change at the beginning of treatment with his or her stage of change at various subsequent time points (e.g., every 3 months, halfway through treatment, at the end of treatment). When examining groups of patients, the investigator may want to compare the percentage of patients who are at different stages of changes at the beginning of treatment versus at subsequent time points. Another way to measure the change process is to assess the more general concept of readiness to change. Readiness to change is a way of thinking about all of the stages in a fluid way, with patients in precontemplation being lowest in readiness to change and patients in maintenance being highest in readiness to change. Standardized measures to assess the change process are described in Table 16–3. Most of these measures are fairly short and are easy to administer and score.

In-session progress also can be examined for individuals and for groups, though this is often a much more time-consuming and difficult task. In-session progress may be assessed by looking at the language that patients use in session, for there is evidence that patient language is a good indicator of behavior change. To assess patient language, it may be necessary to audiotape or videotape sessions.

How Is Motivational Interviewing Different When Used Clinically and in Research?

This chapter has covered many aspects important in the science of Motivational Interviewing. Research requires the ability to distinguish between Motivational Interviewing and other types of interventions. In addition, many studies have shown that Motivational Interviewing is an effective intervention for behavioral health problems including alcohol abuse and/or illicit drug use or misuse of prescription drugs, disordered eating, lack of exercise, and medication nonadherence. There is some evidence that Motivational Interviewing works by increasing patients' readiness to change, as measured by increased change talk during sessions.

Regarding the use of Motivational Interviewing in clinical practice versus research, one of the main differences is that research requires the delivery of a standardized intervention. Standardization means that all study clinicians are conducting the same intervention. This begins with clinician training. Some clinicians may not become proficient enough in Motivational Interviewing soon enough to participate in a research study, for Motivational Interviewing can be time-consuming to learn. However, many people from various professional backgrounds have been successfully trained in Motivational Interviewing. In addition to training, treatment fidelity must be ensured. In research, this is often measured by raters who complete standardized assessments but rarely provide feedback to study clinicians. Study clinicians usually receive intensive audiotaped or videotaped supervision throughout the study alongside ongoing, rigorous assessment of their performance.

In addition to differences in the delivery of the intervention, research usually examines change in groups of patients, as opposed to change in individual patients. To attribute change to the Motivational Interviewing intervention, researchers often compare the Motivational Interviewing group with another group of patients who receive a different type of intervention (a comparison group) or no intervention at all (a control group). Research also requires special permission and oversight from institutional committees called Institutional Review Boards. These boards review all study procedures to make sure that patients who participate in the study will be treated ethically. Ethical treatment of research participants includes having the participant give informed consent and being sure that the potential benefits of participating in the study outweigh the risks. Informed consent means that participants know about study procedures, study duration, and risks and benefits of being in the study. Finally, research differs from clinical practice in the ability to share findings with a broader audience of clinicians and researchers.

Summary

The science behind Motivational Interviewing contains a number of important findings. Nearly all studies have been focused on AMIs, with most including both the counseling style and some form of personalized feedback and not the pure clinical method described in the Motivational Interviewing books. Motivational Interviewing is superior to no treatment and its efficacy is equivalent to that of other active treatments despite its relative brevity, implying that there may be cost-effectiveness advantages to using Motivational Interviewing. The measurement of intervention fidelity is growing among clinical trials, but is lacking in many trials that claim to use Motivational Interviewing but do not present evidence of its competent use or fidelity to its spirit and methods. Lastly, the study of process-outcome relationships in Motivational Interviewing is in its early stages. As more information about process-outcome relationships in Motivational Interviewing accumulates, it will inform the development of an empirically based model of Motivational Interviewing and perhaps of related psychotherapies.

References

Amrhein PC, Miller WR, Yahne CE, et al: Client commitment language during motivational interviewing predicts drug use outcomes. J Consult Clin Psychol 71:862–878, 2003

Beck AT, Steer RA, Brown GK: BDI-II, Beck Depression Inventory: Manual, 2nd Edition. San Antonio, TX, Psychological Corporation, 1996

Burke BL, Arkowitz H, Menchola M: The efficacy of motivational interviewing: a meta-analysis of controlled clinical trials. J Consult Clin Psychol 71:843–861, 2003

Carroll KM, Nich C, Sifry RL, et al: A general system for evaluating therapist adherence and competence in psychotherapy research in the addictions. Drug Alcohol Depend 57:225–238, 2000

Catley D, Harris KJ, Mayo MS, et al: Adherence to principles of motivational interviewing and patient within-session behavior. Behav Cogn Psychother 34:43–56, 2006

Hettema J, Steele J, Miller WR: Motivational interviewing. Annu Rev Clin Psychol 1:91–111, 2005

Knight K, Holcom M, Simpson DD: TCU Psychosocial Functioning and Motivation Scales: Manual on Psychometric Properties. Fort Worth, TX, Texas Christian University Institute of Behavioral Research, 1994

Lane C, Huws-Thomas M, Hood K, et al: Measuring adaptations of motivational interviewing: the development and validation of the behavior change counseling index (BECCI). Patient Educ Couns 56:166–173, 2005

Madson MB, Campbell TC, Barrett DE, et al: Development of the Motivational Interviewing Supervision and Training Scale. Psychol Addict Behav 19:303–310, 2005

McConnaughy EN, Prochaska JO, Velicer WF: Stages of change in psychotherapy: measurement and sample profiles. Psychotherapy: Theory, Research and Practice 20: 368–375, 1983

Miller WR, Mount KA: A small study of training in motivational interviewing: does one workshop change clinician and patient behavior? Behav Cogn Psychother 29:457–471, 2001

Miller WR, Moyers TB: Eight stages in learning motivational interviewing. Journal of Teaching in the Addictions 5:3–17, 2006

Miller WR, Rollnick S: Motivational Interviewing: Preparing People to Change Addictive Behavior. New York, Guilford, 1991

Miller WR, Rollnick S: Motivational Interviewing: Preparing People for Change, 2nd Edition. New York, Guilford, 2002

Miller WR, Tonigan JS: Assessing drinkers' motivation for change: the Stages of Change Readiness and Treatment Eagerness Scale (SOCRATES). Psychol Addict Behav 10:81–89, 1996

Miller WR, Benefield RJ, Tonigan JS: Enhancing motivation for change in problem drinking: a controlled comparison of two therapist styles. J Consult Clin Psychol 61:455–461, 1993

Miller WR, Yahne CE, Moyers TB, et al: A randomized trial of methods to help clinicians learn motivational interviewing. J Consult Clin Psychol 72:1050–1062, 2004

Moyers TB, Martin TM: Associations between patient and therapist behaviors: partial validation of the motivational interviewing approach. Paper presented at the annual meeting of the College on Problems of Drug Dependence, Fort Lauderdale, FL, June 2003

Moyers TB, Martin T: Therapist influence on patient language during motivational interviewing sessions. J Subst Abuse Treat 30:245–251, 2006

Moyers T, Martin T, Catley D, et al: Assessing the integrity of motivational interviewing interventions: reliability of the motivational interviewing skills code. Behav Cogn Psychother 31:177–184, 2003

Moyers TB, Martin T, Manuel JK, et al: Assessing competence in the use of motivational interviewing. J Subst Abuse Treat 28:19–26, 2005a

Moyers TB, Miller WR, Hendrickson SML: How does motivational interviewing work? Therapist interpersonal skill predicts client involvement within motivational interviewing sessions. J Consult Clin Psychol 73:590–598, 2005b

Moyers TB, Martin T, Christopher PJ, et al: Client language as a mediator of motivational interviewing efficacy: where is the evidence? Alcohol Clin Exp Res 31(10 suppl):40s–47s, 2007

Patterson GR, Forgatch MS: Therapist behavior as a determinant for patient noncompliance: a paradox for the behavior modifier. J Consult Clin Psychol 53:846–851, 1985

Prochaska JO, DiClemente CC: Stages and processes of self-change of smoking: toward an integrative model of change. J Consult Clin Psychol 51:390–395, 1983

Project MATCH Research Group: Project MATCH: rationale and methods for a multisite clinical trial matching patients to alcoholism treatment. Alcohol Clin Exp Res 17:1130–1145, 1993

Rubak S, Sandboek A, Lauritzen T, et al: Motivational interviewing: a systematic review and meta-analysis. Br J Gen Pract 55:305–312, 2005

Strang J, McCambridge J: Can the practitioner correctly predict outcome in motivational interviewing? J Subst Abuse Treat 27:83–88, 2004

Thrasher AD, Golin CE, Earp JA, et al: Motivational interviewing to support antiretroviral therapy adherence: the role of quality counseling. Patient Educ Couns 62:64–71, 2006

Tollison SJ, Lee CM, Neighbors C, et al: Questions and reflections: the use of motivational interviewing microskills in a peer-led brief alcohol intervention for college students. Behav Ther 39:183–194, 2008

Velicer WF, DiClemente CC, Prochaska JO, et al: Decisional balance measure for assessing and predicting smoking status. J Pers Soc Psychol 48:1279–1289, 1985

Velicer WF, Fava JL, Prochaska JO, et al: Distribution of smokers by stage in three representative samples. Prev Med 24:401–411, 1995

Movie Library

Alcohol

The Answer Man (2009)
Crazy Heart (2009)
I can do bad all by myself (2009)
Julia (2008)
Rachel Getting Married (2008)
La Vie en Rose (*La Môme*) (2007)
There Will Be Blood (2007)
Bobby (2006)
Capote (2005)
In Her Shoes (2005)
Walk the Line (2005)
Family Portrait (2004)
Spider-Man 2 (2004)
Bad Santa (2003)
House of Sand and Fog (2003)
Old School (2003)
Something's Gotta Give (2003)
Better Luck Tomorrow (2002)
Changing Lanes (2002)
Evelyn (2002)
Far From Heaven (2002)
Skins (2002)
Sweet Sixteen (2002)

Two Weeks Notice (2002)
All Over the Guy (2001)
Big Bad Love (2001)
Chelsea Walls (2001)
Heartbreakers (2001)
28 Days (2000)
Bounce (2000)
Dancing at the Blue Iguana (2000)
DUI: Dead in 5 Seconds (2000)
Pay It Forward (2000)
The Perfect Son (2000)
Shadow Hours (2000)
Spent (2000)
Angela's Ashes (1999)
Girl, Interrupted (1999)
Liberty Heights (1999)
Alcohol: Brain Under the Influence (1998)
My Name Is Joe (1998)
Affliction (1997)
Man About Town (1997)
Nil by Mouth (1997)
Trees Lounge (1996)
Drunks (1995)
Leaving Las Vegas (1995)

Alcohol *(continued)*

Once Were Warriors (1994)
When a Man Loves a Woman (1994)
Bad Lieutenant (1992)
Scent of a Woman (1992)
Shakes the Clown (1991)
Barfly (1987)
Blind Date (1987)
Hoosiers (1986)
Mommy Dearest (1981)
Only When I Laugh (1981)
The Rose (1979)
National Lampoon's Animal House (1978)
Days of Wine and Roses (1962)
What Ever Happened to Baby Jane? (1962)
Cat on a Hot Tin Roof (1958)
The Bad Seed (1956)
The Lost Weekend (1945)
A Star is Born (1937)

Amphetamines

Rock Bottom (2006)
Spun (2002)
Requiem for a Dream (also listed under "Opioids") (2000)

Caffeine

Coffee and Cigarettes (2003)
Caffeination (2002)
Sixty Cups of Coffee (2000)

Cannabis

Pineapple Express (2008)
Harsh Times (2005)

Strangers With Candy (2005)
Harold and Kumar Go to White Castle (2004)
It Runs in the Family (2003)
The Good Girl (2002)
Y Tu Mamá También (2001)
Amores Perros (2000)
American Beauty (1999)
Grass (1999)
Around the Fire (1998)
True Romance (1993)
Fast Times at Ridgemont High (1982)
Cheech and Chong's Up in Smoke (1978)
Assassin of Youth (1937)
Marihuana (1936)
Reefer Madness (1936)

Cocaine

Half Nelson (2006)
Layer Cake (2004)
Better Luck Tomorrow (2002)
City of God (Cidade de Deus) (2002)
Love and Diane (2002)
New Best Friend (2002)
Blow (2001)
O (2001)
Tart (2001)
Burnt Money (Plata Quemada) (2000)
Traffic (2000)
Cruel Intentions (1999)
Boogie Nights (1997)
Sweet Nothing (1996)
Boyz n the Hood (1991)
New Jack City (1991)
The Boost (1988)
Bright Lights, Big City (1988)
Clean and Sober (1988)
Less Than Zero (1987)
Scarface (1983)

Hallucinogens

White Sound (*Das weiss Rauschen*)
  (2002)
Fear and Loathing in Las Vegas (1998)
In the Name of the Father (1993)
The Doors (1991)
Naked Lunch (1991)
Jacob's Ladder (1990)
Altered States (1980)
The People Next Door (1970)
Performance (1970)
Easy Rider (1969)
I Love You, Alice B. Toklas (1968)
Psych-Out (1968)
The President's Analyst (1967)
The Trip (1967)
The Tingler (1959)

Inhalants

Love Liza (2002)
Citizen Ruth (1996)
Blue Velvet (1986)

Nicotine

Good Night, and Good Luck (2005)
Thank You for Smoking (2005)
*Scene Smoking: Cigarettes, Cinema
  and the Myth of Cool* (2001)
The Last Cigarette (directed by
  Roger Ireton) (1999)
The War of the Roses (1989)

Opioids

American Gangster (2007)
Eastern Promises (2007)

Little Miss Sunshine (2006)
SherryBaby (2006)
Dope Sick Love (2005)
Rent (2005)
Maria Full of Grace (2004)
Ray (2004)
What the #$! Do We (K)now!?* (2004)
21 Grams (2003)
The Barbarian Invasions
  (*Les Invasions Barbares*) (2003)
Union Square (2003)
Veronica Guerin (2003)
Wonderland (2003)
Igby Goes Down (also listed under
  "Sedatives, Hypnotics, Anxiolyt-
  ics") (2002)
Sister Helen (2002)
Novocaine (2001)
Riding in Cars With Boys (2001)
Requiem for a Dream (also listed
  under "Amphetamines") (2000)
Brokedown Palace (1999)
Jesus' Son (1999)
Another Day in Paradise (1998)
Broken Vessels (1998)
Gia (1998)
High Art (1998)
Permanent Midnight (1998)
Velvet Goldmine (1998)
Why Do Fools Fall In Love (1998)
Gridlock'd (1997)
Basquiat (1996)
Dog Run (1996)
Pusher (1996)
Trainspotting (1996)
The Basketball Diaries (1995)
Georgia (1995)
Rush (1991)
Drugstore Cowboy (1989)
Sid and Nancy (1986)
Once Upon a Time in America (1984)
Liquid Sky (1982)

Opioids *(continued)*

Christiane F (1981)
French Connection II (1975)
The Panic in Needle Park (1971)
Joe (1970)
Trash (1970)
Chelsea Girls (1966)
The Man With the Golden Arm (1955)
Narcotic (1933)

Phencyclidine

Desperate Lives (1982)
Blue Sunshine (1976)

Sedatives, Hypnotics, Anxiolytics

The Orphanage (*El Orfanato*) (2007)
Igby Goes Down (also listed under "Opioids") (2002)
I'm Dancing as Fast as I Can (1982)
Beyond the Valley of the Dolls (1970)
Valley of the Dolls (1967)

Club Drugs

The Hangover (2009)
Party Monster (2003)
24 Hour Party People (2002)
25th Hour (2002)
When Boys Fly (2002)
The Anniversary Party (2001)
Circuit (2001)
Ivan's xtc (2000)
Go (1999)
Party Monster: The Shockumentary (1999)
Living Out Loud (1998)
Kids (1995)
Family Plot (1976)

Other Substances

Finding Nemo [fish] (2003)
The Attack of the Giant Moussaka [moussaka] (1999)
Female Trouble [liquid eyeliner] (1974)

Helpful Internet Sites

The Addiction Institute of New York

www.addictioninstituteny.org

The Addiction Institute of New York Web site provides information on addiction treatment, training, and research, as well as Internet links to many national addiction organizations. It also maintains an active list of addiction-related films, which may be used in lectures and presentations.

Alcohol Medical Scholars Program

http://alcoholmedicalscholars.org

The Alcohol Medical Scholars Program promotes education in medical schools regarding the identification and treatment of alcohol use disorders and other substance-related problems.

American Academy of Child and Adolescent Psychiatry

http://aacap.org/cs/expert_interviews/substance_abuse

This site contains videos by experts in the field regarding substance abuse in children and adolescents, aimed at medical professionals. Topics include prevention, dual diagnosis, and recognition of signs of substance abuse.

American College of Physician Executives

www.acpe.org

The American College of Physician Executives is the primary organization for education, networking, and career development of physicians in administrative and managerial positions.

Association for Applied Sport Psychology

http://appliedsportpsych.org

The Association for Applied Sport Psychology provides consultations, education, training, and advocacy on sport and exercise psychology.

Association for Humanistic Psychology

www.ahpweb.org

The Web site of the Association for Humanistic Psychology provides information on the humanistic psychology tradition, including the work of Carl Rogers.

The George Washington Institute for Spirituality and Health

www.gwish.org

This site offers practical suggestions on how to ask patients about spiritual issues and how to discuss spirituality with trainees.

The Internet Movie Database

www.imdb.com

The Internet Movie Database is the most comprehensive Web site for television shows and films. It provides information on hundreds of thousands of movies including plotlines, synopses, reviews, trivia, and "goofs."

Motivational Interviewing

www.motivationalinterview.org

This is a Web site with comprehensive information on motivational interviewing.

National Association for Alcoholism and Drug Abuse Counselors (NAADAC), the Association for Addiction Professionals

www.naadac.org

This Web site offers a helpful online course, Blending Solutions: Integrating Motivational Interviewing with Pharmacotherapy (on the home page, click on Education; in the drop-down menu, click on Blending Solutions).

National Council on Aging, Center for Healthy Aging

www.healthyagingprograms.org

The National Council on Aging's Center for Healthy Aging Web site includes resources on many chronic diseases, including alcoholism and substance abuse.

National Institute on Alcohol Abuse and Alcoholism

www.niaaa.nih.gov/Publications

Visit NIAAA's Web site for various helpful publications. Order and download the very well-researched and well-presented brochure *Helping Patients Who Drink Too Much: A Clinician's Guide* (also located at: www.niaaa.nih.gov/Publications/EducationTrainingMaterials/guide.htm). This guide provides copies of the Alcohol Use Disorders Identification Test (AUDIT) in both English and Spanish.

National Institute on Drug Abuse—NIDA for Teens

http://teens.drugabuse.gov

Here teenagers who may be interested in learning more about practical facts about drugs can find appropriate resources. The site has links to games, testimonials, videos, and topics for discussion for teens and their families. This is a good resource for the contemplation-stage teen, who would like to learn more practical information about drugs and their effects.

National Institute on Drug Abuse—Prevention

http://drugabuse.gov/Prevention

This site features *Preventing Drug Use Among Children and Adolescents: A Research-Based Guide for Parents, Educators, and Community Leaders,* 2nd Edition, which offers valuable information on prevention of drug use and abuse in adolescents with practical strategies for parents, educators, and other authority figures in an adolescent's life. This can also be a practical guide for providing information to adolescents who may have already experimented with drugs and alcohol.

Prism Awards

www.prismawards.com

The Prism Awards, cosponsored by the Substance Abuse and Mental Health Services Administration, are designed to recognize the accurate depiction of alcohol, drug, and tobacco use in the popular media.

Substance Abuse and Mental Health Services Administration (SAMHSA)

http://ncadi.samhsa.gov

SAMHSA's National Clearinghouse for Alcohol and Drug Information offers free publications on a variety of addiction topics.

Answer Guide

Chapter 2

1. Motivational Interviewing is most closely related to:

    A. Psychoanalysis.
    B. Behaviorism.
    C. Humanistic psychology.
    D. The 12-step tradition.

    Correct answer: **C**

    Motivational Interviewing is deeply grounded in humanistic psychology, especially Carl Rogers's client-centered approach.

2. The spirit of Motivational Interviewing lies in:

    A. Criticism, elucidation, and analysis.
    B. Creativity, expansion, and advocacy.
    C. Confrontation, education, and authority.
    D. Collaboration, evocation, and autonomy.

    Correct answer: **D**

    In Motivational Interviewing, clinicians collaborate with the patient, evoke the patient's resources and strengths that support change, and respect the patient's autonomy.

3. A clinician who has mixed feelings about seeking supervision for Motivational Interviewing and has not yet planned to contact a supervisor is likely to be in which of the following stages of change?

    A. Precontemplation.
    B. Contemplation.
    C. Preparation.
    D. Relapse.

    Correct answer: **B**

Though ambivalent, the clinician is contemplating change but has not yet developed a plan for change or taken action.

4. Motivational Interviewing often can be successfully combined with other therapeutic modalities. This statement is:

   A. False, because any association with other therapies will confuse the patient.
   B. True, because Motivational Interviewing is compatible with many approaches.
   C. Dangerous, because clinicians should always be passionate advocates of only one psychotherapeutic school.
   D. Irrelevant, because competent clinicians spontaneously know what to do without the need to learn Motivational Interviewing.

   Correct answer: **B**

   Motivational Interviewing is consistent with many other psychotherapeutic modalities, and it can be used as a prelude to them, a permeating factor used alongside other approaches, or a fallback position whenever motivational issues reemerge in treatment.

5. Teaching and supervision of Motivational Interviewing:

   A. Is best done in an accepting and collaborative manner.
   B. Is best done through confrontation to emphasize contrast with the style of Motivational Interviewing.
   C. Requires that the student undergo his or her own motivational therapy.
   D. Should focus on convincing the student that Motivational Interviewing is better than other therapies.

   Correct answer: **A**

   Teaching and supervision are best done in a supportive and collaborative manner that is consistent with the spirit of Motivational Interviewing.

Chapter 3

1. The primary goal of working with a client in the precontemplation stage of change is:

   A. Breaking down the client's denial through confrontation.
   B. Engaging the client in the treatment process.
   C. Helping the client to identify triggers.
   D. None of the above.

Correct answer: **B**

The primary goal is to engage the client in the treatment process. Beyond this simple goal, the treatment is geared toward helping the client to set realistic goals and to help the client identify strategies for attaining those goals.

2. Which of the following statements is false?

   A. Motivational Interviewing does not rely on a confrontational style.
   B. When working with a client in the precontemplation stage, the clinician should focus primarily on engaging the client.
   C. One should ask yes-or-no questions when using Motivational Interviewing.
   D. Motivational Interviewing should reinforce the client's locus of control.

   Correct answer: **C**

   One should concentrate on asking open-ended questions rather than yes-or-no questions.

3. When using a Motivational Interviewing approach to treating substance use issues, the clinician should:

   A. Encourage the client to accept responsibility for his or her successes and failures.
   B. Help the client identify goals.
   C. Focus on helping the client move toward a greater sense of self-efficacy.
   D. All of the above.

   Correct answer: **D**

   All of these are important in working within the Motivational Interviewing model.

4. Which of the following statements is true of clients in the precontemplation stage?

   A. By definition, people in this stage do not seek treatment.
   B. When in this stage, people might seek treatment due to pressure from outside sources.
   C. People in this stage usually move to another stage quickly.
   D. None of the above.

   Correct answer: **B**

Clients might seek treatment but usually do so under pressure from family, friends, or outside sources of authority such as the legal system, workplace, or school.

5. In the precontemplation stage, resistance to change can be characterized by:

A. Reluctance.
B. Rebellion.
C. Resignation.
D. All of the above.

Correct answer: **D**

All of the above. In addition, resistance to change can be characterized by rationalization.

Chapter 4

1. All of the following are true about the contemplation stage, EXCEPT:

A. Ambivalence is very common.
B. Most people move into the preparation stage within days of beginning to contemplate.
C. Most people have many more pros for changing than cons against.
D. Health care practitioners can often help patients contemplate behavior change.

Correct answer: **B**

Contemplation can take a long time for many individuals.

2. Which of the following is NOT generally an effective technique used by clinicians to help a patient contemplate behavior change?

A. Provision of feedback.
B. Inducing guilt.
C. Use of a decisional balance sheet.
D. Provision of factual information.

Correct answer: **B**

In general, purposeful attempts to induce guilt in a patient are not seen as effective interventions.

3. Which is NOT a scale used to help assess an individual's readiness to change a behavior?

A. The University of Rhode Island Change Assessment (URICA).
B. The Readiness Ruler.
C. The Stages of Change Readiness and Treatment Eagerness Scale (SOCRATES).
D. The Princeton Level of Attention to Treatment Obstacles (PLATO).

Correct answer: **D**

The PLATO is not a real scale.

4. All of the following are generally seen as primary goals of the clinician working with a patient in the contemplation stage, EXCEPT:
A. Helping the patient to recognize and work through ambivalence.
B. Helping the patient to recognize the benefits of change.
C. Helping the patient to achieve a sense of self-efficacy.
D. Helping the patient to regain things he or she has lost as a result of the addiction.

Correct answer: **D**

The clinician may eventually assist the patient in regaining things lost through addiction but that is generally not seen as a primary goal in the contemplation stage.

5. All of the following are typical phenomena seen in individuals in the contemplation stage, EXCEPT:
A. Rationalization.
B. Procrastination.
C. Dissociation.
D. Ambivalence.

Correct answer: **C**

Dissociation is not a common defense mechanism in the contemplation stage of behavior change.

Chapter 5

1. Rashad is a 40-year-old male with a history of heavy nicotine addiction for over 20 years. His lover, who has been a smoker for over 35 years, was recently rushed to the emergency room and was diagnosed with emphysema. Rashad is aware of his nicotine dependence and has tried numerous times to quit. He attributes this addiction to his partner. After hearing the em-

physema diagnosis, Rashad immediately went on the Internet to research nicotine cessation. He scheduled an appointment with his doctor to discuss his nicotine dependence. Rashad is also searching for a support group. Rashad is in what stage of change?

A. Precontemplation.
B. Contemplation.
C. Preparation.
D. Action.

Correct answer: **C**

Rashad made a commitment to a time and a plan to address his nicotine dependence. He informed himself by using the Internet for nicotine cessation information. He has taken steps by partnering with his doctor to discuss his nicotine dependence and is actively searching for a support group.

2. Charles is a 40-year-old married male with a 9-year-old daughter. He works as an executive in a busy, high-pressure accounting firm. He denies any alcohol or drug use. He verbalized being sexually dissatisfied with his wife. He spends much time searching pornographic Web sites on his laptop. In fear of being discovered by his wife, he started using his laptop in the basement. At first, he would spend an hour after work surfing the Internet, then it grew to 4 hours. Now, it has consumed him so that he is surfing the Internet for porn during business hours. Two weeks ago, his assistant walked in on Charles sniffing a thong while watching pornographic material during lunch. Embarrassed, Charles quickly turned off his computer and hid the thong in his desk drawer and threatened to fire the assistant if she were to mention this to anyone. The assistant promises to keep his secret in confidence. In order for Charles to be in the preparation stage, which of the following statements is correct?

A. "Who, me? I have no problem. I can stop surfing the Internet for pornographic Web sites whenever I want to. Besides, I am a top executive in this company. Anyway, nobody monitors my computer because I am the boss."
B. "I think I might have a problem controlling my urges and surfing the Internet for pornographic Web sites. It was really embarrassing that my assistant caught me in the act. What if my wife knew?"
C. "I have a problem controlling my urges and surfing the Internet for porn. I could lose my job if my assistant reports me to human resources. My wife will find out, divorce me, and not let me see my daughter. Tomorrow, I will take a day off from work and will seek professional help."

D. "It was really embarrassing that my assistant caught me. Since then, my wife and I have attended couples counseling and I see a psychiatrist who has prescribed medication for me."

Correct answer: **C**

Charles acknowledges that he has a problem and focuses on a timetable and a specific course of action. This is the preparation stage.

3. What is the most important component in moving a patient from contemplation into the preparation stage so that the patient can be successful in dealing with his or her problem?

   A. The patient believes and understands that he or she has a problem and plans to do something about it in the future.
   B. The patient identifies the pros and cons of change.
   C. The patient describes a plan in detail and follows it as part of his or her regular activity.
   D. The patient expresses feelings about how much the change has actually improved the patient's life and reflects on the long-term goal.

   Correct answer: **A**

   Choice A is the preparation stage. The patient understands that change is needed. In turn, the patient reaches a deal for a start date. Choice B is the contemplation stage, in which the patient begins to show an openness about discussing the problem and evaluating the advantages and disadvantages of the need to change. Choice C is the action stage, in which the patient shows a commitment to follow a plan and incorporates it in his or her daily activities. Choice D is the maintenance stage, in which the patient had completed the change and is witnessing the improvement in his or her life. The patient is then focusing on the long-term goal to prevent relapse.

4. How can a clinician know if the patient is ready to move from the preparation stage to the action stage and be successful?

   A. Feedback from the patient regarding the treatment plan and whether he or she is ready to move from the preparation state to the action stage is the best indicator.
   B. Using urine toxicology is the best way to assess the stage of change and readiness to move forward.
   C. The scope of the treatment plan determines the appropriate time to move to the next stage.
   D. The preparation stage typically lasts for 6 months, after which the patient transits to the action stage.

Correct answer: **A**

Although the clinician can never definitely know, the patient's statements are the best barometer of motivation and change.

5. Which patient characteristic best increase the chances of success when entering the preparation stage?

    A. The patient realizes that he or she is substance dependent and is aware of the negative consequences of his or her behavior. Therefore, the patient plans to set a date in the future to change the behavior.
    B. The patient believes that there are fewer opportunities when he or she stops using drugs and thinks, for example, "We are all going to die anyway, might as well die high."
    C. Younger substance abusers have fewer established negative behavioral patterns than older users; they are better candidates for substance use cessation.
    D. The patient is being forced by society to change his or her behavior; for example, a heroin-dependent teenager is mandated by the court to attend a drug treatment program.

    Correct answer: **A**

    This patient is very aware of his or her substance dependency and plans to address the issue in the future.

Chapter 6

1. A patient's wife giving a warm embrace and encouragement when her partner comes home from an AA meeting is an example of:

    A. Positive reinforcement.
    B. Negative reinforcement.
    C. Community reinforcement.
    D. Contingency management.

    Correct answer: **A**

    Positive reinforcement is the addition of something that will strengthen a specific behavior. The hug, warmth, and praise reinforce the specific behavior of the husband going to the AA meeting and do increase the chance that he will go again. Once again, helping patients to generate their own internal reinforcements is even better. Saying "You really seem proud that you've been going to regular AA meetings lately" is better than saying "I'm really proud of you for going regularly to AA meetings."

2. When a person says, "I can't have fun at a party without alcohol":

A. This is a cognition that needs to be accepted.
B. This indicates that parties always need to be avoided.
C. This is an assumption that is testable.
D. All of the above.

Correct answer: **C**

The cognition that someone cannot have fun at a party is an assumption. Cognitive restructuring involves critically looking at the evidence that supports and does not support this assumption. Then more balanced cognitions can be practiced, such as "Alcohol made it easier to feel comfortable at parties, but if I do some relaxation exercises beforehand and remind myself that I'm not here to meet my future wife, I might find some interesting people to talk to."

3. If a trigger cannot be avoided, some useful techniques to cope or manage the person's response to triggers include:

A. Assertive refusal.
B. Imaginal flooding with negative consequences, such as vomiting.
C. Contacting a healthy social support.
D. All of the above.

Correct answer: **D**

Creating an armamentarium of options to deal with triggers increases the likelihood of avoiding the substance. These options may be very creative.

4. When someone stops using a substance, which of the following is most likely to occur?

A. Most areas in the person's life now become stable and fulfilling.
B. Many people, at least temporarily, have difficulty adjusting to life without substance use.
C. Most relationships, damaged as a result of substance abuse, are repaired.
D. Patients have a new clarity and realize that the substance was the cause of most of their difficulties.

Correct answer: **B**

Once a person stops using a substance, many of his or her difficulties still exist. It often takes time and practice for roles to change and for relationship patterns to be replaced. Often, there is a void left by the absence of all the substance use–related activities that occupied so much of a patient's time and energy. It may not be the case that substance use caused certain problems, and insight into the contribution of a substance to the person's difficulties isn't necessarily related to abstinence.

5. With regard to a patient's social network:

   A. Only family members should be included in the treatment.
   B. The individual being treated is the patient, and he or she needs to recover without interference from network members.
   C. Often, network members have negatively contributed to a patient's substance use or to the dysfunctional relationship. Involving such a person is a risk for relapse.
   D. Substance use usually involves interpersonal issues. Involving the network can greatly enhance the treatment.

   Correct answer: **D**

   Although it is important to first evaluate who will be healthy supports, it is rare that a caring member of a person's network will be unable to make changes that support the patient's abstinence. Involving the network can provide much needed support, feedback, the opportunity to practice relationship skills in the office, the ability to educate the network, and so forth. It is seen as an invaluable part of the patient's treatment.

Chapter 7

1. Which of the following correctly describes the maintenance stage of change?

   A. A period during which patients are unaware of having a problem behavior.
   B. A period of abstinence in which the desired behavior change has become sustained.
   C. A period during which patients consider changing their behavior.
   D. A period during which patients take concrete steps to change their behavior.

   Correct answer: **B**

   Maintenance marks the completion of behavior change with an ongoing awareness of the possibility of relapse.

2. Which of the following is NOT a Motivational Interviewing style of response to a patient who has acknowledged a lapse into drinking?

A. "You should have known better than to make a mistake like that."
B. "Can you tell me more about what thoughts and emotions you were having before you took the drink?"
C. "What can we learn from the episode of drinking that will help you in the future?"
D. "Having a slip is a common setback that patients experience, but it is not a failure."

Correct answer: **A**

In Motivational Interviewing the clinician engages in a collaborative effort with the patient, whose autonomy is respected, and intrinsic motivation is evoked. Accusatory statements are not consistent with the spirit of Motivational Interviewing.

3. Which of the following is NOT a recommended coping skill in relapse prevention?

A. A patient attends anger management classes to learn how to deal with this emotion.
B. An alcoholic patient repeatedly returns to a bar where he or she used to drink to desensitize himself or herself to cravings.
C. A patient carries around an index card with a list of reminders about the negative consequences of drinking.
D. A patient decides to begin a new hobby that he or she enjoys.

Correct answer: **B**

Relapse prevention involves identifying and coping with high-risk situations and urges to use. Deliberately evoking cravings by putting oneself in a high-risk situation is not a helpful coping mechanism.

4. In beginning treatment with patients, it is recommended that therapists do all of the following EXCEPT:

A. Provide the patient with a clear explanation of the goals of treatment.
B. Establish a therapeutic connection.
C. Make clear to the patient that any deviation from therapy goals could be grounds for termination.
D. Explore the patient's expectations from treatment.

Correct answer: **C**

In the style of Motivational Interviewing, the agenda is elicited from the patient rather than being rigidly set by the clinician.

5. A *lapse* is defined as:

    A. A strong craving to use alcohol or drugs.

    B. A period of time between the action and maintenance stages of change.

    C. A full-blown return to the previous pattern of behavior.

    D. A brief return to drinking or drug use after a period of abstinence.

    Correct answer: **D**

    A lapse is a brief return to use that does not necessarily progress to relapse, which is a full-blown return to previous behavioral patterns.

Chapter 8

1. A patient resumes drinking alcohol for a month after attaining 1 year of sobriety. He visits his therapist to discuss the relapse. The patient could be in which of the following stages of change as identified by Prochaska and DiClemente (1984)?

    A. Precontemplation.

    B. Contemplation.

    C. Action.

    D. Any of the above.

    Correct answer: **D**

    A patient who relapses can be in any of the first four stages of change (precontemplation, contemplation, preparation, or action) after the relapse.

2. During a relapse, a patient tells the clinician who is working with her that "I should just keep on drinking. I've lost my sobriety now." This patient is most likely in which of the following stages of change?

    A. Precontemplation.

    B. Contemplation.

    C. Preparation.

    D. Maintenance.

    Correct answer: **A**

    The patient has returned to the precontemplation state.

3. With the abstinence violation effect:

   A. Patients attribute their loss of sobriety to factors beyond their control.
   B. Patients maintain their confidence that they can return to abstinence.
   C. Patients view their return to substance use as a learning experience.
   D. Patients remain in the maintenance stage of change.

   Correct answer: **A**

   With the abstinence violation effect, patients see their relapse as stemming from factors beyond their control, which leads them to abandon their abstinence attempt.

4. Which of the following is NOT an example of a common pitfall for clinicians in working with patients who have relapsed?

   A. Having a judgmental attitude toward the patient.
   B. Having self-critical thoughts about how you, the clinician, could have prevented the relapse.
   C. Expressing your (the clinician's) desire for the patient's immediate return to a state of abstinence.
   D. Having an open-minded viewpoint about the patient's motivation to change his or her behavior.

   Correct answer: **D**

   Only answer D emphasizes a patient-centered, motivational approach to treatment.

5. Which of the following is NOT an example of a motivational approach for the clinician to take with patients who relapse?

   A. Identify the possible factors that may have led to the relapse.
   B. Use a decisional matrix to analyze the pros and cons of continuing to use the substance.
   C. Determine additional supports for patients to help them reestablish their abstinence.
   D. Tell patients that the relapse shows how powerful their disease is and that they will need to be stronger next time.

   Correct answer: **D**

   Answers A through C are possible motivational approaches to treating a patient who relapses. Answer D is an example of a judgmental and nonmotivational statement.

Chapter 9

1. What percentage of patients in either mental health or addiction treatment settings has a co-occurring disorder?

   A. 10%.
   B. 25%.
   C. 50%.
   D. 90%.

   Correct answer: **C**

   The prevalence of individuals with co-occurring disorders is elevated from a baseline of 3%–4% of individuals in the community to 40%–60% in mental health treatment settings and 50%–60% in substance abuse treatment settings.

2. Regarding prognosis and longitudinal outcome, in comparison with patients with only a mental illness or an SUD, those with co-occurring disorders:

   A. Have a more favorable course of illness.
   B. Have an approximately equal course of illness.
   C. Have a less favorable course of illness only in terms of poorer treatment engagement.
   D. Have a less favorable course of illness in multiple domains of psychosocial functioning.

   Correct answer: **D**

   In comparison with patients with only a mental illness or an SUD, those with co-occurring disorders have greater severity of illness and a worse longitudinal course of illness in multiple domains, such as increased risk for psychiatric and substance use relapses, higher levels of psychological distress, worse overall psychosocial functioning, poorer treatment engagement, worse treatment retention, and higher rates of violence, suicide, legal difficulties, and medical problems, among others.

3. Motivational Interviewing is a:

   A. Noncoercive, intrinsically oriented treatment.
   B. Coercive, intrinsically oriented treatment.
   C. Coercive, extrinsically oriented treatment.
   D. Noncoercive, extrinsically oriented treatment.

   Correct answer: **A**

Motivational Interviewing is a noncoercive cognitive and experiential method whereby the therapist helps the patient explore and resolve ambivalence in order to increase internal motivation to change behavior.

4. Motivation to change within the AA program can best be characterized by:

A. Peer coercive approaches.
B. Group cohesion.
C. Spiritually oriented approaches such as connection to a "higher power."
D. All of the above.

Correct answer: **D**

In 12-step mutual-help recovery programs, peer coercion and group cohesion combine with a spiritually based treatment approach to motivate change toward the maintenance of abstinence.

5. Which of the following is *not* associated with improved treatment outcomes in patients with co-occurring disorders?

A. Employment.
B. Greater length of time in treatment.
C. Participation in 12-step mutual-help programs.
D. A serial system of care model.

Correct answer: **D**

From a treatment delivery system perspective, integrated treatment models for patients with co-occurring disorders—where treatment for all problem domains (i.e., addiction, psychiatric, and medical) occurs in a single setting—are superior to either serial or parallel treatment models.

Chapter 10

1. Which of the following statements is true, regarding when a patient engaged in Motivational Interviewing psychotherapy should be presented with the option of psychopharmacological treatment?

A. The patient needs to be ready for change first.
B. The patient needs to be in the preparation stage to be able to use the information about medication.
C. The patient needs to be at least in the contemplation stage.
D. The patient can be in any stage of change.

Correct answer: **D**

The option of psychopharmacological treatment can be presented at any stage of change regardless of the patient's readiness, willingness, and ability to change; however, every stage has certain particularities in terms of interactions between Motivational Interviewing and psychopharmacological treatment that should be considered.

2. Which statement best describes the relationship between Motivational Interviewing and psychopharmacological treatment?

   A. Motivational Interviewing may be used to improve medication adherence.
   B. Medication may facilitate transition from one stage of change to the next.
   C. Both A and B are true.
   D. Neither A nor B are true.

   Correct answer: **C**

   There is a reciprocal relationship between psychopharmacological treatment and Motivational Interviewing: psychotherapy influences medication adherence and medication may influence progress in psychotherapy.

3. Which statement is true about the relationship between medication and the Motivational Interviewing principle of supporting self-efficacy?

   A. Medication may increase self-efficacy.
   B. Medication may decrease self-efficacy.
   C. Medication may decrease or increase self-efficacy depending on the circumstances.
   D. Medication rarely affects self-efficacy.

   Correct answer: **C**

   Medication may affect self-efficacy in either direction: it may increase it if adherence to treatment is looked at as an accomplishment or it may decrease it if, for example, the patient perceives medication as taking away his or her control over the process of change.

4. Which statement is false about the following FDA-approved medications for the treatment of alcohol dependence?

   A. Disulfiram can be helpful when administered to patients who want to remain in a state of enforced sobriety.
   B. Naltrexone may be helpful for those with a strong family history of substance abuse.

    C. Acamprosate is believed to increase feelings of discomfort associated with abstinence from alcohol.

    D. Naltrexone treatment can be started when a patient is not abstinent.

    Correct answer: **C**

    Acamprosate is believed to prevent feelings of discomfort associated with abstinence from alcohol.

5. Which of the following is false regarding patients' ambivalence?

    A. Ambivalence is normal in the process of change, and it is helpful for treaters to accept it.

    B. In the context of medication use, ambivalence is a sign of treatment failure.

    C. A patient ready, willing, and able to change may still remain ambivalent.

    D. No stage of change can be expected to be ambivalence free.

    Correct answer: **B**

    Ambivalence is a natural process that may involve a patient's relationship with medication. A patient's ambivalence does not mean that treatment has been unsuccessful, but not allowing the patient to express ambivalence may jeopardize the therapeutic process. Therefore, poor adherence to medication treatment should prompt more exploration of ambivalence in therapy.

Chapter 11

1. The best screening tool for harmful and hazardous drinking to use in primary care practices is the:

    A. DAST.

    B. AUDIT.

    C. CAGE questionnaire.

    D. MAST.

    Correct answer: **B**

    The AUDIT was developed by the World Health Organization as a screening tool for use in primary care and is designed to identify patients with harmful and hazardous levels of alcohol consumption. The CAGE questionnaire is best at identifying those with alcohol abuse and alcohol dependence.

2. According to the National Institute on Alcohol Abuse and Alcoholism recommendations, effective screening for alcohol problems can be accomplished with as little as:

    A. One question.
    B. Two questions.
    C. Three questions.
    D. Four questions.

    Correct answer: **A**

    The National Institute on Alcohol Abuse and Alcoholism provides the option of initiating screening with the following question: "How many times in the past year have you had X or more drinks in a day?" (X = 5 for men and 4 for women.)

3. In attempting to assess a patient's motivation and elicit motivational statements, it is important to ask, "What is your current level of motivation on a scale of 1–10 to remain sober?" If the patient provides an answer indicating partial motivation, such as "6," the clinician should follow up with:

    A. "Why is it so high?"
    B. "Why is it 6 and not 2?"
    C. "Why is it 6 and not 10?"
    D. "It sounds like you are not really that motivated."

    Correct answer: **B**

    By asking the patient why the patient's motivation isn't lower, the therapist is likely to elicit some of the reasons the patient is motivated to change his or her behavior. These reasons can then be reflected back to the patient.

4. The REDS acronym stands for:

    A. Reject resistance, Express empathy, Develop discrepancy, accept ambivalence, and Support sobriety.
    B. Rock and roll, Experience, Drugs, alcohol, System.
    C. Recognize responsibility, Express empathy, Develop discrepancy, advice giving, and Support self-efficacy.
    D. Roll with resistance, Express empathy, Develop discrepancy, and Support self-efficacy.

    Correct answer: **D**

    This is one of the mnemonics to help remember the key principles of Motivational Interviewing.

5. Methadone and buprenorphine:

    A. Can both be provided for treatment of opioid dependence from physicians' offices.

    B. Are only used for detoxification.

    C. Are effective against both opioids and cocaine.

    D. Both result in 40%–70% abstinence from opioids at 3–6 months.

    Correct answer: **D**

    Methadone that is provided for treatment of opioid dependence must be dispensed from a specialized opioid treatment program or clinic. Methadone and buprenorphine can be used for both detoxification and maintenance treatment but are only effective against opioids.

Chapter 12

1. The following is NOT an example of a mutual/self-help group for patients with substance use disorders:

    A. AA.

    B. SMART Recovery.

    C. Women for Sobriety.

    D. Recovery International.

    Correct answer: **D**

    Recovery International (formerly known as Recovery, Inc.) is a mutual/self-help group for people with psychiatric disorders such as depression, bipolar disorder, and schizophrenia.

2. The following BEST describes mutual/self-help:

    A. Substance use disorder treatment.

    B. AA.

    C. Peer support that functions as an adjunct to formal substance use disorder treatment.

    D. A social club.

    Correct answer: **C**

    Remember that mutual/self-help groups are not formal treatment. And although AA is one type of these groups, there are others that offer alternatives to the 12-step format of AA, such as Women for Sobriety and SMART Recovery.

3. The best way to handle a patient who declares "AA is too religious for me" is to:

    A. Roll with resistance and explore further why the patient feels this way.

    B. Reply, "AA is not religion."

    C. Insist that the patient attend 90 meetings in 90 days, as prescribed by AA.

    D. Insist the patient attend SMART Recovery meetings instead.

    Correct answer: **A**

    Remember that mutual/self-help works best when patients attend such meetings voluntarily. Mandating attendance is against the spirit of AA because it is a program of mutual attraction, not coercion. Insisting that a patient attend any group meeting is coercion. By exploring a patient's resistance, you can help facilitate his or her awareness of discordant feelings.

4. The following is a statement that is an example of expressing empathy in response to a patient telling you that he or she is not interested in AA because he or she is not religious:

    A. "I know how you feel. I don't believe in God, either."

    B. "I can understand that because you felt mistreated by nuns in grade school you are skeptical of anything that has to do with God."

    C. "You shouldn't let the past influence your choices now."

    D. "Try SMART Recovery instead."

    Correct answer: **B**

    The statement uses reflective listening to express understanding of how the patient is feeling. The first statement may be seen as an attempt to be empathic; however, it is not focused on the patient's experience. Rather, it is based on the biased opinion of the clinician. Answers C and D are directive statements, not empathic ones. Telling patients what to do is against the spirit of Motivational Interviewing.

5. The following statement is true:

    A. Ninety-five percent of people worldwide believe in God.

    B. Over 90% of physicians endorse the statement, "I believe in God."

    C. Over 90% of Americans endorse the statement, "I believe in God."

    D. One hundred percent of SMART Recovery participants believe in God.

    Correct answer: **C**

Gallup poll data over the past 60 years have consistently found this statistic. Worldwide beliefs in God are more variable. Data on physicians' beliefs are also more variable. Although 12-step program attendees are more likely to believe in God, endorsement of this statement is lower among individuals participating in the SMART Recovery program than among the general population.

Chapter 13

1. Which of the following is NOT a sign of resistance?

    A. Arguing.
    B. Questioning.
    C. Ignoring.
    D. Minimizing.

    Correct answer: **B**

    As a teenager recognizes the need for change, he or she will begin to question his or her own motives as well as soliciting the opinion of others as seen fit.

2. According to Erik Erikson, the developmental stage that hallmarks adolescence is:

    A. Trust versus mistrust.
    B. Initiative versus guilt.
    C. Identity versus role confusion.
    D. Integrity versus despair.

    Correct answer: **C**

    Adolescence introduces the challenges of establishing an identity distinct from the family of origin, as well as developing meaningful relationships with peer groups.

3. Teenagers verbalize self-efficacy in each of the following ways, EXCEPT:

    A. Expressing concern for a problem or effects of the problem.
    B. Expressing optimism for overcoming the problem.
    C. Recognizing the presence of a problem.
    D. Being told the expert opinion on a topic by a clinician.

    Correct answer: **D**

The idea of self-efficacy is reflected in a teenager's own identification of a problem and eliciting assistance on his or her own terms. Giving an expert opinion on a topic without first seeking the teen's input runs the risk of alienating the patient.

4. Motivational Interviewing/MET has been studied in work with adolescents with all of the following disorders, EXCEPT:
   A. Adolescent substance abuse.
   B. Pediatric obsessive-compulsive disorder (OCD).
   C. Adolescent HIV transmission prevention.
   D. Avoidance of dental care.

   Correct answer: **B**

   Cognitive-Behavioral Therapy and psychopharmacological intervention are appropriate evidence-based treatment modalities for pediatric OCD.

5. All of these are signs that a teenager is ready to change, EXCEPT:
   A. Asking more questions.
   B. Labeling substance use as problematic.
   C. Being argumentative.
   D. Increasing talk about the future.

   Correct answer: **C**

   Being argumentative is a sign of resistance and not a sign that someone is ready to change. The other answers are all indicative of a teen's acknowledgment of areas of potential change.

Chapter 14

1. NIAAA guidelines recommend that a healthy male older than age 65 drink:
   A. No more than 4 drinks in a day.
   B. No more than 14 drinks in a week.
   C. No more than 3 drinks in a day, and no more than 7 drinks in a week.
   D. No alcohol whatsoever under any circumstances.

   Correct answer: **C**

   NIAAA guidelines recommend that healthy men over age 65 (and healthy women of any age) drink no more than 3 drinks in a day and no more than 7 drinks in a week. Lower limits are indicated for individuals who take medications that interact with alcohol and individuals who have health conditions exacerbated by alcohol.

2. A 66-year-old male reports drinking 1 mixed drink after dinner most nights, sometimes 2 or 3 on weekend evenings or special occasions, never totaling more than 7 per week. He has adequately controlled diabetes. On multiple occasions he has driven his car home after parties where he has consumed 3 drinks, but denies any traffic accidents. Based on this information, the patient has a diagnosis of:

   A. Moderate drinking.
   B. At-risk drinking.
   C. Problem drinking.
   D. Alcohol dependence.

   Correct answer: **B**

   This patient meets criteria for at-risk drinking. Although he does not exceed the NIAAA-recommended limits for a healthy male of his age, he has a medical problem that could be exacerbated by alcohol use and has engaged in the risky behavior of driving under the influence of alcohol. Although he has not experienced negative consequences from alcohol use, his current level of use puts him at risk.

3. Which of the following older adult patients is most likely to require acute medical care?

   A. A 78-year-old female drinking 2 drinks daily. She has no medical or psychiatric problems.
   B. A 72-year-old female drinking 1 drink every second day to help her fall asleep. She lives with her supportive husband and reports a history of anxiety and diabetes, for which she is in treatment.
   C. A 67-year-old male drinking 4–5 drinks daily. He reports a past history of heavy daily drinking and withdrawal seizures as well as delirium tremens.
   D. A 68-year-old female being treated with medications for hypertension, mild depression, and insomnia. She reports drinking 1 drink nightly. She denies negative consequences from alcohol use.

   Correct answer: **C**

   Patient C has a diagnosis of alcohol dependence and is at risk of potentially life-threatening medical complications from withdrawal, requiring acute medical care. Patient A meets criteria for at-risk drinking based on her consumption of more than 7 drinks weekly. Patients B and D are drinking below the NIAAA recommended limits for a healthy older adult; however, their psychiatric and medical comorbidities plus the likely use of multiple prescription medications put them at risk for adverse consequences. There are, however, no acute safety concerns in patients A, B, and D.

4. Which of the following screening tools for substance abuse was specifically developed for use in older adults?

   A. CAGE.
   B. AUDIT.
   C. MAST-G.
   D. All of the above.

   Correct answer: **C**

   Although all of these screening tools can be used in older adults, only the MAST-G was developed specifically for use in this population.

5. Which of the following should trigger further evaluation of drinking and drug use behavior in an older adult?

   A. A complaint of insomnia.
   B. Unexplained bruising.
   C. Poor hygiene.
   D. All of the above.

   Correct answer: **D**

   All of the above complaints or observations are red flags for the possibility of a new or worsening substance use problem. Refer to Table 14–2 for a more complete list.

Chapter 15

1. A Greek family rethinks its cooking strategies. On one hand, the health benefits of a lower-fat diet are well understood and appreciated. On the other, *fasolakia ladera* are not really *ladera* unless they happily swim in a sea of olive oil. Ambivalence and tension reign in the family. What's the stage of change?

   A. Precontemplation.
   B. Contemplation.
   C. Preparation.
   D. Action.

   Correct answer: **B**

The family members actively consider their options and analyze the proposed change in terms of trade-offs between life with and life without *ladera*—they are in the contemplation stage of change. Given that ambivalence has been well established, the family system is past the precontemplation stage but has not yet resolved to take the next step in preparation of having a healthier diet.

2. Confucius said: "Our greatest glory is not in never falling but in rising every time we fall." This quote is most helpful in:

   A. Preparation.
   B. Action.
   C. Maintenance.
   D. Relapse.

   Correct answer: **D**

   In relapse, people and systems are confronted with the pain of falling off the desired path; rising and reengaging in the process of change is the Confucian "greatest glory." Although the possibility of recurrence may be discussed (and anticipated) during earlier stages of change, the quote speaks directly to relapse.

3. Three friends are stranded in an elevator without their cell phones. One of them keeps buzzing the alarm bell and screams for help while another looks for a way out. The third friend waits for the other two to figure it out. This is an example of the:

   A. Hawthorne effect.
   B. Pygmalion effect.
   C. Self-determination effect.
   D. All of the above.

   Correct answer: **C**

   The self-determination theory of human motivation focuses on the choices people make with their own free will; individual behavior is self-endorsed and self-determined. According to this theory, the three friends behave differently because of their autonomy. In contrast, social psychology theories, which form the basis for the Hawthorne and Pygmalion effects, point to environmental and social pressures as the main determinants of human behavior. According to social psychology, had we examined our subjects in a variety of social settings, we would be more impressed by the similarities than by the differences in the behavior of individuals under similar stressful conditions—such as being stranded in an elevator.

4. According to Jim Collins's analysis of successful companies, a leader's charisma is:

   A. More likely to be a liability than an asset.
   B. More likely to be an asset than a liability.
   C. Irrelevant to success or failure.
   D. More important than the facts in motivating people.

   Correct answer: **A**

   Charismatic leadership tends to promote a culture where the truth is not heard and the brutal facts are not confronted. An effective leader often succeeds despite his or her charisma—not because of it. Trying to motivate people on vision alone and ignoring the facts of the situation are a waste of time.

5. Margaret Mead said: "Never doubt that a small group of thoughtful, committed citizens can change the world. Indeed, it is the only thing that ever has." This attitude is most consistent with:

   A. Theory W.
   B. Theory X.
   C. Theory Y.
   D. Theory Z.

   Correct answer: **C**

   Assuming that people are thoughtful, committed, self-actualized, and self-motivated is the hallmark of Douglas McGregor's Theory Y. Theory X views people as lazy, not particularly intelligent, and responding only to external coercion. "Theory Z" is a term used for later derivatives of Theory Y. There is no Theory W.

Index

*Page numbers printed in **boldface** type refer to tables or figures.*